DEJA REVIEW™

USMLE Step 1

NOTICE

Medicine is an ever-changing science. As new research and clinical experience broaden our knowledge, changes in treatment and drug therapy are required. The authors and the publisher of this work have checked with sources believed to be reliable in their efforts to provide information that is complete and generally in accord with the standards accepted at the time of publication. However, in view of the possibility of human error or changes in medical sciences, neither the authors nor the publisher nor any other party who has been involved in the preparation or publication of this work warrants that the information contained herein is in every respect accurate or complete, and they disclaim all responsibility for any errors or omissions or for the results obtained from use of the information contained in this work. Readers are encouraged to confirm the information contained herein with other sources. For example and in particular, readers are advised to check the product information sheet included in the package of each drug they plan to administer to be certain that the information contained in this work is accurate and that changes have not been made in the recommended dose or in the contraindications for administration. This recommendation is of particular importance in connection with new or infrequently used drugs.

DEJA REVIEW™
USMLE Step 1
Second Edition

John H. Naheedy, MD

Fellow, Pediatric Radiology
Department of Radiology
Children's Hospital Boston
Harvard Medical School
Boston, Massachusetts

Daniel A. Orringer, MD

Chief Resident
Department of Neurosurgery
University of Michigan Medical School
Ann Arbor, Michigan

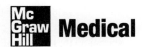 **Medical**

New York   Chicago   San Francisco   Lisbon   London   Madrid   Mexico City
Milan   New Delhi   San Juan   Seoul   Singapore   Sydney   Toronto

Déjà Review™ USMLE Step 1, Second Edition

4 5 6 7 8 9 0   DOC/DOC   14 13 12

ISBN 978-0-07-162718-4
MHID 0-07-162718-9

This book was set in Palatino by Glyph International.

The editors were Kirsten Funk and Peter J. Boyle.

The production supervisor was Catherine H. Saggese.

Project management was provided by Harleen Chopra,
Glyph International.

RR Donnelley was printer and binder.

This book is printed on acid-free paper.

Library of Congress Cataloging-in-Publication Data

Naheedy, John H.
  Deja review. USMLE step1/John H. Naheedy, Daniel A.
Orringer.—2nd ed.
      p.; cm. —(Deja review)
  Other title: USMLE step 1
  Includes index.
  ISBN-13: 978-0-07-162718-4 (pbk. : alk. paper)
  ISBN-10: 0-07-162718-9 (pbk. : alk. paper)
  1. Internal medicine—Examinations, questions, etc.
  2. Physicians—Licenses—United States—Examinations—Study
  guides. I. Orringer, Daniel A. II. Title. III. Title: USMLE
  step 1. IV. Series: Deja review.
  [DNLM: 1. Clinical Medicine—Examination Questions.
  WB 18. 2 N153d 2010]
RC58.N344 2010
616.0076—dc22

                                                    2010003180

To my family and friends,
for their love and encouragement;
and to my parents,
for being an example of everything I want to be.
—John

To my mother and my family.
—Dan

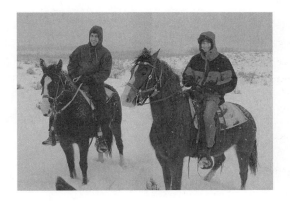

Contents

Contributors

Alexander Choo
Medical Student
Class of 2010
University of California, San Diego
La Jolla, California
*Chapters: Pulmonary, Skin and Connective
Tissues, Musculoskeletal*

Charlotte Gore
Medical Student
Class of 2010
University of California, San Diego
La Jolla, California
*Chapters: Basic Principles, Neuroscience,
Gastroenterology, Hematology and Oncology,
Behavioral Science, Make the Diagnosis*

Kristen A. Kipps
Medical Student
Class of 2010
University of California, San Diego
La Jolla, California
*Chapters: Immunology, Microbiology and
Infectious Diseases*

Brian S. Pugmire
Medical Student
Class of 2010
University of California, San Diego
La Jolla, California
Chapter: Renal and Genitourinary

Krishna C. Ravi
Medical Student
Class of 2010
University of California, San Diego
La Jolla, California
Chapter: Cardiovascular

Omeed Saghafi
Medical Student
Class of 2010
University of California, San Diego
La Jolla, California
Chapter: Reproduction and Endocrinology

Student Reviewers

Betty Chung
MD/PhD Candidate
University of Medicine and Dentistry
    of New Jersey
School of Osteopathic Medicine
Class of 2012

Sarah Fabiano
SUNY Upstate Medical University
Class of 2010

Ali Rizvi, MPH
Lake Erie College of Osteopathic Medicine
Class of 2010

Preface

Déjà Review™ *USMLE Step 1* has been scrutinized and edited to produce a second edition that is even higher yield and easier to use than the first. Outstanding medical students who have recently taken Step 1 have revised the original text to ensure the material covered herein is complete and current. The authors, now with a combined 30 years of experience in the medical field, have also edited the manuscript to emphasize the relevant core concepts covered in the USMLE Step 1 examination. We are confident that our efforts have produced one of the most useful guides for Step 1 review available today.

The main objective of a medical student preparing for Step 1 of the United States Medical Licensing Examination (USMLE) is to commit a vast body of knowledge to memory. Having recently prepared for Step 1, we realize how daunting this task can be. We feel there are two main principles that will allow you to be successful in your preparations for Step 1: (1) repetition of key facts and (2) using review questions to gauge your comprehension and memory. The Déjà Review™ series is a unique resource that has been designed to allow you to review the essential facts and determine your level of knowledge on the subjects tested on Step 1. We also know, from experience, that building a solid foundation in the basic sciences will allow you to make a smooth transition into the clinical years of medical school.

ORGANIZATION

All concepts are presented in a question and answer format that covers the key facts on hundreds of commonly tested USMLE Step 1 topics. The material is divided into chapters organized by body systems. Special emphasis has been placed on the molecular and genetic basis of pathology, as this area has become increasingly emphasized in recent examinations.

This question and answer format has several important advantages:
- It provides a rapid, straightforward way for you to assess your strengths and weaknesses.
- It allows you to efficiently review and commit to memory a large body of information.
- It offers a break from tedious, convoluted multiple-choice questions.
- The "Make the Diagnosis" section exposes you to the prototypic presentation of diseases classically tested on the USMLE Step 1.
- It serves as a quick, last-minute review of high-yield facts.

The compact, condensed design of the book is conducive to studying on the go, especially during any downtime throughout your day.

HOW TO USE THIS BOOK

This text has been sampled by a number of medical students who found it to be an essential part of their preparation for Step 1, in addition to their course examinations. Remember, this text is not intended to replace comprehensive textbooks, course packs, or lectures. It is simply intended to serve as a supplement to your studies during your first 2 years of medical school and throughout your preparation for Step 1. We encourage you to begin using this book early in your first year to reinforce topics covered in your course examinations. We also recommend having the book spiral bound to make it more portable and easier to use outside of the library or classroom. You may cover up the answers with the included bookmark and quiz yourself or even your classmates. For a greater challenge, try covering up the questions!

However you choose to study, we hope you find this resource helpful throughout your preclinical years and during your preparation for the USMLE Step 1. Best of luck!

John H. Naheedy, MD
Daniel A. Orringer, MD

Acknowledgments

The authors would like to thank the following individuals for their invaluable contributions to this text and their efforts in making this a useful, accurate resource for students:

Stephen M. Baird, MD
Professor Emeritus of Pathology
School of Medicine
University of California, San Diego
Veterans Affairs San Diego Healthcare
   System
La Jolla, California

Vi Q. Bowman, MD
Fellow, Department of Internal Medicine
Division of Infectious Diseases
University of California San Diego,
   Medical Center
San Diego, California

David L. Clark, PhD
Associate Professor
Division of Anatomy
College of Medicine
Ohio State University
Columbus, Ohio

John J. Curry III, PhD
Director, Problem-Based Learning Pathway
Associate Professor, Departments of
   Physiology & Obstetrics and Gynecology
College of Medicine
Ohio State University
Columbus, Ohio

Robert M. DePhilip, PhD
Associate Professor
Division of Anatomy
College of Medicine
Ohio State University
Columbus, Ohio

Richard Fertel, PhD
Associate Professor
Department of Pharmacology
College of Medicine
Ohio State University
Columbus, Ohio

Heather L. Hofflich, DO
Department of Internal Medicine
Division of Endocrinology, Diabetes and
   Metabolism
University of California, San Diego
La Jolla, California

John H. Hughes, PhD
Associate Professor
Department of Molecular Virology,
   Immunology, and Medical Genetics
College of Medicine
Ohio State University
Columbus, Ohio

Carolyn J. Kelly, MD
Professor
Department of Internal Medicine
Associate Dean for Admissions and Student
   Affairs
University of California, San Diego
La Jolla, California

David E. Krummen, MD
Assistant Professor of Medicine
Division of Electrophysiology
University of California San Diego
Veterans Affairs San Diego Healthcare
   System
La Jolla, California

Nora D. Laiken, PhD
Assistant Dean of Educational Support
   Services
School of Medicine
University of California, San Diego
La Jolla, California

Jess Mandel, MD
Professor
Department of Internal Medcine
Division of Pulmonary & Critical Care
Associate Dean for Undergraduate Medical
    Education
University of California, San Diego
La Jolla, California

Khashayar Mohebali, MD
Chief Resident, Clinical Instructor
Division of Plastic and Reconstructive
    Surgery
Department of Surgery
University of California, San Francisco
San Francisco, California

Alexandra Schwartz, MD
Associate Clinical Professor
Department of Orthopedic Surgery
University of California, San Diego Medical
    Center
San Diego, California

Pal L. Vaghy, MD
Associate Professor
Department of Molecular and Cellular
    Biochemistry
College of Medicine
Ohio State University
Columbus, Ohio

The authors would like to recognize the faculty and staff at the Ohio State University College of Medicine and dedicate this edition to the memory of the late Dr. John M. Stang, for his constant encouragement and his endless commitment to education. We would also like to thank the students who used this text in preparation for their boards and provided critical feedback. Finally, a special thanks to Lilly Ghahremani of Full Circle Literary for her guidance, and to our managing editor Kirsten Funk for her patience and guidance throughout this project.

CHAPTER 1

Basic Principles

MOLECULAR BIOLOGY, BIOCHEMISTRY, AND GENETICS

DNA, Genes, and Chromosomes

Which nucleotide bases are purines and which are pyrimidines?	"**CUT** the **PY**": Cytosine, Uracil, and Thymine = **PY**rimidines; "**PUR**e As Gold": **PUR**ines = adenine and guanine
Which proteins make up the core of a nucleosome?	Histones: H2A, H2B, H3, and H4
Which proteins are associated with DNA between nucleosomes?	Histone H1

Name the type of mutations described below:

Type of mutation that does not result in a change in amino acid sequence	Silent
Type of mutation that results in a change in amino acid sequence	Missense
Type of mutation that results in a stop codon	Nonsense "NO sense"
Type of mutation that changes the reading frame	Frameshift
Type of mutation in which a portion of DNA is lost	Deletion
Type of mutation in which a single base is exchanged	Point

Name the type of cytogenetic disorders described below:

Failure of chromosomes to disjoin properly during cell division

Nondisjunction

Loss of a portion of a chromosome

Deletion

Two internal chromosomal breaks with inverted reincorporation of a portion of the chromosome

Inversion

Single breaks in two chromosomes resulting in the exchange of segments between chromosomes without loss of genetic material

Balanced reciprocal translocation

Single breaks in two acrocentric chromosomes resulting in one large chromosome and one small chromosome accompanied by the loss of some genetic information, hereditary form of Down syndrome

Robertsonian translocation

Mitotic error in early development leading to the development of two karyotypically distinct populations of cells in an organism

Mosaisicm

What term is used to describe the AT-rich sequences in the genome where DNA replication begins?

Origin of replication

DNA Replication, Transcription, and Translation

Name the protein(s) involved in replication or DNA repair with the functions listed below:

Stabilize single-stranded DNA

Single-stranded DNA-binding proteins

Recognition of AT-rich sequences at the origin of replication and separation of DNA strands in bacteria (prokaryotes)

DnaA protein

Unwinding DNA double helix

DNA helicases

Prevention of supercoiling during replication

DNA topoisomerases

Placement of RNA primer at site where replication is initiated

Primase, and an RNA polymerase

Removal of RNA primers from DNA synthesized discontinuously

DNA polymerase I (specifically, the 5'-3' exonuclease activity)

DNA chain elongation in prokaryotes	DNA polymerase III
Proofreading of newly synthesized DNA strand	DNA polymerase III (specifically, the 3'-5' exonuclease activity)
Repair UV damage to DNA	UV-specific endonuclease, exonuclease, and DNA ligase
Removal of damaged bases from DNA	Apurinic or apyrimidinic endonuclease, exonuclease, and DNA ligase
What term is used to describe the DNA strand synthesized continuously toward the replication fork?	Leading strand
What term is used to describe the DNA strand synthesized discontinuously away from the replication fork?	Lagging strand
What are the three stop codons?	UGA, UAA, UAG (**U** Go Away, **U** Are Away, **U** Are **G**one)
In which direction are DNA and RNA synthesized?	5' → 3'
What is the start codon?	AUG
Name the type of RNA responsible for each of the following functions:	
Largest RNA molecule	mRNA
Most abundant type of RNA	rRNA
Smallest RNA molecule	tRNA
Portion of RNA transcript encoding information for protein synthesis	Exons ("exons are expressed")
Portion of RNA transcript that is found between sequences of RNA encoding information for protein synthesis	Introns
Type of RNA covalently bound to a single amino acid	tRNA
Name the term used to describe the region of genomic DNA where RNA polymerase and transcription factors bind to regulate transcription:	Promoter
Name the term used to describe the region of genomic DNA where transcription factors activators bind to enhance transcription:	Enhancer

Name the term to describe the region of genomic DNA where repressors bind.	Silencer

Name the enzyme responsible for each of the following functions:

Synthesis of rRNA	RNA polymerase I
Synthesis of mRNA	RNA polymerase II
Synthesis of tRNA	RNA polymerase III

Name three major regulatory mechanisms of transcription in eukaryotes:	1. Regulation by transcription factors at the level of the promoter 2. Regulation by histones binding to specific genomic regions 3. Regulation of DNA structure (including methylation, gene rearrangement, and amplification)

What genetic structure regulates transcription in prokaryotes?	An operon

Name the elements of an operon responsible for each of the following functions:

Region where proteins bind to enable transcription	Promoter region
Molecule that binds at the promoter	Activator or repressor
Sequence in DNA where regulatory protein bind	Operator
Molecule that binds the operator to regulate transcription	Repressor

What are three modifications made to an RNA transcript before it leaves the nucleus?	1. 5′ Capping with 7-methylguanosine 2. 3′ Polyadenylation 3. Splicing of introns
Which small molecule provides the energy for charging a tRNA with its amino acid?	Adenosine triphosphate (ATP)
Which small molecule provides the energy for binding tRNA to the ribosome and for translocation?	Guanosine triphosphate (GTP)
Which molecules, central to the discipline of molecular biology, recognize and cleave specific sequences of a DNA molecule?	Restriction enzymes

Molecular Biology Techniques

Name the molecular biology techniques
described below:

Method of separating molecules based on movement through a gel placed in an electric field	Gel electrophoresis
Technique for detecting specific DNA sequences using restriction enzymes and a radiolabeled DNA probe	Southern blot
Technique for detecting specific RNA sequences using restriction enzymes and a radiolabeled DNA probe	Northern blot
Technique for detecting specific protein sequences using radiolabeled antibodies	Western blot
A rapid technique for amplifying a specific DNA sequence in vitro	Polymerase chain reaction
Technique for detecting different alleles at a gene of interest using restriction enzymes	Restriction fragment length polymorphism analysis
Technique for detecting the presence of antigen or antibody using radiolabeled antibodies	Radioimmunoassay (RIA)
Technique for detecting the presence of antigen or antibody using antibodies linked to enzymes with detectable activity	Enzyme-linked immunosorbent assay (ELISA)

Inherited Diseases

Name inheritance patterns described
below:

Twenty-five percent of offspring from two carrier parents affected	Autosomal recessive (AR)
Commonly cause defects in structural genes	Autosomal dominant (AD)
Commonly cause defects in enzymes	AR
Defect seen in multiple generations in both sexes	AD
Defects not typically seen in consecutive generations	AR

Disease is not observed in females.	X-linked (XL) recessive
Disease is transmitted by mother.	Mitochondrial inheritance
Half of male offspring from affected mother will manifest disease.	XL recessive
Disease manifestations commonly present after puberty.	AD

What are the conditions for a population to be in Hardy-Weinberg equilibrium?

1. No mutation at locus of interest
2. No selection for allele at locus of interest
3. Random mating
4. Closed population (no migration)

What are the two Hardy-Weinberg equations?

1. $p^2 + 2pq + q^2 = 1$
2. $p + q = 1$ (p and q are separate alleles and pq is the heterozygote frequency)

Name the disease or condition associated with each of the following statements:

Lack of UV-specific endonuclease causing dry skin and malignant melanoma	Xeroderma pigmentosa
Lack of aldolase B causing hypoglycemia, jaundice, and cirrhosis	Fructose intolerance
Lack of fructokinase causing fructosemia and fructosuria	Essential fructosuria
Lack of galactose-1-phosphate uridyltransferase causing cataracts, hepatosplenomegaly (HSM), and mental retardation	Galactosemia
Deficiency of lactase causing bloating, flatulence, and diarrhea on consumption of dairy products	Lactose intolerance
Lactic acidosis and neurologic deficits in an alcoholic	Pyruvate dehydrogenase deficiency
Hemolytic anemia in patients of Mediterranean descent after eating fava beans or taking antimalarial medication	Glucose-6-phosphate dehydrogenase deficiency
Hemolytic anemia due to deficiency in glycolysis	Hexokinase, glucose-phosphate isomerase, aldolase, triose-phosphate isomerase, phosphate glycerate kinase, enolase, or pyruvate kinase deficiency

Inappropriate hepatocellular accumulation of glycogen caused by a deficiency of glucose-6-phosphatase, associated with severe fasting, hypoglycemia, lactic acidosis, hyperlipidemia, and impaired fructose metabolism	von Gierke disease/type I glycogen storage disease
Inappropriate accumulation of glycogen in the liver, heart, and muscle caused by a deficiency of lysosomal α-1,4-glucosidase, resulting in cardiomegaly	Pompe disease/type II glycogen storage disease
Inappropriate accumulation of glycogen in liver and heart due to deficiency of α-1,6-glucosidase, a debranching enzyme often leading to muscular hypotonia	Cori disease/type III glycogen storage disease
Inappropriate accumulation of glycogen in skeletal muscle fibers due to deficiency of glycogen phosphorylase, leading to myalgia and myoglobinuria with exercise	McArdle disease/type V glycogen storage disease
Defect in cystathione synthase leading to the presence of homocysteine in the urine	Homocystinuria
Defect of renal tubular amino acid transporter for cysteine, ornithine, lysine, and arginine	Cystinuria
Inadequate catabolism of branched-chain amino acids (Ile, Val, and Leu) due to lack of α-ketoacid dehydrogenase leading to mental retardation	Maple syrup urine disease
Lack of phenylalanine hydroxylase (PAH) leading to a buildup of phenylalanine resulting in mental retardation, hypopigmentation, eczema, and a mousy odor	Phenylketonuria (can also get Phe buildup due to deficiency of tetrahydrobiopterin, BH4, cofactor of PAH)
Lack of homogentisic acid oxidase leading to a buildup of homogentisate, causing darkening of the urine and connective tissues	Alkaptonuria
Lack of tyrosinase leading to a lack of melanin	Albinism

Lack of adenosine deaminase inhibits DNA synthesis by causing the accumulation of metabolites in the purine salvage pathway; one of the causes of severe combined immunodeficiency syndrome	Adenosine deaminase deficiency
Lack of hypoxanthine-guanine phosphoryltransferase (HGPRTase) causing an overproduction of uric acid leading to neurologic deficits, hyperuricemia, and behavioral abnormalities, including self-mutilation	Lesch-Nyhan Syndrome (Lacks Nucleotide Salvage)
Trisomy 21 → mental retardation, slanted palpebral fissures, hypertelorism, macroglossia, atrial septal defect (ASD), duodenal atresia, early-onset Alzheimer disease, and multiple visceral anomalies	Down syndrome
Expansion of unstable region of X chromosome (abnormal *FMR1* gene with CGG expansion) leading to mental retardation, enlarged testes, and craniofacial anomalies	Fragile X syndrome
XL recessive deficiency of α-galactosidase A → buildup of ceramide trihexoside which causes pain in the extremities, ocular abnormalities, angiokeratomas, cardiovascular disease, and renal failure	Fabry disease
AR deficiency of galactosylceramide β-galactosidase leading to cerebral accumulation of galactocerebroside, which causes progressive neurologic degeneration	Krabbe disease (aka globoid cell leukodystrophy)
AR deficiency of β-glucocerebrosidase leading to the accumulation of glucocerebroside in the brain, bone marrow, liver, spleen → HSM, aseptic necrosis of femur, and neurologic dysfunction	Gaucher disease

AR deficiency of sphingomyelinase on Chromosome 11 leading to buildup of sphinogmyelin and cholesterol in histiocytes of the liver, spleen, and lymphatic system, resulting in cortical atrophy, cherry red spot on macula, HSM	Niemann-Pick disease
AR deficiency of hexosaminidase A on Chromosome 18, leading to the accumulation of GM_2 ganglioside within lysosomes resulting in neurologic degeneration and developmental delay, and cherry red spot on macula	Tay-Sachs disease
AR deficiency of arylsulfatase A, leading to an accumulation of cerebroside sulfate and dysfunction and demyelination of the central and peripheral nervous systems resulting in ataxia and dementia	Metachromatic leukodystrophy
XL recessive deficiency of iduronate sulfatase, leading to an accumulation of heparan and dermatan sulfate resulting in mental retardation, coarse facial features, and short stature	Hunter syndrome
AR deficiency of α-l-iduronidase, leading to the accumulation of partially degraded glycosaminoglycans within lysosomes resulting in dysmorphic, gargoyle-like facies, corneal clouding, HSM, and skeletal abnormalities	Hurler syndrome
AR deficiency of UDP-*N*-acetylglucosamine: *N*-acetylglucosaminyl-L-phosphotransferase, loss of protein tagging with mannose-6-phosphate, leading to defective trafficking of enzymes into lysosomes → developmental delay and coarse facial features	I-cell disease (mucolipidosis type II)

Name the genetic disease associated with each of the following clinical or pathologic findings:

Cherry red spot of the macula	Tay-Sachs disease and Niemman-Pick disease
Cells containing "crinkled paper" cytoplasm and glycolipid-laden macrophages	Gaucher disease
Corneal clouding	Hurler syndrome

Carbohydrate, Protein, and Lipid Metabolism

Name the major metabolic pathway regulated by the following enzymes:

Isocitrate dehydrogenase	Citric acid cycle
Phosphofructokinase	Glycolysis
Fructose-1,6-bisphosphatase	Gluconeogenesis
Glycogen synthase	Glyconeogenesis
Glycogen phosphorylase	Glycogenolysis
Glucose-6-phosphate dehydrogenase	Pentose phosphate pathway
Acetyl-coenzyme A (CoA) carboxylase	Lipogenesis
Carnitine acyltransferase	Lipolysis (β-oxidation)
HMG-CoA reductase	Cholesterol synthesis

Name the major activators and/or inhibitors for each of the following enzymes:

Citrate synthase	Activator: no major activator
	Inhibitors: ATP, NADH, succinyl-CoA, and acyl-CoA derivatives of fatty acids
Phosphofructokinase-1	Activator: AMP, fructose-2,6-bisphosphate (liver)
	Inhibitor: citrate, ATP, and cAMP
Pyruvate dehydrogenase	Activator: CoA, nicotinamide adenine (NAD), adenosine diphosphate (ADP), and pyruvate
	Inhibitor: acetyl-CoA, NADH, and ATP
Pyruvate carboxylase	Activator: acetyl-CoA
	Inhibitor: ADP

Fructose-1,6-bisphosphatase	Activator: cAMP
	Inhibitor: AMP and fructose-2,6-bisphosphate
Glycogen synthase	Activator: glucose-6-phosphate
	Inhibitor: no major inhibitor
Glycogen phosphorylase	Activators: cAMP and Ca^{2+} (muscle)
	Inhibitors: glucose, glucose-6-phosphate, and ATP
Glucose-6-phosphate dehydrogenase	Activator: $NADP^+$
	Inhibitor: NADPH
Acetyl-CoA carboxylase	Activator: citrate
	Inhibitor: malonyl-CoA, palmitoyl-CoA, and cAMP
Carnitine acyltransferase	Activator: no major activator
	Inhibitor: malonyl-CoA
HMG-CoA reductase	Activator: no major activator
	Inhibitor: cholesterol and cAMP

Describe the effect of insulin on the following metabolic processes:

Glycogen synthesis in muscle and liver	Increase
Gluconeogenesis in the liver	Decrease
Glycogenolysis in the liver	Decrease
Glucose uptake in muscle and adipose tissue	Increase
Triacylglycerol degradation	Decrease
Triacylglycerol synthesis	Increase
Protein synthesis	Increase

Describe the effect of glucagon on the following metabolic processes:

Glycogenolysis in the liver	Increase
Gluconeogenesis in the liver	Increase
β-Oxidation of fatty acids in the liver	Increase
Amino acid uptake by liver	Increase

Which small molecule accepts reducing equivalents and is typically involved in catabolic processes?	NAD^+

Which small molecule donates reducing equivalents and is typically involved in anabolic processes?	Nicotinamide adenine dinucleotide phosphate (NADPH)

Name the cellular compartment (cytosol, mitochondria, or both) where each of the following processes occur:

Citric acid cycle	Mitochondria
Fatty acid oxidation	Mitochondria
Fatty acid synthesis	Cytosol
Gluconeogenesis	Both
Glycolysis	Cytosol
Heme synthesis	Both
Hexose monophosphate (HMP) shunt	Cytosol
Protein synthesis	Cytosol (rough ER)
Steroid synthesis	Cytosol (smooth ER)
Urea cycle	Both

Hexokinase or glucokinase?

Found in most tissues	Hexokinase
Found exclusively in the liver and β-islet cells	Glucokinase
High affinity for glucose	Hexokinase
Faster reaction velocity	Glucokinase
Inhibited by glucose-6-phosphate	Hexokinase

Name the molecule(s) that serve as the primary source of energy for the following organs:

Liver	Amino acids, lipids, glucose, fructose, and lactate
Central nervous system (CNS)	Glucose
Heart	Lipids, ketone bodies, lactate, and glucose
Adipose tissue	Glucose and lipids
Type I skeletal muscle fibers (slow twitch, "red")	Lipids and ketone bodies
Type II skeletal muscle fibers (fast twitch, "white")	Glucose

What are the four major enzymes that function in gluconeogenesis?	1. Pyruvate carboxylase 2. PEP carboxykinase 3. Fructose-1,6-bisphosphatase 4. Glucose-6-phosphatase (**P**athway **P**roduces **F**resh **G**lucose)
Name four important cellular processes that require reducing equivalents supplied primarily by the pentose phosphate pathway:	1. Fatty acid and steroid biosynthesis 2. Glutathione-mediated reduction of H_2O_2 3. Cytochrome P-450 system 4. Respiratory burst in phagocytes
Which molecule serves as donor of methyl groups in many metabolic processes?	S-adenosylmethionine
Name four biosynthetic pathways that require methyl group donation by S-adenosylmethionine:	Synthesis of 1. Choline 2. Creatine 3. Epinephrine 4. 7-Methylguanosine
Which metabolic process is responsible for transferring reducing equivalents from RBCs and muscle tissue to the liver?	Cori cycle
Which two amino acids play key roles in the transport of nitrogen from the periphery to the liver?	1. Alanine 2. Glutamine
What are the cofactors for the pyruvate dehydrogenase complex?	B_1, B_2, B_3, B_5, and lipoic acid
Name the eight intermediates of the citric acid cycle:	1. Citrate (**Cindy**) 2. Isocitrate (**Is**) 3. α-Ketoglutarate (**Kinky**) 5. Succinyl-CoA (**So**) 4. Succinate (**She**) 6. Fumarate (**Fornicates**) 7. Malate (**More**) 8. Oxaloacetate (**Often**)
Name a toxin that directly blocks the flow of electrons through the electron transport chain:	Cyanide
Cyanide is a by-product of the metabolism of what antihypertensive?	Nitroprusside

Name a toxin that directly inhibits mitochondrial ATPase:	Oligomycin
Name a toxin that uncouples oxidative phosphorylation by increasing the permeability of the inner mitochondrial membrane:	2,4-Dinitrophenol (DNP)
What are the primary metabolic substrates released by the liver in the fed state and the fasting state?	Very low-density lipoprotein (VLDL) (fed); glucose and ketone bodies (fasting)

Name the apolipoprotein or lipoprotein responsible for each of the following functions:

Activates lecithin-cholesterol acyltransferase	Apolipoprotein A-I
Binds to low-density lipoprotein (LDL) receptor, mediates VLDL secretion	Apolipoprotein B-100
Delivery of cholesterol from the tissues to the liver	High-density lipoprotein (HDL)
Delivery of cholesterol produced by the liver to the tissues	LDL
Delivery of triglycerol absorbed in the small intestine to tissues	Chylomicron
Delivery of triglycerol produced by the liver to tissues	VLDL
Mediates chylomicron remnant uptake	Apolipoprotein E
Serves as a cofactor for lipoprotein lipase	Apolipoprotein C-II

Which enzyme, found in the liver and bone marrow, catalyzes the rate-limiting step of heme synthesis?	Aminolevulinate synthase
What are the major intermediates in the degradation of heme?	Heme → biliverdin → bilirubin → bilirubin diglucuronide (conjugated bilirubin)
Conjugated bilirubin is excreted in which bodily fluid?	Bile

Which compound produced by intestinal bacterial degradation of conjugated bilirubin gives urine its yellow color?	Urobilinogen
Which common physical finding in severe liver disease results from the accumulation of bilirubin (hyperbilirubinemia)?	Jaundice
Name the essential amino acids:	"PriVaTe **TIM HALL**": Phe, Val, Trp, Thr, Ile, Met, His, Arg, Leu, Lys
Which amino acids (AAs) are exclusively ketogenic?	Leu and Lys
Which AAs can be ketogenic or glucogenic?	Tyr, Ile, Phe, and Trp
Which AAs are exclusively glucogenic?	All the amino acids not listed in the above two items
Which AAs are negatively charged at physiologic pH (7.4)?	Asp, Glu (the two acidic AAs)
Which AAs are positively charged at physiologic pH (7.4)?	Arg, Lys (the two basic AAs), His also basic but weakly charged at pH 7.4
Which AA is used to carry ammonium from the muscles to the liver?	Alanine
Which small molecule, essential to the excretion of ammonium, is derived from the removal of ammonium from glutamine?	α-Ketoglutarate
What are the intermediates of the urea cycle?	1. Ornithine (**Ordinarily**) 2. Carbamoyl phosphate (**Careless**) 3. Citrulline (**Crappers**) 4. Aspartate (**Are**) 5. Arginosuccinate (**Also**) 6. Fumarate (**Frivolous**) 7. Arginine (**About**) 8. Urea (**Urination**)
What is the limiting reagent for hepatic ethanol (EtOH) catabolism?	NAD^+
Which metabolic abnormality in chronic alcoholics results from depletion of NAD^+ in the liver?	Hypoglycemia (due to inhibition of gluconeogenesis)

Depletion of NAD$^+$ inhibits which two major metabolic processes?	1. The conversion of pyruvate to lactate 2. Oxaloacetate to malate
In what metabolic state does the liver commonly produce ketone bodies?	During starvation (or diabetic ketoacidosis)

G Proteins

What class of G protein is associated with the following cell surface receptors:

α_1	Q
α_2	I
β_1	S
β_2	S
M_1	Q
M_2	I
M_3	Q
M_4	S
D_1	S
D_2	I
H_1	Q
H_2	S
V_1	Q
V_2	S

Which two second messengers are increased by the activation of a G_q protein?	1. IP_3 2. Diacylglycerol (DAG)
Which enzyme is induced by the activation of a G_q protein?	Protein kinase C
Which enzyme is induced by the activation of a G_s protein?	Protein kinase A
Which second messenger is increased by the activation of a G_s protein?	cAMP
Which enzyme is inhibited by the activation of a G_i protein?	Protein kinase A
Which second messenger is decreased by the activation of a G_i protein?	cAMP

Enzymes

What is the shape of the plot of reaction velocity against substrate concentration for enzymes following Michaelis-Menten kinetics?	Hyperbolic
For an enzyme following Michaelis-Menten kinetics, how does halving enzyme concentration affect $V_{max?}$?	V_{max} will be halved. (V_{max} is directly proportional to enzyme concentration for all substrate concentrations.)
What is the shape of a plot of reaction velocity against substrate concentration for enzyme with a single allosteric regulator?	Sigmoid or "S" shaped
Name two important parameters of the cellular environment that directly affect enzyme kinetics:	1. pH 2. Temperature
The inverse of V_{max} ((the maximum reaction velocity) for a given enzyme is represented by what point on a Lineweaver-Burk plot?	The y intercept
The inverse of K_m (the Michaelis-Menten constant) for a given enzyme is represented by what point on a Lineweaver-Burk plot?	The x intercept
An enzyme with a small K_m will have a high or low affinity for its substrate?	High affinity ($K_m = 1/2V_{max}$)
How does a competitive inhibitor affect K_m?	Increases
How does a noncompetitive inhibitor affect K_m?	No effect
How does a competitive inhibitor affect V_m?	No effect
How does a noncompetitive inhibitor affect K_m?	Decreases

Cell Cycle

Name the phase of the cell cycle
associated with each of the following
cellular events:

Quiescence	G_0
Centrosome duplication	S
RNA, protein, organelle synthesis	G_0
DNA, RNA, histone synthesis	S
Release of E2F from Rb	G_1/S transition
Cyclin-dependent kinase (Cdk)-cyclin A and Cdk-cyclin B are active.	G_2/M transition
Cdk-cyclin D and Cdk-cyclin E are active.	G_1/S transition
Chromatin condensation, mitotic spindle formation	M: prophase
Kinetochore assembly	M: prometaphase
Centrosomes move to opposite poles.	M: prophase
Nuclear envelope and nucleolar disappearance	M: prometaphase
Chromosome alignment at metaphase plate	M: metaphase
Kinetochore separation	M: anaphase
Nuclear envelope and nucleolar formation	M: telophase
Cytoplasmic division (cytokinesis)	M: cytokinesis
Most variable phase of cell cycle	G_1

Which two important molecules are involved in the G_1 to S checkpoint?	Rb, p53
What is the significance of p53?	Allows cell to detect DNA defects and repair them before proceeding with replication

Cell Membranes

What are the major categories of molecules that make up the cell membrane?	Cholesterol, phospholipids, sphingolipids, glycolipids, and proteins

Where in the cell membrane are glycoproteins found?

Exclusively in the noncytoplasmic side

What is the effect of increasing the cholesterol content of a cell membrane?

Membrane fluidity is decreased.

NUTRITION

Name the fat-soluble vitamins:

Vitamins A, D, E, and K

Where are these vitamins absorbed?

Ileum

What conditions cause fat-soluble vitamin deficiencies?

Malabsorption syndromes (eg, cystic fibrosis, celiac disease, ileal disease, ileal resection)

Why do toxicities occur more commonly with fat-soluble vitamins?

Fat-soluble vitamins can accumulate in fatty tissues; varying fat content with age leads to different thresholds of toxicity for children versus elderly.

Which prolonged dietary deficiency of protein and calories is characterized by retarded growth and cachexia in children?

Marasmus

Which disease, characterized by protein deficiency with adequate caloric intake, results in retarded growth, anemia, and severe edema?

Kwashiorkor

Name the vitamin(s) associated with each of the following statements:

Composes NAD^+ and $NADP^+$

Vitamin B_3 (niacin)

Remains in the body with stores lasting up to 3 to 5 years

Vitamin B_{12} (cobalamin)

Important in purine/pyrimidine synthesis

Folate

Important part of visual pigments and epithelial cell differentiation

Vitamin A (retinol)

Antioxidant that delays cataracts and atherosclerosis

Vitamin E (α-tocopherol)

Component of CoA and fatty acid synthase

Vitamin B_5 (pantothenate)

Cofactors for pyruvate-dehydrogenase complex	Vitamins B_1 (thiamine), B_2 (riboflavin), B_3 (niacin), and B_5 (pantothenic acid)
Found only in animal products; Schilling test used to detect deficiency	Vitamin B_{12} (cobalamin)
Cofactor for norepinephrine (NE) synthesis and collagen cross-linkage; ↑ Fe absorption	Vitamin C (ascorbic acid)
Cofactor in transamination reactions	Vitamin B_6 (pyridoxine)
Toxicity causes nausea, stupor, and hypercalcemia	Vitamin D
Important in methionine synthesis and isomerization of methylmalonyl-CoA	Vitamin B_{12} (cobalamin)
Toxicity causes skin changes, arthralgias, and premature epiphyseal closure, the first sign of toxicity usually CNS changes from edema.	Vitamin A (retinol)
Catalyzes γ-carboxylation of coagulation factors, synthesized by GI flora	Vitamin K
The most toxic vitamin in overdose	Vitamin D
The most common vitamin deficiency in the United States	Folate

Name the vitamin deficiency associated with each of the following findings:

Wernicke-Korsakoff syndrome, beriberi	Vitamin B_1 (thiamine); B_1 = Ber1Ber1
Rickets, osteomalacia, and hypocalcemic tetany	Vitamin D
Neonatal hemorrhage and ↑ prothrombin time (PT)	Vitamin K
Megaloblastic anemia with neurologic dysfunction	Vitamin B_{12} (cobalamin)
*D*ermatitis, *d*iarrhea, and *d*ementia (pellagra)	Vitamin B_3 (niacin)
Deficiency caused by long-term raw egg ingestion	Biotin (avidin in egg whites binds biotin)
Megaloblastic anemia without neurologic dysfunction	Folate
Dry skin, dry eyes, and night blindness	Vitamin A (retinol)
Hemolysis (from RBC fragility) and ataxia	Vitamin E (α-tocopherol)

EEG abnormalities and peripheral neuropathy; caused by isoniazid (INH) and oral contraceptives	Vitamin B_6 (pyridoxine)
Cheilosis, corneal vascularization, and angular stomatitis	Vitamin B_2 (riboflavin)
Neural tube defects during pregnancy	Folate
Scurvy, hemorrhages, and impaired wound healing	Vitamin C (ascorbic acid)
Deficiency caused by *Diphyllobothrium latum* infection, sprue, pernicious anemia, and Crohn's disease	Vitamin B_{12} (cobalamin)

Name the trace element associated with each of the following statements:

Important in protein synthesis; deficiency causes acrodermatitis and ↑ sense of taste/smell	Zinc
Involved in hemoglobin synthesis; excess caused by ceruloplasmin deficiency	Copper
Cofactor for glutathione peroxidase; deficiency causes cardiomyopathy	Selenium
Involved in collagen cross-linkage; excess causes pulmonary fibrosis	Silicon
Involved in methionine metabolism; deficiency mimics vitamin B_{12} deficiency	Cobalt (constituent of cobalamin)
Reduces insulin resistance, glucose tolerance factor	Chromium

GENERAL EMBRYOLOGY

Name the embryonic structure described below:

Consists of the inner cell mass which ultimately gives rise to the fetus	Embryoblast
Consists of the outer cell mass which ultimately gives rise to the placenta	Trophoblast
Derived from embryoblast; clefts form the amniotic cavity	Epiblast

Derived from embryoblast; ultimately forms the yolk sac	Hypoblast
Border between future mouth and pharynx; formed by both hypoblast and epiblast cells	Buccopharyngeal membrane
Produces β-human chorionic gonadotropin (hCG)	Syncytiotrophoblast
Forms the lining of the cytotrophoblast	Extraembryonic somatic mesoderm
Consists of the syncytiotrophoblast, cytotrophoblast, and extraembryonic somatic mesoderm	Chorion
Forms the covering of the yolk sac	Extraembryonic visceral mesoderm

The following developmental milestones occur how long after contraception?

Implantation	Within 1 week
Bilaminar disc	Within 2 weeks
Gastrulation	Within 3 weeks
Formation of the primitive streak and neural plate	Within 3 weeks
Organogenesis, peak of susceptibility to teratogens	Weeks 3 to 8
Limb formation	Week 4
Cardiac contractions begin	Week 4
Male and female genitals can be distinguished.	Week 10

Name the abnormality/abnormalities caused by the following teratogens:

Angiotensin-converting enzyme (ACE) inhibitors	Renal dysgenesis → oligohydramnios, pulmonary hypoplasia, and limb contractures
Tetracycline	Yellow teeth and enamel hypoplasia
Aminogylcosides	Eighth cranial nerve damage → deafness
Oral hypoglycemics	Neonatal hypoglycemia
Warfarin	Craniofacial (nasal hypoplasia) and CNS defects, stillbirth
Dilantin	Fetal hydantoin syndrome: craniofacial and limb defects, mental deficiencies
Valproic acid	Spina bifida

Lithium	Cardiac (Ebstein) anomaly
Isotretinoin	Craniofacial (small ears), CNS, cardiac, and thymus defects
Indomethacin	Constriction of ductus arteriosus
Diethylstilbesterol (DES)	Clear cell vaginal cancer and cervical/uterine malformations in female offspring
Thalidomide	Limb reduction defects
Alcohol	Fetal alcohol syndrome: craniofacial defects (absent philtrum, flattened nasal bridge, and microphthalmia), growth restriction, and brain, cardiac, and spinal defects
Tobacco	Growth restriction, prematurity, low birth weight
Radiation	Growth restriction, CNS defects, and leukemia

Name the embryonic layer that gives rise to each of the following tissues:

Adrenal cortex	Mesoderm
Anterior pituitary	Ectoderm (oral ectoderm/Rathke pouch)
Aorticopulmonary septum	Ectoderm (neural crest)
Autonomic nerves	Ectoderm (neural crest)
Long bones and vertebrae	Mesoderm
Facial bones	Ectoderm (neural crest)
CNS neurons and astrocytes	Ectoderm (neural tube)
Connective tissue	Mesoderm
Epidermis	Ectoderm (surface ectoderm)
Epithelial lining of the GI tract	Endoderm
Myocardium	Mesoderm
Kidneys	Mesoderm
Lens of eye	Ectoderm (surface ectoderm)
Liver parenchyma	Endoderm
Mammary glands	Ectoderm (surface ectoderm)
Melanocytes	Ectoderm (neural crest)
Striated muscle	Mesoderm
Nucleus pulposus	Mesoderm (notochord)

Pancreas	Endoderm
Parafollicular cells of the thyroid	Ectoderm (neural crest)
Retina	Ectoderm (neural tube)
Schwann cells	Ectoderm (neural crest)
Spleen	Mesoderm
Parathyroid	Endoderm
Posterior pituitary	Ectoderm (neural tube)
Thymus	Endoderm
Thyroid	Endoderm
Kidneys, ureters, and gonads	Mesoderm

BASIC PATHOLOGY

Cellular Adaptations

Give the appropriate term for each of the following definitions:

Complete failure of cell production	Aplasia
Relative decrease in cell production	Hypoplasia
Increase in cell size	Hypertrophy
Replacement of one adult (differentiated) cell (epithelial or mesenchymal) type with another adult cell type	Metaplasia
Decrease in cell substance results in a decrease in cell size; may result in decreased tissue/organ size.	Atrophy
Increase of organ/tissue size due to an increase in the number of cells	Hyperplasia

Cell Injury

Name the mechanism of cell injury characterized by each of the following statements:

Mitochondrial dysfunction →↓ cellular ATP → failure of Na$^+$/K$^+$ ATPase, failure of protein synthesis	Ischemic/hypoxic cell injury
Dissociation of ribosomes and polysomes	ATP depletion

Causes lipid peroxidation of membranes	Reactive oxygen species (O_2-free radicals)
Associated with ionizing radiation, UV light, and reperfusion after ischemic injury	Reactive oxygen species (O_2-free radicals)
Prevented by enzymes such as glutathione peroxidase, catalase, and superoxide dismutase	Generation of reactive oxygen species (O_2-free radicals)
Which molecules are released in response to mitochondrial damage?	Cytochrome c and H^+
Cytoskeletal abnormalities, ATP depletion, and cell swelling are associated with what key event in cell injury?	Defective membrane permeability
What is the effect of increased cytoplasmic calcium ions in a cell undergoing apoptosis or necrosis?	Activation of ATPase, endonuclease, phospholipase, and proteases

Necrosis/Apoptosis

Classify the following as features of apoptosis or necrosis:

Cellular blebbing and cell shrinkage	Apoptosis
Involves many contiguous cells	Necrosis
Physiologic, programmed cell removal	Apoptosis
Active form of cell death (requires energy consumption)	Apoptosis
Gross, irreversible cellular injury	Necrosis
Involves single cells or groups of cells	Apoptosis
Involution and shrinkage of affected cells and fragments	Apoptosis
Marked inflammatory reaction	Necrosis
Inhibited by *bcl-2*; facilitated by *bax*, *p53*	Apoptosis

State the function of each of the following molecules during apoptosis:

Caspases (cysteine protease)	Protein cleavage
Endonucleases	DNA cleavage

Phosphatidylserine and thrombospondin	Cell surface molecules recognized by phagocytes
Tumor necrosis factor (TNF)-α receptor and FAS (CD95)	Death receptors
Bcl-2 and Bcl-x	Major antiapoptotic proteins
Bad and Bax	Major proapoptotic proteins
Cytochrome c	Activation of procaspase 9
Apoptosis-activating factor-1 (Apaf-1)	Cytoplasmic receptor for cytochrome c
TNF-α	Bindings of this ligand to its receptor induce association with a death domain.
Granzyme B	Activation of the caspase cascade (released by cytotoxic T cells)

Name the type of necrosis characterized by each of the following features:

Enzymatic degradation of tissue seen in abscesses	Liquefactive necrosis
Commonly seen in tuberculous granulomas	Caseous necrosis
Fibrin-like, proteinaceous deposition in arterial walls	Fibrinoid necrosis
Lipase-induced autodigestion of adipose tissue → saponification	Fat necrosis
Interruption of blood supply to organs supplied by end arteries; architecture well preserved	Coagulative necrosis
Results from vascular occlusion; most commonly affects lower extremities or bowel	Gangrenous necrosis

Cell Changes/Accumulations

What type of cellular change is characterized by excess accumulation of intracellular triglycerides?	Fatty change (steatosis)
What type of calcification is caused by hypercalcemia?	Metastatic calcification
What type of calcification occurs in previously damaged tissues?	Dystrophic calcification

Name four endogenous pigments that accumulate in cells:	1. Melanin 2. Bilirubin 3. Hemosiderin 4. Lipofuscin
Name four diseases associated with protein misfolding:	1. Alzheimer disease 2. α-1-Antitrypsin deficiency 3. Cystic fibrosis 4. Amyloidosis
Name the cellular pigment described below:	
Accumulates in jaundice	Bilirubin
Identified with Prussian blue dye; can result in organ damage or simple deposition	Hemosiderin
Yellowish, fat-soluble "wear-and-tear" pigment	Lipofuscin
Formed in the epidermis from tyrosine	Melanin

Inflammation

Which three classes of adhesion molecules are involved in inflammation?	1. Selectins (E, P, and L) 2. Immunoglobulin (Ig) family (intercellular adhesion molecule [ICAM], platelet cell adhesion molecule [PCAM]) 3. Integrins
What are the five steps in the extravasation of inflammatory leukocytes?	1. Margination 2. Pavementing 3. Tumbling (rolling) 4. Adhesion 5. Transmigration
Which two groups of cell adhesion molecules pair mediate tumbling?	1. Selectins on endothelial cells 2. Sialylated glycoproteins (eg, sialyl-Lewis-X) on leukocytes
Which two groups of cell adhesion molecules pair mediate leukocyte adhesion to endothelial cells?	1. ICAM and vascular cell adhesion molecule (VCAM) (Ig superfamily) on endothelial cells 2. Integrins on leukocytes

Which factors induce endothelial expression of P-selectin?

Platelet activation factor (PAF), histamine, and thrombin

Which factors induce endothelial expression of ICAM and VCAM?

Interleukin (IL)-1 and TNF

Name five chemotactic factors for neutrophils:

1. Bacterial products
2. C5a
3. LTB_4
4. Chemokines (IL-8)
5. Fibrin split (degradation) products

Name five functional responses of leukocytes following their activation:

1. Eicosanoid production
2. Cytokine secretion
3. Generation of reactive oxygen species
4. Degranulation
5. Altered cell adhesion molecule expression
6. Upregulation of receptors (toll-like, G protein-coupled, opsonin, cytokines)

Name two receptors that function in binding and phagocytosis of bacteria:

1. Mannose
2. Scavenger receptors

What term is used to describe the process of coating substances (with Ig or C3b) to facilitate phagocytosis?

Opsonization

Which neutrophil intracellular microbicidial mechanism uses the HMP shunt to generate an oxidative burst?

H_2O_2-myeloperoxidase (MPO)-halide system of bacterial killing

Name two processes associated with impaired leukocyte adhesion:

1. Recurrent bacterial infections
2. Altered wound healing

Decide whether each of the following substances causes vasoconstriction or vasodilation:

Bradykinin

Vasodilation

Thromboxane (TXA)

Vasoconstriction

Prostacyclin (PGI$_2$)

Vasodilation

Leukotrienes (LTC$_4$, LTD$_4$, and LTE$_4$)

Vasoconstriction

Prostaglandins (PGD$_2$, PGE$_2$, and PGF$_2$)

Vasodilation

Remember: most substances also cause analogous effects on bronchial tone.

Name seven substances that increase vascular permeability:	1. Histamine 2. Serotonin 3. C3a and C5a 4. Leukotrienes (LTC_4, LTD_4, and LTE_4) 5. Bradykinin 6. Nitric oxide (NO) 7. PAF (low concentration)
Which two enzymes stimulate the release of arachidonic acid from membrane phospholipids?	1. Phospholipase A_2 2. Phospholipase C
What are the two major pathways in arachidonic acid metabolism?	1. Cyclooxygenase (COX) 2. Lipoxygenase
What signaling molecules are produced by the COX pathway?	TXA_2 (in platelets), PGI_2 (in endothelial cells), and other prostaglandins (in other tissues)
What are the two major enzymes involved in prostaglandin production?	1. COX-1 2. COX-2
Which cycloxygenase enzyme serves in homeostatic functions?	COX-1
What products does the lipooxygenase pathway produce?	HPETEs and leukotrienes
Which arachidonic acid metabolite is thought to sensitize nerve endings to pain mediators?	PGE_2 ($\downarrow$ PGE_2 → analgesic effects)
Name four acute-phase responses of inflammation.	1. Systemic effects (fever and leukocytosis) 2. Hepatic synthesis of acute-phase reactants (C-reactive protein [CRP] ferritin, complement, and prothrombin) 3. Synthesis of adhesion molecules 4. Neutrophil degranulation
Which substance links the kinin, coagulation, plasminogen, and complement systems?	Factor XIIa (Hageman factor)
Which group of plasma proteins participates in immune-mediated lysis of cells?	Complement system

Which substance produced by endothelial cells relaxes smooth muscle and inhibits platelet aggregation?

Nitric oxide (NO)

Which factor is a pyrogen and causes fever?

IL-1 $\rightarrow$ PGE$_2$

Name four possible outcomes of acute inflammation:

1. Complete resolution
2. Abscess/ulcer/fistula formation
3. Healing by fibrosis and scarring
4. Progression to chronic inflammation

Which pattern of chronic inflammation is characterized by nodular collections of epithelioid histocytes and multinucleated giant cells?

Granulomatous inflammation

Name three etiologies of granulomatous inflammation:

1. Infectious (*Mycobacterium tuberculosis*, *Histoplasma*, catscratch disease, leprosy, syphilis)
2. Foreign bodies
3. Idiopathic (eg, sarcoidosis, Crohn's disease)

Tissue Repair

What are the four factors determining the size of a cell population?

1. Proliferation
2. Cell death
3. Cell differentiation
4. Replacement by stem cells

What are the three categories of cells based on their inherent proliferative activity?

1. Permanent (cardiac myocytes, neurons)
2. Quiescent (hepatocytes, endothelial cells, lymphocytes)
3. Labile (epidermis, GI, and respiratory tract epithelial cells; bone marrow; hair follicles)

Name five factors that mediate cellular proliferation during the process of tissue repair:

1. Platelet-derived growth factor (PDGF)
2. Epidermal growth factor (EGF) and transforming growth factor-alpha (TGF-α)
3. Fibroblast growth factors (FGFs)
4. Hepatyocyte growth factor
5. Vascular endothelial growth factor (VEGF)

What highly vascular, newly formed connective tissue fills defects left by removal of cellular debris?	Granulation tissue
What are the four key components to the orderly formation of a scar?	1. Angiogenesis and granulation tissue formation 2. Fibroblast emigration and proliferation 3. Deposition of extracellular matrix 4. Maturation and remodeling → scar
Name five factors that delay or impede tissue repair:	1. Impaired circulation 2. Persistent infection 3. Retention of debris or foreign body 4. Nutritional deficiency (eg, protein and vitamin C) 5. Metabolic disorders (eg, diabetes mellitus)

Hemodynamic Dysfunction

Name five causes of edema:	1. ↑ Hydrostatic pressure 2. ↑ Capillary permeability 3. ↓ Oncotic pressure 4. ↑ Na+ retention (renal disorders or congestive heart failure [CHF]) 5. Lymphatic obstruction
Describe the contents of a transudate.	Low-protein content (SG <1.012), few cells, and little protein
What type of fluid accumulation forms as a result of increased vascular permeability due to endothelial cell destruction?	Exudate
What is the composition of exudate?	High protein (SG >1.020) ↑ inflammatory leukocytes, and ↑ protein
Name two organs commonly affected by chronic passive congestion and their related pathologic findings:	1. **Lungs:** hemosiderin-laden macrophages or "heart-failure cells" (from left heart failure) 2. **Liver:** nutmeg liver (from right heart failure)
Name the two types of infarcts and several examples of each:	1. Anemic (white) infarcts: heart, spleen, and kidneys 2. Hemorrhagic (red) infarcts: lungs, testes, and GI tract (occurs in areas with collateral circulation)

Thrombosis

What is Virchow triad?	The three primary influences on thrombus formation: 1. Endothelial injury 2. Stasis 3. Hypercoagulability
Name the three components necessary for hemostasis:	1. Vascular endothelium 2. Platelets 3. Coagulation cascade
Name five factors that promote platelet aggregation:	1. ADP 2. Thrombin 3. TXA_2 4. Collagen 5. Platelet-activating factor
Which product of the COX pathway limits further platelet aggregation?	PGI_2
Where are proteins C and S made?	Endothelial cells

Classify the following as features of the extrinsic or the intrinsic pathway:

Involves activation of factor VII	Extrinsic pathway
Clinically monitored by the PT	Extrinsic pathway
Initiated by activation of factor XII	Intrinsic pathway
Monitored by partial thromboplastin time (PTT)	Intrinsic pathway

Name the component(s) of the coagulation cascade associated with each of the following features:

Vitamin K-dependent coagulation factors	Factors II, VII, IX, X, proteins C and S
Ion necessary for proper function of the coagulation cascade	Calcium
Factors inhibited by antithrombin III (AT III)	Thrombin, factors IX, X, XI, and XII

Complex that activates proteins C and S	Thrombomodulin-thrombin complex
The most important fibrinolytic protease	Plasmin
Converts plasminogen to plasmin	Tissue plasminogen activator (t-PA), also urokinase plasminogen activator
Cleaved by activated protein C (APC) → inhibition of coagulation	Factors Va and VIIIa
Which molecule dramatically enhances the activity of AT III?	Heparin
What is the most frequent cause of hereditary thrombophilia?	Factor V (Leiden) mutation (2%-15% of white population)
Hereditary thrombophilia can also be caused by deficiency of what major antithrombotic proteins?	AT III, protein C, and protein S
How does the Leiden mutation confer hypercoagulability?	Renders mutant factor V resistant to cleavage by APC
Which prothrombotic disorder is characterized by autoantibodies that induce platelet activation?	Antiphospholipid antibody syndrome
Name the type of thrombus associated with each of the following:	
Reddish-blue cast; usually in lower extremities	Venous thrombosis
Lines of Zahn	Arterial thrombus
Sterile vegetations of heart valves in patients with hypercoagulable states	Nonbacterial thrombotic endocarditis
Noninfective heart valve vegetations from circulating immune complexes	Verrucous (Libman-Sacks) endocarditis

Embolism

Name the type of embolism described by each of the following statements:	
Venous thrombus that gains access to arterial circulation through a right-to-left shunt	Paradoxical embolus

Associated with decompression sickness	Air embolus
Occurs at parturition; can lead to disseminated intravascular coagulation (DIC) and death	Amniotic fluid embolus
Embolus obstructing the bifurcation of the pulmonary artery	Saddle embolus
Often arises from one wall of a heart chamber, especially in the context of atrial fibrillation	Mural thrombus → arterial emboli
Important cause of death in immobilized, post-op patients	Pulmonary embolus
Occur after severe, multiple long bone fractures	Fat emboli

Shock

Name the type of shock described by each of the following statements:

Associated with gram-negative endotoxemia	Septic shock
Circulatory collapse from pump failure of left ventricle (LV)	Cardiogenic shock
IgE-mediated systemic vasodilation with ↑ vascular permeability	Anaphylactic shock
Caused by severe hemorrhage or fluid loss	Hypovolemic shock
Associated with severe trauma causing reactive peripheral vasodilation	Neurogenic shock
Which two mediators are associated with systemic vasodilation in septic shock?	1. NO 2. PAF

Name the characteristic manifestations of shock on each of the following organs:

Lungs	Pulmonary edema
Liver	Steatosis and centrilobular necrosis
Colon	Patchy mucosal hemorrhages
Adrenals	Lipid depletion of cortex
Kidneys	Acute tubular necrosis

BASIC PHARMACOLOGY

Absorption/Distribution

In which part of the GI tract are most oral drugs absorbed?	Duodenum
Name three factors that influence absorption of drugs:	1. Chemical properties (active transport vs passive diffusion) 2. pH (percent of drug in the uncharged state determines rate of absorption) 3. Physical factors (blood flow, surface area, and contact time with absorptive surfaces)
What is first-pass metabolism?	Hepatic degradation/alteration of an oral drug after absorption, before it enters the general circulation

Complete the following formulas:

(Rate of drug elimination)/ (plasma drug concentration) =	Clearance (CL)
(Amount of drug in body)/ (plasma drug concentration) =	Volume of distribution (V_d)
$(C_p \times V_d)/F =$	Loading dose (also defined as the amount of drug necessary to rapidly raise a desired plasma concentration of the drug)
$(C_p \times CL)/F =$	Maintenance dose (also defined as the amount of drug necessary to maintain a desired plasma concentration of the drug)
$(0.693 \times V_d)/CL =$	Half-life ($t_{1/2}$)

C_p= target plasma concentration, F = bioavailability

If a patient were known to be a rapid metabolizer, would the loading dose or maintenance dose have to be adjusted to maintain a desired plasma concentration of the drug?	The loading dose would be unchanged; the maintenance dose would need to be increased.
How do dosage calculations change for patients with impaired renal/hepatic function?	Loading dose stays the same, maintenance dose decreases.

List four conditions that alter drug distribution:	1. Edematous state (eg, CHF and nephrotic syndrome) 2. Pregnancy ($\uparrow$ intravascular volume) 3. Obesity (accumulation of lipophilic agents in fat cells) 4. Hypoalbuminemia (no albumin to bind drugs $\rightarrow\uparrow$ availability)
Name the key mechanism of drug-drug interactions:	Drug displacement from albumin (combined administration of classes I and II drugs)

Metabolism/Elimination

Name four clinical situations that would result in increased drug half-life.	1. Prerenal state ($\downarrow$ renal plasma flow) 2. Renal disease $\rightarrow$ decreased extraction ratio 3. Adding a second drug that displaces the first from albumin, thus $\uparrow V_d$ 4. $\downarrow$ Metabolism (hepatic insufficiency or drug interaction)

Classify each of the following statements as characteristic of phase I or phase II metabolism:

Produces slightly polar, water-soluble metabolites	Phase I
Involves mixed-function oxidase (P-450)	Phase I
Involves conjugation reactions (acetylation, glucuronidation, and sulfation)	Phase II
Produces very polar, inactive metabolites that are excreted by the kidneys	Phase II
Reduction, oxidation, and hydrolysis	Phase I
Phase that may be compromised first in geriatric patients	Phase I
Phase that may be compromised in neonates	Phase I

Classify each of the following statements as characteristic of first- or zero-order drug elimination:

Constant *fraction* of drug eliminated per unit of time	First-order elimination
Constant *amount* of drug eliminated per unit of time	Zero-order elimination

Plasma concentration decreases linearly with time	Zero-order elimination
Plasma concentration decreases exponentially with time	First-order elimination
Elimination rate is independent of concentration	Zero-order elimination

Pharmacodynamics

What term describes the maximum effect a drug can produce?	Efficacy
What term describes the measure of the amount of drug needed to produce a given result?	Potency
What term describes the dose of a drug that produces the desired effect?	Effective dose (ED)
What term describes the dose of a drug that produces death?	Lethal dose (LD)
What term describes the measure of the safety of a drug?	Therapeutic index
How is therapeutic index calculated?	LD_{50}/ED_{50} (LD_{50} = dose lethal in 50% of the population, ED_{50} = dose effective in 50% of the population)
How does a competitive antagonist affect the dose-response curve?	Shifts it to the right ($\uparrow ED_{50}$)
How does a noncompetitive antagonist affect the dose-response curve?	Shifts it downward ($\downarrow$ maximal response)
How does a partial agonist differ from a full agonist?	Acts like an agonist when an agonist is not present; acts like an antagonist if an agonist is present

Drug Development

Name the phase of drug development described by each of the following statements:	
Measures effect of the drug in patients with a disease	Phase II clinical testing
Measures whether the drug is safe in healthy volunteers	Phase I clinical testing

Postmarketing surveillance	Phase IV
Large, multicenter clinical trials to prove efficacy and safety	Phase III clinical trials

Toxicology

Name the antidote for each of the following toxins:

Iron	Deferoxamine
Copper/gold/arsenic	Penicillamine
Lead	CaEDTA, succimer, dimercaprol (BAL in oil), and oral penicillamine
Arsenic/mercury	Dimercaprol
Carbon monoxide	100% O_2 and hyperbaric O_2
Cyanide	Nitrite, vitamin B_{12}, and thiosulfate
Methemoglobin	Methylene blue
Methanol/ethylene glycol	ETOH, fomepizole, and dialysis
Acetaminophen (Tylenol)	N-acetylcysteine
Aspirin (salicylates)	Alkalinze urine (promotes excretion) and dialysis
Opioids	Naloxone (IV, IM, and SQ) or naltrexone (PO)
Benzodiazepines	Flumazenil
Organophosphates, anticholinesterases	Atropine and pralidoxime (PAM)
Heparin	Protamine sulfate
Warfarin	Vitamin K, fresh frozen plasma (FFP) for acute reversal
tPA	Aminocaproic acid
Digitalis	Antidig F_{ab} fragments (first stop drug and stabilize K^+, Mg^{2+}, and lidocaine)
Cyclophosphamide	Mesna

P-450

Classify each of the following drugs as inhibitors or inducers of P-450:	Inducers: "Queen Barb takes Phen-phen and Refuses Greasy Carbs"
	Inhibitors: "Inhibitors Stop Cyber-Kids from Eating Grapefruits"

Barbiturates	Inducer
INH	Inhibitor
Spironolactone	Inhibitor
Rifampin	Inducer
Cimetidine	Inhibitor
Ketoconazole	Inhibitor
Phenytoin and carbamazepine	Inducer
Quinidine	Inducer
Disulfiram	Inhibitor
Sulfonamides	Inhibitor
Steroids	Inhibitor
Macrolides (erythromycin)	Inhibitor
Chloramphenicol	Inhibitor
Griseofulvin	Inducer
Grapefruit	Inhibitor
Verapamil	Inhibitor
Chronic EtOH use	Inducer
Acute EtOH use	Inhibitor

CHAPTER 2

Immunology

IMMUNOLOGY BASICS

Cells of the Immune System

Name the type of immune cell that
fits each description given below:

Major cells involved in innate immunity	Monocytes, macrophages, neutrophils, natural killer (NK) cells
Cell-mediated immune response	T lymphocyte
Humoral immunity	B lymphocyte
Primary phagocytic cell in acute inflammation	Neutrophil
Type of cell necessary for transplant rejection	T lymphocyte
Contains myeloperoxidase and lysozyme	Neutrophil
Major mediator of a type 1 hypersensitivity reaction	Mast cell
Major mediator of the antiparasitic response	Eosinophil
Granules contain histamine and heparin	Basophil and mast cells
Major antigen-presenting cells in tissues	Macrophages, dendritic cells, and B cells
Demonstrates a multilobed ("hypersegmented") nucleus in vitamin B_{12} or folate deficiency	Neutrophil
Secretes interleukin (IL)-1 to promote T cell activity	Macrophage
Expresses IgE receptors on its cell membrane to mediate the allergic response	Basophil

Expresses high levels of major histocompatibility complex (MHC) class II on its cell membrane	Macrophage
Macrophage precursor	Monocyte
Cell type increased in atopic asthma	Eosinophil
Recognizes antigen presented in the context of MHC class II molecules	T-helper cell
Antibody-producing cell with abundant rough endoplasmic reticulum	Plasma cell
Major source of IL-2 production	T-helper cell (specifically T_H1 cells)
Major cell of the humoral immune response	B lymphocyte

Immunoglobulins

Name the type of immunoglobulin (Ig) associated with the following features:

Most abundant type of Ig	IgG
First class of Ig produced in an immune response upon exposure to antigen	IgM
Able to fix complement	IgG and IgM
Found on the lining of mucous membranes and in secretions, including breast milk and saliva	IgA
Able to cross placenta	IgG
Type of Ig commonly occurring as a dimer	IgA
Type of Ig commonly occurring as a pentamer	IgM
Ig elevated in patients with asthma and allergies	IgE
Responsible for long-term immunity	IgG
Causes mast cells and basophils to release histamine when triggered by antigen	IgE
Type of Ig found embedded in the cell membrane of developing B cells	IgD

Total levels and concentration of this antibody can be estimated using radioimmunosorbent test (RIST) and radioallergosorbent test (RAST).	IgE
What term is used to describe the portion of a molecule that serves as an antigenic determinant?	Epitope
What term is used to describe a small molecule that can serve as an antigenic determinant only if it is attached to a larger carrier molecule?	Hapten
What type of chemical bonds are critical in linking the heavy and light chains of Igs?	Disulfide bonds
Which products result when papain digests an Ig?	Two Fab fragments (each capable of binding antigen) and one F_c fragment
Which products are produced following pepsin digestion of an Ig?	One $F(ab')_2$ fragment and one F_c fragment
What term is used to describe the region in an antibody that determines antigen specificity?	The hypervariable region or complementarity determining region (CDR)
Name five mechanisms by which antibody diversity is created:	1. Mutations in the genes encoding the CDR region
	2. Random VJ recombination in light chains
	3. Random VDJ recombination in heavy chains
	4. Random assembly of light and heavy chains
	5. Imperfect recombination of VDJ genes

T Cells

Name the T-lymphocyte cell surface protein associated with the following features:	
Antigen-specific receptor on 95% of T cells	$\alpha\beta$ T-cell receptor ($\alpha\beta$ TCR)
Antigen-specific receptor on 5% (or less) of T cells	$\gamma\delta$ T-cell receptor ($\gamma\delta$ TCR)

Signal transduction protein always associated with TCR	CD3
T-cell marker expressed in immature T cells	CD2
Responds to MHC class II molecule expressed by antigen-presenting cells	CD4
Responds to MHC class I molecule expressed on all cells	CD8
Found specifically on T-helper cells	CD4
Found specifically on cytotoxic T cells	CD8
Cells with this surface marker ↓ in HIV/AIDS	CD4
Type of T cell that destroys virally infected cells	CD8

HLA Subtypes

Name the HLA haplotype(s) associated with the following diseases:

Ankylosing spondylitis	HLA-B27
Type 1 diabetes mellitus	HLA-DR3/DR4
Multiple sclerosis	HLA-DR2
Rheumatoid arthritis	HLA-DR4
Screening for abacavir hypersensitivity	HLA-B*5701

Cytokines

Name the cytokine described below:

Endogenous pyrogen	IL-1 (produced by macrophages)
Promotes IgA synthesis	IL-5
Induces IL-2 production by T cells	IL-1
High concentrations induce cell death in some tumors and cause cachexia.	Tumor necrosis factor (TNF)-α
Induces T- and B-cell activity during the initial stages of an immune response	IL-1

Induces production of IgE and IgG	IL-4 (produced by T-helper cells)
Induces differentiation of eosinophils and promotes growth in B cells	IL-5 (produced by T-helper cells)
Chemotactic factor for neutrophils	IL-8 (produced by monocytes and endothelial cells)
Secreted by activated T cells and induces maturation of bone marrow stem cells	IL-3
Inhibits production of interferon-gamma (IFN-γ) by T-helper cells	IL-10 (produced by T_H2 cells)
Inhibits production of IFN-γ	IL-4
Inhibits differentiation of T_H1 cells	IL-10
Stimulates T_H1 differentiation	IL-12 (produced by macrophages and B cells)
Activates T-helper, T-cytotoxic, natural killer, and B cells	IL-2 (produced by T-helper cells)
Promotes production of IFN-γ T-helper cells	IL-12
Low concentrations promote neutrophil activity and IL-2 receptor expression.	TNF-α
Inhibits growth and function of T and B cells and promotes collagen secretion during tissue repair	Transforming growth factor-beta (TGF-β)

Gel and Coombs Hypersensitivity Reactions

Name the Gel and Coombs hypersensitivity reaction described below:

Mediated by IgE bound to mast cells and basophils	Type 1 (immediate or anaphylactic hypersensitivity)
Antibody-mediated cytotoxic reaction	Type 2 (cytotoxic reaction)
Occurs in response to environmental allergies	Type 1
Antigen-sensitized T cells release cytokines, which induce an inflammatory response up to 48 hours after initial contact with antigen.	Type 4 (delayed-type hypersensitivity)

Associated with the release of histamine, platelet-activating factor, leukotrienes, prostaglandins, and thromboxanes	Type 1
Binding of cytotoxic T cells or complement to F_c portion of antibody causes target cell lysis	Type 2
Immune complex deposition in tissues results in an inflammatory response	Type 3 (immune complex reaction)

Name the type of hypersensitivity reaction responsible for the following diseases or conditions:

Arthus reaction	Type 3
Asthma	Type 1
Chronic transplant rejection	Type 4
Contact dermatitis, reaction to poison ivy	Type 4
Drug allergies	Type 1
Environmental allergies	Type 1
Erythroblastosis fetalis	Type 2
Goodpasture syndrome	Type 2
Graves disease	Type 2
Hemolytic anemia	Type 2
Immune complex-mediated glomerulonephritis	Type 3
Lambert-Eaton	Type 2
Myasthenia gravis	Type 2
Multiple sclerosis	Type 4
Pernicious anemia	Type 2
Purified protein derivative (PPD)/tuberculin skin test	Type 4
Rheumatic fever	Type 2
Rheumatoid arthritis	Type 3
Systemic anaphylaxis	Type 1
Serum sickness	Type 3
Systemic lupus erythematosus (SLE)	Type 3
Transfusion reaction due to ABO incompatibility	Type 2

Complement

Which class of bacteria is particularly susceptible to complement-mediated lysis?	Gram-negative organisms
Which antibody isotypes activate the classic pathway of the complement cascade?	IgG and IgM
Which molecules activate the alternative pathway of the complement cascade?	Aggregated IgA, endotoxin, and other components of the bacterial cell wall

Name the component(s) of the complement cascade responsible for the following functions:

Neutralization of viruses	C1 to C4
Opsonization	C3b
Neutrophil and macrophage chemotaxis	C5a
Synthesis of membrane attack complex (MAC)	C5b to C9
Formation of C3 convertase	C3b, Bb (alternative pathway) or C4b, C2b (classic pathway)

Name the disease or condition caused by a deficiency of the following complement components:

C1 esterase inhibitor	Hereditary angioedema
C3	Sinus and upper respiratory tract infections
C5b to C9	Recurrent *Neisseria* infections
Decay accelerating factor	Paroxysmal nocturnal hemoglobinuria

Transplant Rejection and MHC Molecules

For each of the following descriptions, name the type of transplant rejection:

Preformed antibodies in host react against graft antigens	Hyperacute rejection (minutes to hours)
Activation of previously sensitized T cells	Accelerated rejection (hours to days)

Involves T-cell activation, differentiation, and antibody production	Acute rejection (days to weeks)
Immune complex deposition combined with subacute cell cytotoxicity	Chronic rejection (months to years)
What are the four different classes of grafts?	1. Autograft (from self) 2. Syngeneic (from identical twin or clone) 3. Allograft (from same species) 4. Xenograft (from different species)
The activity of cytotoxic T cells against tumor or virally infected cells requires which cell surface receptor for antigen presentation?	MHC class I
The activity of cytotoxic T cells against pathogens phagocytosed by macrophages requires which cell surface receptor for antigen presentation?	MHC class II

PATHOLOGY IMMUNE SYSTEM

Autoantibodies

Describe the disease associated with the following autoantibodies:

Antinuclear antibodies (ANA)	SLE (sensitive but not specific for SLE)
Antiacetylcholine esterase (ACh)	Myasthenia gravis
Antibasement membrane	Goodpasture disease
Anticentromere	**CREST** syndrome (**C**alcinosis, **R**aynaud, **E**sophageal dysmotility, **S**clerodactyly, **T**elangiectasias)
Anti-dsDNA	SLE (highly specific for SLE)
Antiepithelial cell	Pemphigus vulgaris
Antigliadin	Celiac sprue
Antihistone	Drug-induced lupus
Anti-IgG F$_c$ (rheumatoid factor)	Rheumatoid arthritis
Anti-Jo1	Myositis
Antimicrosomal	Hashimoto thyroiditis

Antimitochondrial	Primary biliary cirrhosis
Antinuclear ribonucleoprotein (nRNP)	Mixed connective tissue disease
Antiplatelet	Idiopathic thrombocytopenic purpura
Anti-Scl-70 (DNA topoisomerase 1)	Systemic sclerosis
Anti-Smith	SLE (highly specific for SLE)
Anti-SS-A (Ro) and anti-SS-B (La)	Sjögren syndrome
Antithyroglobulin	Hashimoto thyroiditis
Anti-thyroid-stimulating hormone receptor (TSHr)	Graves disease
Anti-voltage-gated calcium channel	Lambert-Eaton syndrome
Cytoplasmic pattern of antineutrophil cytoplasmic antibodies (c-ANCA)	Wegener granulomatosis
Perinuclear pattern of antineutrophil cytoplasmic antibodies (p-ANCA)	Microscopic PolyANgiitis, Polyarteritis Nodosa (PAN), and Churg-Strauss syndrome
List the four types of nuclear antigens against which ANAs are directed:	1. DNA 2. Histones 3. Nonhistone proteins 4. Nucleolar antigens

Systemic Lupus Erythematosus

What pathologic finding is common to all tissues affected by SLE?	Acute necrotizing vasculitis of small arteries and arterioles caused by immune complex deposition
Describe the effect of SLE on each of the following organs:	
Skin	Malar rash, discoid rash, photosensitivity
Joints	Arthritis and arthralgias
Brain	Neuropsychiatric changes or seizures (2° to cerebral vasculitis), cognitive dysfunction
Eyes	Cotton-wool spots, retinal hemorrhages
Heart	Pericarditis, Libman-Sacks Endocarditis (SLE → LSE)
Lungs	Pleuritis, pulmonary fibrosis
Gastrointestinal (GI)	Oral and nasopharyngeal ulcers

Spleen	Splenomegaly and onion skinning of splenic vessels
Kidneys	Wire-loop glomerular lesions and mesangial immune complex deposits $\rightarrow$ glomerulonephritis
Hematology	Hemolytic anemia, leukopenia, thrombocytopenia, antiphospholipid antibody syndrome
Blood vessels	Raynaud phenomenon
Libman-Sacks endocarditis causes sterile vegetations to form on both sides of which cardiac valve?	Mitral valve
Name five medications capable of inducing a lupus-like syndrome:	1. Hydralazine 2. Isonicotinic acid (INH) 3. Phenytoin 4. Procainamide 5. Penicillamine
Name the disease related to SLE that is characterized by immune complex deposition at the dermal-epidermal junction:	Discoid lupus erythematosus

Immunodeficiencies

Name the immunodeficiency associated with the following clinical and pathologic features:

B-cell deficiency causing recurrent respiratory tract bacterial infections in boys >6 months of age	X-linked (XL) agammaglobulinemia
T-cell deficiency due to failure of development of the third and fourth pharyngeal pouches	Thymic aplasia (DiGeorge syndrome)
Defective B and T cells, most cases caused by XL recessive mutation in γ-chain of cytokine receptors *or* autosomal recessive (AR) mutation in adenosine deaminase	Severe combined immunodeficiency
AR disease characterized by IgA deficiency, cerebellar dysfunction, and conjunctival telangiectasias	Ataxia-telangiectasia

XL deficiency of nicotinamide adenine dinucleotide phosphate (NADPH) oxidase activity, resulting in an impaired neutrophil respiratory burst and leading to increased bacterial and fungal infections	Chronic granulomatous disease
Recurrent bacterial infections early in life due to a defect in CD40 ligand that prevents B-cell class switching	Hyper-IgM syndrome
AR microtubule defect resulting in decreased phagocytosis, partial albinism, and neuropathy	Chediak-Higashi disease
AR syndrome characterized by failure of neutrophil chemotaxis-associated eczema, elevated IgE, noninflamed staphylococcal abscesses	Job (hyper-IgE) syndrome
XL recessive disease characterized by recurrent infections, thrombocytopenia, eczema	Wiskott-Aldrich syndrome
Mutation of the *Btk tyrosine kinase* gene resulting in the underproduction of all classes of antibodies	XL agammaglobulinemia
Defect in the receptor for IL-7	Severe combined immunodeficiency
Associated with *Staphylococcus aureus, Streptococcus pneumoniae,* and *Haemophilus influenzae* respiratory infections and persistent *Giardia lamblia* infections	XL agammaglobulinemia
Associated with recurrent GI and pulmonary infections	Isolated IgA deficiency
Frequent viral and fungal infections in a patient with hypocalcemia due to low PTH levels	Thymic aplasia (DiGeorge syndrome)
Associated with tetany and congenital defects of the heart and aorta	Thymic aplasia (DiGeorge syndrome)
Small thymus devoid of lymphocytes, hypoplastic lymph nodes, and splenic white pulp	Severe combined immunodeficiency
↑ IgA, normal IgE, and ↓ IgM levels	Wiskott-Aldrich syndrome
Hypogammaglobulinemia commonly due to failure of T-cell-mediated B-cell maturation	Common variable immunodeficiency

Autoimmune Connective Tissue Disorders

Name the autoimmune disease
of connective tissue associated with
the following clinical and pathologic
findings:

Keratoconjunctivitis sicca or xerophthalmia, xerostomia, and evidence of other connective tissue disease	Sjögren syndrome
Autoimmune inflammatory disorder associated with malignancy; frequently caused muscle weakness	Polymyositis
Heliotrope rash	Dermatomyositis
Rapidly progressive diffuse fibrosis of skin and involved organs including the heart, GI tract, kidney, lung, muscle, and skin	Diffuse scleroderma
CREST syndrome of calcinosis, Raynaud phenomenon, esophageal dysfunction, sclerodactyly, telangiectasias	Localized scleroderma
↑ Serum creatine kinase (CK) levels	Polymyositis

What is the most common cause
of death due to scleroderma?

Renal crisis (accounts for 50% of deaths related to scleroderma)

Which autoimmune disease
of connective tissue lacks renal
involvement?

Mixed connective tissue disease

Amyloidoses

Name the group of disorders
characterized by extracellular deposition
of protein in a β-pleated sheet
conformation.

Amyloidoses

Which stain is used to identify the
presence of amyloid in tissue that
exhibits apple green bifringence
under polarized light?

Congo red

Which molecular configuration
is common to all forms of amyloid?

Cross-β-pleated sheet

Name the effect of amyloidosis on each of the following organs:

Kidneys	Glomerular, peritubular, and vascular hyalinization
Spleen	Sago spleen (tapioca-like amyloid deposits in follicles) or lardaceous spleen (amyloid deposition in splenic pulp)
Liver	Hepatomegaly with amyloid deposition in the space of Disse
Heart	Restrictive cardiomyopathy
Tongue	Hypertrophy due to amyloid deposition

CHAPTER 3

Microbiology and Infectious Diseases

BACTERIOLOGY

Taxonomy

Name two genera of gram-positive cocci:	1. *Streptococcus* 2. *Staphylococcus*
Name four genera of gram-positive bacilli:	1. *Clostridium* 2. *Listeria* 3. *Bacillus* 4. *Corynebacterium*
Which of these gram-positive bacilli are spore forming?	*Clostridium* and *Bacillus*
Which gram-positive cocci are catalase positive (+)?	*Staphylococcus*
Which of these is also coagulase (+)?	*Staphylococcus aureus*
Name the streptococci that typically show the following pattern of hemolysis:	
α **(green/partial hemolysis)** *"αlmost hemolytic"*	*Streptococcus pneumoniae* and viridans group (eg, *Streptococcus mutans*)
β **(clear hemolysis)** *"βetter hemolysis"*	Group A (*Streptococcus pyogenes*) and group B (*Streptococcus agalactiae*)
γ **(no hemolysis)**	Group D (*Enterococcus* and *Peptostreptococcus*)

Laboratory Evaluation of Gram-Positive Bacteria

How are *S. pneumoniae* and viridans streptococci differentiated in the laboratory?

Streptococcus pneumoniae is bile soluble and optochin sensitive.

How can capsulated *S. pneumoniae* bugs be detected in the laboratory?

Quellung positive (capsule swells when antisera is added)

What determines the Lancefield grouping of streptococci?

C-carbohydrate in the bacterial cell wall

How are groups A and B differentiated in the laboratory?

Group A is bacitracin sensitive.

How are spores from gram-positive rods killed?

Autoclave (spores are resistant to heat and most chemicals)

Name the gram-negative organisms associated with each of the following statements:

Three pathogenic gram-negative cocci

1. *Neisseria meningitides*
2. *Neisseria gonorrhea*
3. *Moraxella catarrhalis*

Six gram-negative coccobacilli

1. *Haemophilus influenzae*
2. *Pasteurella*
3. *Brucella*
4. *Bordetella pertussis*
5. *Francisella*
6. *Legionella*

Three clinically important gram-negative rods that are typically lactose fermenting

1. *Enterobacter*
2. *Escherichia coli*
3. *Klebsiella* (all implicated in urinary tract infections [UTIs])

Two obligate intracellular organisms

1. *Chlamydia* (steals adenosine triphosphate [ATP] from host)
2. *Rickettsia* (lacks coenzyme A [CoA] and nicotinamide adenine [NAD] → cannot produce own ATP)

Four obligate aerobes

1. *Nocardia*
2. *Pseudomonas*
3. *Mycobacterium tuberculosis*
4. *Bacillus*

Three obligate anaerobes

1. *Clostridium*
2. *Bacteroides*
3. *Actinomyces* (no catalase and/or superoxide dismutase → susceptible to oxidative damage)

How are the pathogenic *Neisseria* species differentiated in the laboratory?

Neisseria meningitidis ferments maltose.

How can *Pseudomonas* be rapidly differentiated from many lactose nonfermenters in the laboratory?

Pseudomonas is oxidase positive.

Provide culture requirements or conditions for each of the following bacteria:

Corynebacterium diphtheriae

Tellurite agar or Loeffler media

Bordetella pertussis

Bordet-Gengou potato blood agar

Neisseria gonorrhoea

Thayer-Martin (VCN—vancomycin, colistin, and nystatin) and a selective medium

Legionella pneumophila

Charcoal yeast agar with iron and L-cysteine

Mycoplasma pneumoniae

Eaton agar

Mycobacterium tuberculosis

Lowenstein-Jensen agar

Vibrio species

Thiosulfate-Citrate-Bile Salts-Sucrose (TCBS) agar

Enterococcus

40% bile and 6.5% NaCl

Haemophilus influenzae

Chocolate agar (contains factor V [NAD] and X [hematin])

Lactose-fermenters (*Klebsiella, Escherichia,* etc)

MacConkey agar → pink colonies

Fungi

Sabouraud agar

Bacteriology Basics

Which cell membrane structure is unique to gram-positive organisms?

Teichoic acid

Which molecule, unique to the bacterial cell wall, provides rigid support and resistance against osmotic pressure?

Peptidoglycan

Which heat-stable lipopolysaccharide (LPS) is found in the cell wall of gram-negative bacteria?

Endotoxin

Which is the only gram-positive organism with LPS-lipid A?

Listeria monocytogenes

Name five important systemic effects of endotoxin (particularly, lipid A):

1. ↑Interleukin (IL)-1 → fever
2. ↑ Tissue necrosis factor (TNF) → hemorrhagic tissue death
3. ↑ Nitric oxide → hypotension and shock
4. Activation of alternate complement pathway →↑ C3a (edema) and C5a (polymorphonuclear [PMN] chemotaxis)
5. Activation of factor XII → coagulation cascade → DIC

Which has a higher toxicity, endotoxins or exotoxins?

Exotoxins: fatal dose on the order of 1 µg (vs hundreds of micrograms for endotoxins)

Name the mechanism of DNA transfer characterized by the following statements:

DNA is taken up directly from the environment by competent cells

Transformation (can occur in eukaryotic cells, too)

Medically important natural transformers: **HHSNG**: "**H**ere, **H**ave **S**ome **N**ew **G**enes": *H. pylori, H. influenzae, S. pneumoniae, N. gonorrhoea*

Plasmid or chromosomal DNA transferred from one bacterium to another via cell-to-cell contact

Conjugation

DNA transferred by a virus from one cell to another; can be generalized or specialized

Transduction

DNA segments able to excise and reincorporate into different locations

Transposons

Name the bacterium whose exotoxin has the following effects:

Superantigen that induces IL-1 and IL-2 synthesis in toxic shock syndrome; also leads to food poisoning

Staphylococcus aureus

α-Toxin is a lecithinase → gas gangrene

Clostridium perfringens

Prevents the release of the neurotransmitter (NT) glycine from Renshaw cells in spinal cord → paralysis

Clostridium tetani

↑ Adenylate cyclase by adenosine diphosphate (ADP) ribosylation → whooping cough	*Bordetella pertussis*
Exotoxin encoded by β-prophage; α subunit → inactivates elongation factor 2 (EF-2) halting protein synthesis; β subunit → permits entry into cardiac and neural tissue	*Corynebacterium diphtheriae*
Erythrogenic superantigen → rash in scarlet fever	*Streptococcus pyogenes*
Prevents release of acetylcholine (ACh) → central nervous system (CNS) paralysis; spores in canned food and honey, construction sites	*Clostridium botulinum*
Heat-stable toxin ↑ guanylate cyclase; heat-labile toxin ↑ adenylate cyclase by ADP ribosylation of G protein → watery diarrhea	*Escherichia coli*
Inactivates the 60S ribosome → kills intestinal cells	*Shigella dysenteriae*
Permanent ADP ribosylation of G protein →↑ adenylate cyclase →↑ Cl⁻ and H₂O in gut → voluminous stools	*Vibrio cholerae*
Exotoxin A inhibits protein synthesis by blocking EF-2	*Pseudomonas*
Which virulence factor allows organisms to colonize mucosal surfaces?	IgA protease (eg, *S. pneumoniae* and *H. influenzae*)

Name the bacterial structure associated with each antigenic classification given below:

K-antigen	Capsule (related to virulence of the bacteria)
	K = Kapsule
O-antigen	Outer portion of the polysaccharide of endotoxin
	O = Outer
H-antigen	Flagella (seen in motile species)

Name the key virulence factor(s) associated with each of the following organisms:

Group A streptococcus	M-protein, streptokinase, and hyaluronidase
Staphylococcus aureus	Protein A (prevents complement fixation and phagocytosis), penicillinase, and hyaluronidase
Streptococcus viridans	Extracellular dextran → helps bind to heart valves
Yersinia pestis	F1 capsular antigen (antiphagocytic) and protease (degrades clots)
Haemophilus influenzae	Capsule: six types (a-f) and IgA protease
Borrelia	Antigenic variation
Mycobacterium tuberculosis	Mycosides (cord factor, wax D, and sulfatides)

Infectious Diseases

Name the organism(s) associated with each of the following characteristics:

Gram-positive rods with metachromatic granules	*Corynebacterium diphtheriae*
Three urease (+)	*Helicobacter pylori, Proteus,* and *Ureaplasma urealyticum*
Aerosol transmission from environmental water source (eg, air conditioner)	*Legionella pneumophila*
Contain mycolic acid in membranes	*Mycobacterium* and *Nocardia*
Peptidoglycan wall lacks muramic acid	*Chlamydiae*
Produces pyocyanin (blue-green) pigment	*Pseudomonas aeruginosa*
Produces yellow-gold pigment	*Staphylococcus aureus*
Produces reddish pigment	*Serratia marcescens*
Only bacterial membrane containing cholesterol	*Mycoplasma pneumoniae*
Filamentous, branching rods in a cervicofacial infection	*Actinomyces israelii*
Two forms: elementary and reticulate bodies	*Chlamydiae*

Pleomorphic gram-negative rods in "school of fish" pattern	*Haemophilus ducreyi*
Clue cells on wet mount	*Gardnerella vaginalis*
High titer of cold agglutinins (IgM)	*Mycoplasma pneumoniae*
Two fungi-like bacteria	*Actinomyces israelii* and *Nocardia asteroides*

Name the organism(s) associated with the following pathology:

Fitz-Hugh and Curtis syndrome	*Chlamydia trachomatis* or *N. gonorrhea*
Invades gastrointestinal (GI) mucosa → diarrhea; motile; can disseminate hematogenously	*Salmonella*
Infected dog or cat bites (or scratches)	*Pasteurella multocida*
Ghon complex	*Mycobacterium tuberculosis* (1° tuberculosis [TB]). **Note:** hilar nodes plus Ghon focus usually in lower lobe
Meningitis and pneumonia in neonates	*Haemophilus influenzae*
Atypical pneumonia with avian reservoir	*Chlamydia psittaci*
Gas gangrene in traumatic open wounds	*Clostridium perfringens*
Infects skin and superficial nerves	*Mycobacterium leprae*
Fibrocaseous cavitary lung lesion	*Mycobacterium tuberculosis* (2° TB). **Note:** usually at apex because ↑ affinity for ↑ O_2 environments
Mycobacterium causing disseminated disease in acquired immunodeficiency syndrome (AIDS) patients	*Mycobacterium avium-intracellulare*
Mycobacterium causing cervical lymphadenitis in kids	*Mycobacterium scrofulaceum*

For each of the following clinical findings, name the organism responsible and the drug(s) of choice:

Oral/facial abscesses with sulfur granules in sinus tracts	*Actinomyces israelii*—penicillin G (IV)
Currant jelly sputum	*Klebsiella*—first- or second-generation cephalosporins
Woolsorter's disease	*Bacillus anthracis*—penicillin G or ciprofloxacin
Scarlet fever, impetigo, and pharyngitis	*Streptococcus pyogenes*—penicillin

Pontiac fever	*Legionella pneumophila*—macrolide (erythromycin and azithromycin)
Gram-positive coccus causing sepsis/meningitis in a newborn	*Streptococcus agalactiae*—ampicillin (**Note:** group **B**, think **B**abies)
Acute epiglottitis, meningitis, otitis, and pneumonia	*Haemophilus influenzae*—second-generation cephalosporins (treat meningitis with ceftriaxone, plus rifampin for contacts)
Gastritis and ~90% of duodenal ulcers	*Helicobacter pylori*—triple therapy
Waterhouse-Friderichsen syndrome	*Neisseria meningitidis*—ceftriaxone
Pneumonia in cystic fibrosis and burn patients	*Pseudomonas cepacia*—bactrim or ciprofloxacin
Bacterial vaginosis with discharge and fishy odor	*Gardnerella vaginalis*—metronidazole
Burn and wound infections with fruity odor	*Pseudomonas aeruginosa*—aminoglycoside plus antipseudomonal (eg, piperacillin and tazobactam)
Acute postinfectious glomerulonephritis	*Streptococcus pyogenes*—penicillin G
Pseudomembranous enterocolitis	*Clostridium difficile*—metronidazole or oral vancomycin
Atypical "walking" pneumonia in young adult	*Mycoplasma pneumoniae*—erythromycin or doxycycline
Urethritis/pelvic inflammatory disease (PID), neonatal conjunctivitis, and pneumonia	*Chlamydia trachomatis* types D to K—erythromycin eye drops in neonates, azithromycin for urethritis, pneumonia
Lyme disease	*Borrelia burgdorferi*—doxycycline
Malignant, vesicular papules covered with black eschar → bacteremia and even death	*Bacillus anthracis*—penicillin G or ciprofloxacin
Pneumonia, sepsis, otitis externa, UTIs, hot-tub folliculitis, osteomyelitis	*Pseudomonas aeruginosa*—aminoglycoside plus antipseudomonal piperacillin and tazobactam
Undulant fever, Bang disease	*Brucella* sp.—doxycycline plus gentamicin or rifampin (pasteurize milk to prevent)
Bubonic plague	*Yersinia pestis*—gentamicin
Rocky Mountain spotted fever	*Rickettsia rickettsii*—tetracycline/doxycycline
Trench fever (lasts 5 days; recurs in 5-day cycles)	*Bartonella quintana*—gentamicin/doxycycline
Tabes dorsalis, aortitis, and gummas	*Treponema pallidum* (3° syphilis)—penicillin G

Q fever (acute)	*Coxiella burnetii*—doxycycline
Weil disease	*Leptospira interrogans*—penicillin G
Yaws	*Treponema pertenue*—penicillin G
Pott disease	*Mycobacterium tuberculosis* (disseminated)—four-drug antituberculous therapy, including rifampin plus isoniazid (INH)
Dental caries	*Streptococcus mutans*—amoxicillin or amoxicillin/clavulonic acid (prevention with topical fluoride/chlorhexidine)
Rheumatic fever	*Streptococcus pyogenes*—penicillin G
Scalded skin syndrome and toxic shock syndrome	*Staphylococcus aureus*—penicillin agent (vancomycin if methicillin-resistant *S. aureus* [MRSA])
Hansen disease	*Mycobacterium leprae*—dapsone plus clofazimine or rifampin
What is the differential for a rash affecting the palms and soles?	Rocky Mountain spotted fever, 2° syphilis, hand-foot-and-mouth disease (coxsackie A), and Kawasaki syndrome

Name the mode of transmission and reservoir(s) for each of the following bacteria:

Brucella **sp.**	Contact with animals or dairy products; cows
Francisella tularensis	Tick or deerfly bite; rabbits and deer
Pasteurella multocida	Animal bite/scratch; cats and dogs
Borrelia burgdorferi	Ixodes tick bite; lives on deer and mice
Yersinia pestis	Flea bite; rodents (eg, prairie dogs)
Rickettsia rickettsii	Tick bite; dogs, rabbits, and rodents (endemic to eastern United States)
Rickettsia prowazekii	Human body louse; humans and flying squirrels

Name the laboratory test described below:

Detects antirickettsial antibodies	Weil-Felix reaction (cross-reacts with proteus)
Sensitive for treponemes	Fluorescent treponemal antibody-absorption test (FTA-ABS) (+) (earliest and longest, used as confirmatory test for syphilis if RPR is reactive)
Useful in screening for TB	Purified protein derivative (PPD) test

Name the screening test for syphilis and four biological false positives:

VDRL test
1. Viruses (mononucleosis and hepatitis)
2. Drugs (narcotics)
3. Rheumatoid arthritis/fever
4. Leprosy and lupus

Name the normal, dominant flora for each of the following locations:

Nose	*Staphylococcus aureus*
Oropharynx	Group D streptococci (viridans)
Dental plaques	*Streptococcus mutans*
Colon	*Bacteroides fragilis > E. coli*
Vagina	*Lactobacillus;* colonized by *E. coli* and group B streptococcus
Skin	*Staphylococcus epidermidis*

Name the nosocomial pathogen(s) associated with each of the following:

Urinary catheter	*Escherichia coli* and *Proteus mirabilis*
Respiratory therapy equipment, ventilators	*Pseudomonas aeruginosa*
Wound infections	*Staphylococcus aureus*
Water aerosols	*Legionella* sp.

Tuberculosis

Decide whether each of the following statements is more closely associated with 1° or 2° TB:

Radiographic finding = Ghon complex; classically affects lower lobes	1° TB
Miliary TB	2° TB
Fibrocaseous cavitary lung lesion; classically affects apical lungs (↑ affinity for ↑ O_2 environment)	2° TB
Symptoms of cough/hemoptysis, fever, night sweats, and weight loss	2° TB

What type of hypersensitivity reaction is seen after infection with *M. tuberculosis?*

Type IV or delayed-type hypersensitivity (basis for PPD test)

What unique type of cell is seen in association with caseating granulomas in TB?	Langerhans giant cell
What is the mode of transmission of *M. tuberculosis*?	Respiratory droplets
What term describes the lymphatic and hematogenous spread of TB, causing numerous small foci of infection in extrapulmonary sites?	Miliary TB
Name five common sites of extrapulmonary TB:	1. CNS (tuberculous meningitis) 2. Vertebral bodies (Pott disease) 3. Psoas major muscle → abscess 4. GI tract (liver and cecum) 5. Cervical lymph nodes → scrofuloderma
What is an effective screening tool for latent TB?	PPD test
How is active TB infection diagnosed?	Clinical and radiologic signs of 2° TB and acid-fast bacilli in sputum
What is the management of PPD + latent TB?	Treatment with INH + pyridoxine (vitamin B_6) for 9 months
What is the treatment for active TB?	Respiratory isolation and initial four-drug therapy (**RIPE: R**ifampin, **I**NH, **P**yrizinamide, **E**thambutol)
What is the major toxicity of most TB drugs?	Hepatotoxicity; INH → vitamin B_6 deficiency; ethambutol → optic neuritis

ANTIBIOTICS

Name the drug(s) whose mechanism of action is described below:

Binds penicillin-binding proteins → inhibits transpeptidase → blocks cell wall synthesis; also releases autolytic enzymes (bactericidal)	β-Lactam antibiotics (penicillin, cephalosporins, cephalomycins, carbapenems, and monobactams)
Forms reactive cytotoxic metabolites inside cell	Metronidazole
Binds and inactivate β-lactamase → protects antibiotic	β-Lactamase inhibitors
Inhibits 50S peptidyl transferase	Chloramphenicol

Blocks entry of aa-tRNA to 30S ribosomal complex	Tetracyclines
Blocks transpeptidation of D-ala	Vancomycin
Inhibits dihydrofolate reductase	Trimethoprim (TMP)
Para-aminobenzoic acid (PABA) antimetabolites →↓ dihydropteroate synthase	Sulfonamides
Binds to 30S subunit → block formation of 70S initiation complex → misreading of mRNA	Aminoglycosides
Binds to 50S subunit → inhibit translocase	Macrolides (erythromycin and azithromycin)
Blocks DNA topoisomerase (gyrase)	Quinolones (ciprofloxacin and levofloxacin)
Blocks 50S peptide bond formation	Clindamycin
Inhibits DNA-dependent RNA polymerase	Rifampin
Interferes with mycolic acid synthesis	INH
Bind to bacterial/fungal cell membranes → disrupt osmotic properties	Polymyxins
PABA antagonist → blocks purine synthesis	Sulfones (dapsone and sulfoxone)

Name the antibacterial drug(s) associated with each of the following unique toxicities:

Kernicterus in infants	Sulfonamides and ceftriaxone
Interstitial nephritis	Penicillins
Disulfiram-like reactions	Metronidazole, second-generation cephalosporins
Photosensitivity rash	Doxycycline
Gray baby syndrome	Chloramphenicol
Megaloblastic anemia	TMP
Hemolytic anemia in G6PD-deficient patient	Sulfonamides, chloramphenicol, nitrofurantoin, and INH
Hepatotoxicity, vitamin B_6 deficiency, lupuslike syndrome	INH (**Note:** ↑ $t_{1/2}$ in slow acetylators)
Pseudomembranous colitis	Clindamycin (most common)

Fanconi syndrome	Tetracycline (ingestion of expired drug)
Ototoxicity and nephrotoxicity	Aminoglycosides
Red, pruritic rash on torso with rapid IV infusion (red man syndrome)	Vancomycin
Reversible cholestatic hepatitis; ↑ GI motility	Erythromycin
Achilles tendonitis; cartilage damage in laboratory animals	Fluoroquinolones
Red-orange discoloration of bodily secretions	Rifampin
Discolors teeth; suppresses bone growth in kids	Tetracycline
Aplastic anemia (dose independent)	Chloramphenicol
Neurotoxicity and nephrotoxicity	Polymyxins

Name six uses for metronidazole:	1. Giardia 2. Entamoeba 3. Trichomonas 4. *Gardnerella vaginalis* 5. Anaerobes (*C. difficile*, bacteroides) 6. *Helicobacter pylori* (part of triple therapy)
Which drug is used as solo prophylaxis for TB?	INH
How do organisms develop resistance against vancomycin?	D-lac (or D-ser) replaces terminal D-ala in cell wall → ↓ affinity of vancomycin for cell wall

VIROLOGY

Taxonomy/Basics

Name six medically important DNA viral families:	HHAPPPy: 1. Hepadnaviridae 2. Herpesviridae 3. Adenoviridae 4. Poxviridae 5. Parvoviridae 6. Papovaviridae
Name two families of circular DNA viruses:	1. Papovaviridae 2. Hepadnaviridae
Name the only ssDNA viral genome:	Parvovirus

Name the only DNA virus that replicates in the cytoplasm:

Poxviridae (carries its own DNA-dependent RNA polymerase)

Name three naked DNA viruses:

PAP:
1. Parvo
2. Adeno
3. Papov

Name the only dsRNA viral genome:

Reoviruses (eg, rotavirus)

Name the family of the smallest RNA viruses:

Picornaviruses

Name four families of naked RNA viruses:

CRAP:
1. Calicivirus
2. Reovirus
3. Astrovirus
4. Picornavirus

Name two families of RNA viruses that do not replicate solely in the cytoplasm:

1. Influenza viruses
2. Retroviruses

Where do most enveloped viruses acquire their membranes?

From plasma membrane (except herpesviruses—nuclear membrane)

Name four families of segmented viruses:

BOAR (all RNA viruses)
1. **B**unyaviridae
2. **O**rthomyxoviridae (influenza viruses)
3. **A**renaviridae
4. **R**eoviridae

Name the only diploid viruses:

Retroviruses

What types of nucleic acids do not require special enzymes to be infectious?

Those with same structure as host nucleic acids (eg, positive-stranded ssRNA and most naked dsDNA)

Name the type of viral genetic strategy described below:

The virus contains its own genetic material but is coated with surface proteins from another virus, which determine its infectivity

Phenotypic mixing

Occurs when viruses exchange segments of their genomes

Reassortment

Occurs when a nonmutated virus assists a mutated one by making a functional gene product that serves both itself and the mutated virus

Complementation

Exchanging oligonucleotides by crossing-over within base sequences	Recombination
What type of antigenic change in the influenza virus causes *epidemics*?	Antigenic drift (minor changes from random mutation)
What type of antigenic change in the influenza virus causes *pandemics*?	Antigenic shift (reassortment of genome, including animal acquisition) (**D**rifting is a **S**low Process, **S**hifting is a **R**apid Process)

For each of the following vaccines, state whether it is live attenuated or killed:

Sabin polio	Live attenuated
Salk polio	Killed (Sal**K** = **K**illed)
May revert to virulence	Live attenuated (very rare)
For whom is it dangerous to receive live vaccines?	Immunocompromised hosts (ie, transplant recipients, AIDS patients, and pregnant women)

Infectious Diseases

Name the virus(es) associated with each of the following statements:

Tzanck prep shows multinucleated giant cells	Herpes simplex virus (HSV)-1, HSV-2, and varicella-zoster virus (VZV)
Viral culture with buffy coat	Cytomegalovirus (CMV)
Transmitted by bat, raccoon, and skunk bites	Rabies virus
Transmitted by arthropods	Arboviruses
Cowdry type A inclusion bodies	Herpesviruses (HSV-1, CMV, and VZV)
Number 1 cause of diarrhea in kids <3 years old (y/o)	Rotavirus
Number 1 cause of viral pneumonia in infants <6 months	Respiratory syncytial virus (RSV)
Severe (but rare) seqealae include giant cell pneumonia and subacute sclerosing panencephalitis (SSPE)	Measles virus (rubeola)
Councilman bodies in liver	Yellow fever virus
Reactivation of virus in brain of AIDS patient → demyelination, death	JC virus → progressive multifocal leukoencephalopathy (PML)

Bullet-shaped, helical nucleocapsid; travels up nerve axons to CNS in retrograde fashion	Rabies virus
Koplik spots	Measles virus (rubeola)
Dane particle	Hepatitis B virus
Atypical lymphocytes	Epstein-Barr virus (EBV) and CMV
Nosocomial infection associated with the newborn nursery	CMV and RSV
Negri bodies in neurons	Rabies virus
Incomplete RNA virus → requires envelope	Hepatitis D virus
Positive heterophile antibody test	EBV
Necrosis of large motor neurons in anterior horn spinal cord → flaccid paralysis	Poliovirus

For each of the following clinical findings, name the associated virus:

Shingles	VZV
Suboccipital lymphadenopathy	Rubella virus
Herpangina, hand-foot-and-mouth disease	Coxsackie A virus
Gingivostomatitis, keratitis, and temporal lobe encephalitis	HSV-1
Genital and neonatal infections	HSV-2
Fever, hepatosplenomegaly pharyngitis, and posterior auricular lymphadenopathy; "kissing disease"	EBV (mononucleosis)
Common cold	Rhinoviruses (>100 serotypes; associated with 85% of cases)
PML	JC polyomavirus
Chickenpox	Varicella
Small, pearly, umbilicated papular epidermal growths near genitals	Molluscum contagiosum virus
German measles and congenital infections	Rubella virus
Explosive gastroenteritis; recent epidemics on cruiseships and schools	Norwalk virus

Exanthem subitum (roseola)	Human herpesvirus (HHV)-6
Contains hemagglutinin and neuraminidase virulence factor; undergoes antigenic shift and responsible for pandemics	Influenza A
Fever, black vomitus, and jaundice; transmitted by *Aedes* mosquito	Yellow fever virus
Pericarditis, myocarditis, and pleurodynia	Coxsackie B virus
Acute viral hepatitis	Hepatitis A and B
Mononucleosis, congenital infection, and pneumonia	CMV
Subacute sclerosing panencephalitis (SSPE)	Measles (rubeola) virus
Intussusception from hyperplasia of Peyer patches	Adenoviruses
Kaposi sarcoma	HHV-8
Aseptic meningitis, orchitis, and parotitis	Mumps virus
Barking cough and laryngeal swelling	Parainfluenza viruses (croup)
Hepatitis from IV drug abuse or blood transfusion	Hepatitis C virus
Hydrophobia, seizures, and fatal encephalitis	Rabies virus
Cause of common and genital warts	Human papillomavirus (HPV)
Tropical spastic paresis	Human T-cell leukemia/lymphoma virus (HTLV)
Hepatitis with high mortality rate in pregnant women	Hepatitis E virus
Reye syndrome	Influenza viruses (occurs with aspirin [ASA] ingestion)
Epidemic keratoconjunctivitis; childhood URIs	Adenoviruses
Cough, coryza, and conjunctivitis	Measles (rubeola) virus
Erythema infectiosum (fifth disease); transient aplastic anemic crisis	Parvovirus B19

Name the oncogenic virus associated with the following cancers:

Burkitt lymphoma	EBV
Hepatocellular carcinoma	Hepatitis B and C viruses

Hairy cell leukemia	HTLV-2
Adult T-cell lymphoma	HTLV-1
Nasopharyngeal carcinoma	EBV
Kaposi sarcoma	HHV-8
Cervical, penile, and anal carcinoma	HPV types: 16, 18, 31, 33, and 45

Name the family of viruses characterized by the following:

Smallpox, molluscum contagiosum, and vaccinia	Poxviridae
Hantavirus and California encephalitis	Bunyaviridae
Marburg and Ebola hemorrhagic fever	Filoviridae
Lassa fever and lymphocytic choriomeningitis	Arenaviridae

Human Immunodeficiency Virus

Which continent has the highest incidence (and prevalence) of AIDS?	Africa
What are the three major routes of HIV transmission?	1. Sexual contact 2. Vertical (mother to newborn) transmission 3. Parenteral
What is the most common mode of HIV transmission on a global basis?	Heterosexual contact
What type of virus is HIV?	Human retrovirus of the lentivirus family
What test is used to screen for HIV infection?	Enzyme-linked immunosorbent assay (ELISA) looks for AB to viral proteins; ↑ sensitivity.
What test is used to confirm HIV(+) screening results?	Western blot assay (high false negative within 2 months of infection); ↑ specificity
Which enzyme creates dsDNA from RNA for integration into host genome?	Reverse transcriptase (RT)

What test is used to monitor the effects of antiretroviral therapy?	HIV RT-polymerase chain reaction (RT-PCR) (measures viral load)
What is the strongest measure of disease progression in an HIV(+) patient?	$CD4^+$ T-cell count
Name two key glycoproteins on the surface of the HIV viral envelope:	1. gp41 (fusion) 2. gp120 (attachment) proteins; together = gp160
Name two key HIV viral core proteins:	1. p24 (nucleocapsid) 2. p17 (matrix protein)
Name three key HIV retroviral enzymes contained in the core:	1. RT 2. Integrase 3. Protease (all encoded by *pol* gene)
Which viral antigen peaks within 2 months of infection, then rises again years later?	p24
What are the two cell surface molecules to which gp120 must bind?	1. CD4 2. A chemokine receptor (CCR5 or CXCR4)
HIV infects which three cell types?	1. $CD4^+$ T cells 2. Monocytes/macrophages 3. Dendritic cells
The induction of what cellular transcription factor during an immune response leads to activation of transcription of HIV proviral DNA?	Nuclear factor-kappa B (NF-κB)
Protease inhibitors of HIV prevent cleavage of the protein product of what viral genes?	*Gag* and *pol* genes
What are the three mechanisms by which HIV-infected $CD4^+$ T cells are lost?	1. HIV cytopathic effect 2. Apoptosis 3. HIV-specific cytotoxic T-cell killing
What are the three stages of HIV infection?	1. Acute retroviral infection 2. Chronic phase 3. AIDS
What is the surrogate measure of viral load in an HIV(+) patient?	HIV-1 RNA
What is the strongest measure of disease progression in AIDS?	$CD4^+$ T-cell count

Which tissues are the major reservoirs of HIV-infected T cells and macrophages in patients?	1. Lymph nodes 2. Spleen 3. Tonsils
Which cell type in the brain is infected by HIV?	Microglial cells
List the major immune abnormalities in AIDS:	1. Decreased number of CD4$^+$ T cells 2. Decreased T-cell function 3. Polyclonal activation of B cells 4. Altered macrophage function
What is the clinical picture of direct viral disease from HIV?	Constitutional symptoms (weight loss, fever, fatigue, and night sweats) and/or neurologic symptoms (encephalopathy with dementia and aseptic meningitis)
How is AIDS defined?	CD4$^+$ <200 or AIDS-defining illness, regardless of CD4$^+$ count

Name the common AIDS opportunistic organisms or infections/diseases associated with the following:

Four fungal infections	1. Candidiasis (GI tract) 2. Cryptococcosis (meningitis) 3. Histoplasmosis (disseminated) 4. Coccidioidomycosis (disseminated)
Five bacterial infections	1. *Mycobacterium tuberculosis* (lung/disseminated) 2. *Mycobacterium avium-intracellulare* (lung) 3. *Nocardia* (lung/CNS/disseminated) 4. *Salmonella* (disseminated) 5. Encapsulated organisms
Four viral infections	1. HSV 2. VZV (shingles) 3. CMV (retinitis or colitis) 4. JC virus (PML)
Three protozoal infections	1. *Pneumocystis* (lung or disseminated) 2. *Toxoplasm* (lung/CNS) 3. *Cryptosporidium* (GI)

State the typical CD4$^+$ count associated with each of the following HIV complications:

Opportunistic infections are typically seen, especially *Pneumocystis jiroveci* pneumonia	<200 cells/mL
Mycobacterium avium complex (MAC), CMV, and cryptosporidiosis	<50 cells/mL

Toxoplasmosis	<100 cells/mL
TB becomes more common	<400 cells/mL
List four common neoplasms in patients with AIDS:	1. Kaposi sarcoma 2. Non-Hodgkin B-cell lymphoma 3. CNS lymphoma 4. Squamous cell carcinoma of the cervix or anus
What has been shown to minimize the risk of perinatal HIV transmission?	Zidovudine (AZT) given to pregnant women, cesarean delivery, and avoiding breast feeding

Prions

Which infectious agents lack both DNA and RNA?	Prions (made of proteins only)
What are symptoms of prion diseases?	Rapidly progressing dementia, psychiatric disturbances, and cerebellar symptoms (ataxia, myoclonis). All prion diseases are fatal.
Name four prion diseases:	1. Creutzfeldt-Jacob disease (rapidly progressive dementia) 2. Mad cow disease 3. Kuru 4. Fatal familial insomnia
What type of histopathologic change is seen in these diseases?	Spongiform encephalopathy

ANTIVIRAL AGENTS

For each of the following drugs, provide:

1. The mechanism of action (MOA)
2. Indication(s) (IND)
3. Significant side effects and unique toxicity (TOX) (if any):

Acyclovir and valacyclovir	**MOA:** guanosine analog; activated by herpes thymidine kinase → inhibits viral DNA polymerase **IND:** HSV (treatment and prophylaxis for oral, genital, and ocular herpes), VZV (chickenpox and shingles) **TOX:** neurotoxic (delirium and tremors) and nephrotoxic

Ganciclovir

MOA: guanosine analog; activated by human thymidine kinase → inhibits CMV DNA polymerase

IND: CMV (retinitis, pneumonia, colitis), especially in immunocompromised people

TOX: bone marrow suppression, nephrotoxic, and ↓ spermatogenesis (toxicity > acyclovir because activated by human enzyme)

Foscarnet

MOA: pyrophosphate analog; inhibits viral DNA polymerase (no activation required)

IND: CMV, HSV (refractory infections)

TOX: reversible nephrotoxicity and anemia

Nucleoside RT inhibitors (zidovudine—azidothymidine [AZT], didanosine—ddI, zalcitabine—ddC, lamivudine—3TC, and stavudine—d4T)

MOA: nucleoside analogs; activated by phosphorylation → inhibits RT → prevents incorporation of viral genome into host DNA

IND: part of combination therapy for HIV

TOX: bone marrow suppression, peripheral neuropathy, pancreatitis (especially ddI), lactic acidosis, and macrocytic anemia (AZT)

Nonnucleoside RT inhibitors (nevirapine, delavirdine, and efavirenz)

MOA: binds directly to and inhibits HIV RT → prevents incorporation of viral genome into host DNA

IND: part of combination therapy for HIV

TOX: rash (including Steven-Johnson), ↑ liver enzymes, inhibits P-450, vivid dreams/CNS changes (with efavirenz)

Protease inhibitors (saquinavir, ritonavir, indinavir, nelfinavir, and amprenavir)

MOA: blocks protease enzyme → inhibits assembly of viral core and new viruses
IND: part of combination therapy for HIV

TOX: GI upset, insulin resistance, ↑ lipids, fat redistribution syndromes, interstitial nephritis, and thrombocytopenia (indinavir)

Amantadine and rimantadine

MOA: inhibits viral penetration and uncoating; releases dopamine (DA) from intact nerve terminals

IND: influenza A treatment/ prophylaxis, Parkinson disease

TOX: CNS effects: confusion, ataxia, and slurred speech (less with rimantadine); teratogenesis

Zanamivir and oseltamivir	**MOA:** neuraminidase inhibitor → alters virion aggregation and release **IND:** influenza A and B treatment and prophylaxis (oseltamivir) **TOX:** bronchospasm in patients with asthma/COPD (zanamivir)
Ribavirin	**MOA:** guanosine analog; activated by phosphorylation → inhibits inosine-5'-monophosphate (IMP) dehydrogenase **IND:** RSV, hantavirus, and chronic hepatitis C **TOX:** hemolysis (when given IV)
Interferon-α	**MOA:** human glycoproteins that interfere with ability of viruses to replicate (block protein synthesis and degrade mRNA) **IND:** chronic hepatitis B and C, genital warts, Kaposi sarcoma, and hairy cell leukemia **TOX:** bone marrow suppression
What constitutes highly active antiretroviral therapy (HAART)?	Two nucleoside RT inhibitors and a protease inhibitor or nonnucleoside RT inhibitor. **Note:** no patient should ever be on monotherapy as resistance is invariable.
When is HAART typically initiated?	CD4$^+$ <500 cells/mL or very high viral load
Which drug is used to prevent vertical transmission during pregnancy?	Zidovudine (AZT)

MYCOLOGY

Which four endemic mycoses can mimic TB?	1. Histoplasmosis 2. Coccidioidomycosis 3. Paracocidioidomycosis 4. Blastomycosis
What is a dimorphic fungus?	Lives in two forms: cold = mold (<37°C), heat = yeast

Name the fungus associated with each of the following statements:

"Spaghetti and meatball" appearance on KOH prep	*Malassezia furfur*
Contains cancer-causing aflatoxins	*Aspergillus flavus*
Dimorphic fungus living on rose thorns and splinters	*Sporothrix schenckii*
Urease (+), stains with India ink, and latex agglutination (+)	*Cryptococcus neoformans*
Organism found inside macrophages; spread in pigeon and bat droppings	*Histoplasma capsulatum*
Budding yeast, pseudohyphae; germ tubes at 37°C	*Candida albicans*
Wide angle (>90°) branching of irregular nonseptated hyphae	*Mucor* and *Rhizopus* sp.
Big, broad-based budding dimorphic fungus	*Blastomycosis* **B-B-B-B-B** (Big, Broad-Based Budding Blasto)
45° angle branching and septated hyphae; fruiting bodies	*Aspergillus* sp.
Narrow-based unequal budding yeasts with capsular halo	*Cryptococcus neoformans*
Endemic to Ohio and Mississippi river valleys	*Histoplasma capsulatum*
"Flying-saucer" appearance of silver stain	*Pneumocystis carinii* (also *P. jiroveci*)
"Captain's wheel" appearance; endemic to rural Latin America	*Paracoccidioidomycosis*

For each of the following diseases, name the fungus/yeast responsible and the drug of choice:

Rose gardener disease with ascending lymphangitis	*Sporothrix schenckii*—potassium iodide
Tinea nigra	*Phaeoannellomyces werneckii*—topical salicylic acid
Thrush in an immunocompromised patient	*Candida albicans*—nystatin (swish and swallow) and amphotericin B if systemic infection
San Joaquin (desert valley) fever; endemic to southwest United States, California	*Coccidioides immitis*—fluconazole and amphotericin B

Interstitial pneumonia of the immunocompromised	*Pneumocystis carinii* (or *P. jiroveci*)—TMP-sulfamethoxazole (SMX) or pentamidine (prophylaxis when CD4$^+$ <200 cells/mL)
Tinea (pityriasis) versicolor	*Malassezia furfur*—topical miconazole or selenium sulfide
Meningitis from pigeon droppings	*Cryptococcus neoformans*—amphotericin + flucytosine for 2 weeks followed by fluconazole
Tinea cruris/capitis/corporis/ unguium/pedis	*Trichophyton, Epidermophyton,* or Microsporum sp.—topical miconazole, oral griseofulvin for capitis and unguium
Fungus ball in lungs or invasive disease	*Aspergillus fumigatus*—voriconazole

ANTIFUNGALS

Name the drug whose mechanism of action is described below:

Blocks ergosterol (unique to fungi) synthesis by inhibiting P-450	Azole family (ketoconazole, fluconazole, miconazole, voriconazole, and posaconazole)
Binds ergosterol → produces membrane pores	Amphotericin B and nystatin
Blocks ergosterol synthesis by blocking squalene epoxidase	Terbinafine
Interferes with microtubule formation → inhibits mitosis	Griseofulvin
Converted to 5-fluorouracil (5-FU) → blocks formation of purines	Flucytosine

Name the antifungal drug(s) associated with each of the following unique toxicities:

Rigors, acute febrile reaction, nephrotoxicity, and arrythmias	Amphotericin B—follow BUN/ creatinine daily. **Note:** newer lipid formulations (ie, AmBisome less nephrotoxic)
Photosensitivity, mental confusion, bone marrow suppression, and induces P-450	Griseofulvin

Antiandrogenic effects, adrenal suppression, and liver dysfunction	Azole family (especially ketoconazole)
Bone marrow suppression and alopecia	Flucytosine

PARASITOLOGY

Protozoa

Name the protozoan associated with each of the following statements:

Transmitted by Tsetse fly; shows antigenic variation	*Trypanosoma brucei* (*gambiense* and *rhodesiense*)
Transmitted by *Anopheles* mosquito	*Plasmodium*
Transmitted by Reduviid bug	*Trypanosoma cruzi*
Transmitted by cysts in meat or cat feces	*Toxoplasma*
Transmitted by sandfly	*Leishmania*
Obligate intracellular parasite; cysts on acid-fast stain	*Cryptosporidium*
Maltese "X" cross shape	*Babesia*
Pear-shaped, binucleate, flagellated trophozoite	*Giardia lamblia*
Blood smear shows trophozoites and schizonts	*Plasmodium*
Macrophages containing amastigotes	*Leishmania donovani*

For each of the following clinical findings, name the associated protozoan and the treatment:

Megacolon, megaesophagus, and cardiomegaly (with apical atrophy)	*Trypanosoma cruzii* (Chagas disease)— nifurtimox
Cyclic fever, headache, anemia, and splenomegaly	*Plasmodium*—chloroquine for erythrocyte forms and primaquine for latent forms (*Plasmodium vivax* and *Plasmodium ovale*)
Chloroquine-resistant malaria	*Plasmodium falciparum*—mefloquine or quinine and pyramethamine/ sulfadoxine
Bloody diarrhea with "flask-shaped" ulcers, liver abscesses, and trophozoites in stool	*Entamoeba histolytica*—metronidazole and iodoquinol

Black fever or "kala-azar"	*Leishmania donovani*—sodium stibogluconate (pentavalent antimony)
Severe, watery diarrhea in AIDS patient	*Cryptosporidium*—supportive (hydration, improve immune status)
Flatulence, bloating, and foul-smelling diarrhea	*Giardia lamblia*—metronidazole
African sleeping sickness	*Trypanosoma brucei* (*gambiense* and *rhodesiense*)—suramin (acutely) or melarsoprol (for CNS symptoms)
Encephalitis with brain abscesses in immunocompromised host; congenital defects	*Toxoplasma gondii*—pyrimethamine and sulfadoxine or clindamycin
Vaginitis with foul-smelling, frothy discharge	*Trichomonas vaginalis*—metronidazole
Fever and hemolytic anemia after *Ixodes* tick bite	*Babesia* sp.—quinine and clindamycin
Why are many Africans resistant to *P. vivax* infection?	They carry sickle cell trait and/or they lack antigens Duffy a and b on RBCs.
What causes the cyclic symptoms in malaria?	Immune response to burst RBCs that release merozoites

Helminths

For each of the following clinical findings, name the associated helminth and the treatment:

Larvae penetrate skin of feet; GI infection → anemia	*Ancylostoma duodenale* or *Necator americanus* (hookworms)—mebendazole or pyrantel pamoate
Worms visibly crawling in conjunctiva; spread by deerfly	*Loa loa*—diethylcarbamazine
Fever, periorbital edema, and myositis after ingesting raw pork	*Trichinella spiralis*—thiabendazole
River blindness; spread by female blackflies	*Onchocerca volvulus*—ivermectin (rIVERmectin for RIVER blindness)
Elephantiasis from lymphatic blockage	*Wuchereria bancrofti*—diethylcarbamazine
Larvae penetrate skin → autoinfection; GI infection	*Strongyloides stercoralis* (threadworm)—thiabendazole or ivermectin
Intestinal infection and anal pruritis; ↑ incidence in children; positive "tape test"	*Enterobius vermicularis* (pinworms)—mebendazole or pyrantel pamoate

Fluke associated with squamous cell carcinoma of the urinary tract	*Schistosoma haematobium*—praziquantel
Granulomatous hepatitis and chorioretinitis	*Toxocara canis*—diethylcarbamazine
GI infection; competes for food → malnutrition in children; eggs visible in feces	*Ascaris lumbricoides*—mebendazole or pyrantel pamoate
Inflammation and 2° bacterial infection of lungs from undercooked crab meat	*Paragonimus westermani*—praziquantel
Biliary tract inflammation from undercooked fish	*Opisthorchis (Clonorchis) sinensis*—praziquantel
Undercooked pork larval worm → mass lesions in brain; cysticercosis	*Taenia solium*—praziquantel or niclosamide, albendazole for cysticercosis
Hydatid liver cysts from eggs in dog feces → anaphylaxis if antigens released from cysts	*Echinococcus granulosus*—albendazole, careful surgical removal of cysts (preinjected with ETOH)
Fish tapeworm causing vitamin B$_{12}$ deficiency	*Diphyllobothrium latum*—praziquantel
Cercariae penetrate skin → granulomas and inflammation of liver and spleen; snails are hosts	*Schistosoma sp.*—praziquantel
Which cell count is elevated during many helminth infections and can be detected by routine CBC?	*Eosinophils*
Which is the most common helminth infection in the United States?	*Enterobius vermicularis*

Name the antiparasitic drug(s) associated with each of the following unique toxicities:

Cinchonism	Quinine
Hemolytic anemia in G6PD-deficient person	Chloroquine, primaquine, quinine, and TMP-SMX
Mazzotti reaction (pyrexia, hypotension, and respiratory distress caused by death of parasites)	Diethylcarbamazine (with *Onchocerca*)

CHAPTER 4

Neuroscience

EMBRYOLOGY

Name the structure(s) in the adult nervous system that arise from the following embryonic components:

Alar plate	Sensory neurons
Basal plate	Motor neurons
Telencephalon	Cerebral hemispheres and lateral ventricles
Diencephalon	Thalamus, optic nerves, and third ventricle
Mesencephalon	Midbrain and aqueduct
Metencephalon	Pons, cerebellum, and superior fourth ventricle
Myelencephalon	Medulla and inferior fourth ventricle
Neural crest cells	Peripheral sensory and autonomic nerves and sensory ganglia

What is the level of the conus medullaris in a newborn and in an adult?

L2 or L3 (newborn), L1 (adult)

NEUROANATOMY AND NEUROPHYSIOLOGY

Organization of the Nervous System

What are the divisions of the autonomic nervous system?

Sympathetic, parasympathetic

Where are the preganglionic cell bodies of the sympathetic nervous system?

Intermediolateral horn of the spinal cord from T1 to L3

Where are the preganglionic cell bodies of the parasympathetic nervous system located?	Brainstem (cranial nerve nuclei) and spinal cord from S2 to S4
Which is the primary neurotransmitter (NT) of both sympathetic and parasympathetic ganglia?	Acetylcholine (ACh)
Which is the primary type of cholinergic receptor of both sympathetic and parasympathetic ganglia?	Nicotinic
Which NT mediates the transmission of impulses from sympathetic neurons to effector organs?	Norepinephrine (NE)
Which NT mediates the transmission of impulses from parasympathetic neurons to effector organs?	ACh
Which NT mediates the transmission of impulses from somatic neurons to skeletal muscle?	ACh
What types of receptors are present on the effector organs innervated by the sympathetic nervous system?	α_1, α_2, β_1, and β_2
What type of receptor is present on the effector organs innervated by the parasympathetic nervous system?	Muscarinic
What type of receptor is present on muscle innervated by the somatic nervous system?	Nicotinic

Sympathetic Nervous System

Name the effect of the sympathetic nervous system on the following organ systems and the type of receptor which mediates each effect:	
Eyes	Pupillary dilation (α_1)
Salivary glands	Increased thick, viscous secretions
Bronchioles	Bronchodilation (β_2), ↑ secretions
Heart	Tachycardia (β_1), ↑ contractility (β_1), ↑ AV nodal conduction (β_1)

Vascular smooth muscle	Vasoconstriction of cutaneous mucous membrane and splanchnic vessels (α_1); vasodilation in skeletal muscle (β_2)
Gastrointestinal (GI) tract	$\downarrow$ Muscle motility and tone (β_2), contraction of sphincters (α_1)
Male sex organs	Ejaculation (α_2)
Uterus	Relaxation (β_2), contraction (α_1)
Bladder and ureters	Relaxation of detrusor (β_2), contraction of trigone and sphincter (α_1)
Sweat glands	$\uparrow$ Secretions (muscarinic)
Kidneys	$\uparrow$ Renin secretion
Adipocytes	$\uparrow$ Lipolysis (β_1)
Pancreas	$\downarrow$ Insulin secretion (α_2), $\uparrow$ insulin secretion (β_2)

Parasympathetic Nervous System

What is the effect of the parasympathetic nervous system on the following organ systems:	
Eyes	Pupillary constriction
Bronchioles	Bronchoconstriction
Heart	Bradycardia, $\downarrow$ contractility, $\downarrow$ AV nodal conduction
GI tract	$\uparrow$ Motility, relaxation of sphincters
Male sex organs	Erection
Bladder and ureters	Contraction of detrusor, relaxation of sphincters and trigone
What type of cholinergic receptor mediates all of the effects on the organs above?	Muscarinic

Motor and Sensory Fibers

What type of motor fiber innervates extrafusal muscle fibers?	A-alpha (A-α)
What type of motor fiber innervates intrafusal muscle fibers?	A-gamma (A-γ)

Name the function of each of the following types of sensory fibers:

Ia (A-α)	Proprioception, muscle spindles
Ib	Proprioception, Golgi tendon organs
II (A-β)	Touch, pressure, and vibration; secondary afferents of muscle spindles
III (A-δ)	Touch, pressure, fast pain, and temperature
IV (c)	Slow pain and temperature (unmyelinated)

What types of sensory fibers have the largest diameter and consequently the fastest conduction velocity?

Ia and Ib

What type of motor fibers have the largest diameter and consequently the fastest conduction velocity?

A-α

What type of sensory fibers have the smallest diameter and consequently the slowest conduction velocity?

C

What is the electrochemical effect of an inward Na^+ current on a sensory fiber?

Depolarization

Name the function of each of the following components of a sensory pathway:

Sensory receptor	Translates environmental stimulus into an electrical impulse
First-order neuron	Carries impulse from sensory receptor into central nervous system (CNS)
Second-order neuron	Carries impulse from primary neuron to the thalamus
Third-order neuron	Carries impulse from second-order neuron to the cerebral cortex
Fourth-order neuron	Carries impulses from third-order neurons to appropriate somatosensory area of cerebral cortex

Name the type of mechanoreceptor described below:

Onion-like subcutaneous receptors that respond to vibration and tapping	Pacinian corpuscle

Primary receptors of the dermal papillae that mediate two-point tactile discrimination	Meissner corpuscle
Encapsulated receptor that responds to pressure	Ruffini corpuscle
Disc-shaped touch receptor of the deep dermis	Merkel tactile disc

Rods or cones?

Sensitive to low-intensity light	Rods
Sensitive to high-intensity light	Cones
Receptor used primarily for night vision	Rods
Receptor used primarily for day vision	Cones
Present in fovea	Cones
High visual acuity	Cones
Receptor which adjusts to low light conditions most rapidly	Cones
Receptor capable of color vision	Cones

Name the type of muscle sensor for each of the following functions:

Detection of static and dynamic changes in muscle length	Muscle spindles
Detection of muscle tension	Golgi tendon organs
Detection of vibration	Pacinian corpuscles
Detection of pain	Free nerve endings
What type of motoneuron is responsible for ensuring that a muscle will respond appropriately throughout contraction, despite changes in tension?	γ-Motoneurons
What type of muscle reflex, mediated by type Ia afferent fibers, causes muscle contraction in response to muscle stretch?	Stretch or myotatic reflex
What type of muscle reflex, mediated by type Ib afferent fibers, causes muscle relaxation in response to muscle contraction?	Golgi tendon reflex

What type of muscle reflex, mediated by types II, III, and IV afferent fibers, causes ipsilateral flexion and contralateral extension?

Flexor withdrawal reflex

What are the components of the afferent limb of a myotatic reflex arc?

Muscle spindle receptor → Ia fiber → dorsal root ganglion

What comprises the efferent limb of a myotatic reflex arc?

Ventral motor neuron

For each of the following muscle stretch reflexes, name the muscle group and spinal level tested:

Ankle jerk

Gastrocnemius (S1)

Knee jerk

Quadriceps (L2-L4)

Biceps jerk

Biceps (C5-C6)

Forearm jerk

Brachioradialis (C5-C6)

Triceps jerk

Triceps (C7-C8)

What type of posturing is caused by a transecting lesion above the level of the medulla but below the midbrain?

Decerebrate rigidity

What type of posturing is caused by a transecting lesion above the level of the red nucleus (midbrain)?

Decorticate rigidity

What are the three layers of the cerebellar cortex?

1. Granular layer (innermost)
2. Purkinje layer (middle)
3. Molecular layer (outermost)

Which is the major NT of cerebellar Purkinje cells?

γ-Aminobutyric acid (GABA).

Note: The output of Purkinje cells is always inhibitory.

Meninges

What are the three layers of the meninges?

"The meninges **PAD** the CNS"
1. **P**ia
2. **A**rachnoid
3. **D**ura

What meningeal space, which lies between the pia and arachnoid, contains the cerebrospinal fluid (CSF)?

Subarachnoid space

What structure produces CSF?	The choroid plexus of the lateral, third, and fourth ventricles
What structures reabsorb CSF into venous circulation?	The arachnoid granulations
Trace the flow of CSF from the choroid plexus into venous circulation.	Choroid plexus → lateral ventricles → interventricular foramina (of Monro) → third ventricle → cerebral aqueduct → fourth ventricle → lateral foramina (of Luschka) or median foramen (of Magendie) → subarachnoid space → arachnoid granulations → superior sagittal sinus
What are the three major functions of CSF?	1. To provide support and protection to the CNS 2. To remove metabolic waste products 3. To transport hormones and cytokines throughout the CSF and to the systemic circulation

Vasculature of the Central Nervous System

Name the blood vessel that supplies each of the following structures:

Anterior two-thirds of the spinal cord, the medullary pyramids, medial lemniscus, and root fibers of cranial nerve (CN) XII	Anterior spinal artery
Retina	Central artery of the retina (a branch of the ophthalmic artery)
Lateral geniculate body, globus pallidus, posterior limb of internal capsule	Anterior choroidal artery (an important branch of internal carotid artery)
Hypothalamus and ventral thalamus	Posterior communicating artery
Leg-foot area of motor and sensory cortices	Anterior cerebral artery (ACA)
Anterior putamen, caudate nucleus, and anteroinferior internal capsule	Medial striate arteries (branches of the ACA)
Broca (expressive) and Wernicke (receptive) speech areas, face and arm areas of motor cortices, frontal eye field	Middle cerebral artery (MCA)
Internal capsule, caudate nucleus, putamen, globus pallidus	Lateral striate arteries (branches of the MCA)

Nucleus ambiguus and the inferior surface of the cerebellum	Posterior inferior cerebellar artery
Caudal lateral pontine tegmentum (including portions of the nuclei of CN V, VII) and the inferior cerebellar surface	Anterior inferior cerebellar artery
Superior surface of cerebellum, cerebellar nuclei, and the cochlear nuclei	Superior cerebellar artery
Majority of midbrain, portions of the thalamus, lateral and medial geniculate bodies, occipital lobe, inferior aspect of the temporal lobes, and the hippocampus	Posterior cerebral artery (PCA)
Majority of the dura	Middle meningeal artery
Name the cerebral veins that drain directly into the superior sagittal sinus:	Bridging veins
Name the cerebral vein that drains deep cerebral veins into the straight sinus:	Vein of Galen
CN III, CN V_1, CN V_2, CN VI, postganglionic sympathetic fibers, and both internal carotid arteries all pass through which structure?	Cavernous sinus

Axonal Transport

Name the cytoplasmic structure in the nerve cell body and dendrites that are involved in protein synthesis:	Nissl substance
Name the type of axonal transport described below:	
Transport responsible for delivery of synthesized NTs away from the cell body	Fast anterograde axonal transport
Transport responsible for delivery of cytoskeletal and cytoplasmic components away from the cell body	Slow anterograde transport
Transport responsible for returning material to the cell body for degradation	Fast retrograde transport

Kinesin-dependent transport	Fast anterograde axonal transport
Dynein-dependent transport	Fast retrograde transport
Transport responsible for carrying nerve growth factor, viruses, and toxins to cell bodies	Fast retrograde transport

| Name the process of anterograde axonal and myelin degeneration accompanied by Schwann cell proliferation: | Wallerian degeneration |

Supporting Cells of the Nervous System

Name the type of cell described below:

Primary supportive cell type of the CNS	Astrocyte
Myelin-producing cell type of the CNS	Oligodendrocyte
CNS scavenger cell type	Microglia
CSF-producing cell type	Ependymal cell
Myelin-producing cell type of the peripheral nervous system (PNS)	Schwann cells

| What type of intercellular connections are responsible for maintaining the integrity of the blood-brain barrier? | Tight junctions |

| What proteins are commonly used to identify astrocytes? | Glial fibrillary acidic protein (GFAP) and glutamine synthetase |

Pigments and Inclusions

Name the process or disease associated with the following neuronal histopathologic findings:

Lipofuscin granules	Aging
Depletion of neuromelanin in substantia nigra and Lewy bodies	Parkinson disease
Negri bodies	Rabies
Amyloid plaques and neurofibrillary tangles	Alzheimer disease
Cowdry type A inclusion bodies	Herpes simplex encephalitis

Spinal Tracts

Name the spinal tract responsible
for each of the following functions:

Voluntary control of skeletal muscle   Lateral corticospinal/pyramidal tract

Sensation of pain and temperature   Lateral spinothalamic tract

Two-point discrimination and   Dorsal column-medial lemniscus tract
vibratory sensation

Control of facial muscles   Corticobulbar tract

Coordination of muscle tone, posture,   Dentothalamic tract
balance, and motor activity

Describe the major difference between   Corticobulbar fibers innervate the lower
the innervation of the lower and upper   facial muscles unilaterally, while upper
facial muscles.   facial muscles are innervated bilaterally

Name the structure in the spinal cord   Cuneate fasciculus
composed of ascending fibers of the
dorsal column-medial lemniscus
pathway originating in the upper
extremities:

Name the structure in the spinal cord   Gracile fasciculus (medial to cuneate
composed of ascending fibers of the   fasciculus)
dorsal column-medial lemniscus
pathway originating in the lower
extremities:

At what level of the brainstem do fibers   Caudal medulla
of the dorsal column-medial lemniscus
pathway cross?

What type of receptors provide input   Free nerve endings
to the lateral spinothalamic tract?

At what level do fibers of the   At the same level or 1 to 2 levels
spinothalamic tract cross?   above/below where they enter the
                                               spinal cord

Name the structure where fibers of the   Ventral white commissure/anterior
lateral spinothalamic tract cross   commisure
the midline:

Where do fibers of the dorsal   The sensory cortex (Brodmann areas 3,
column-medial lemniscus pathway,   1, and 2)
the trigeminothalamic, and lateral
spinothalamic tract all terminate?

What part of the cortex gives rise to the fibers of the lateral corticospinal and corticobulbar tracts?

The motor, premotor, and sensory areas of the cortex (Brodmann areas 6, 4, and 3, 1, 2)

Fibers of the lateral corticospinal tract pass through which limb of the internal capsule?

Posterior limb

Name the structure where fibers of the lateral corticospinal tract cross the midline:

Medullary pyramids

Classify each of the following clinical findings as upper motor neuron (UMN) or lower motor neuron (LMN) signs:

Spastic paresis	UMN
Flaccid paralysis	LMN
Babinski sign (upgoing toes)	UMN
Fasciculations and fibrillations	LMN
Areflexia	LMN
Atrophy	LMN
Hyperreflexia	UMN

Cranial Nerves

Name the cranial foramen that each of the cranial nerves below pass through:

I	Cribiform plate
II	Optic canal
III, IV, V$_1$, VI	Superior orbital fissure. **Note:** all of these nerves pass through the cavernous sinus as well.
V$_2$	Foramen **R**otundum
V$_3$	Foramen **O**vale (for divisions of the trigeminal nerve think "**S**tanding **R**oom **O**nly")
VII, VIII	Internal acoustic meatus
IX, X, XI	Jugular foramen
XII	Hypoglossal canal

Name the function(s) for each cranial nerve listed below:

I: olfactory	Smell
II: optic	Vision
III: oculomotor	1. Eye movement 2. "Parasympathetic" ciliary and pupillary sphincter mm **Note:** mm is used as the abbreviation for "muscles".
IV: trochlear	Contraction of superior oblique muscle
V₁: trigeminal—ophthalmic branch	Sensation from nose to forehead
V₂: trigeminal—maxillary branch	Sensation from lateral nose, upper lip, superior buccal area
V₃: trigeminal—mandibular branch	1. Sensation from areas of the lower face not covered by V_1 and V_2 2. Movement of the Muscles of Mastication (Masseter, teMporalis, Medial, and lateral pterygoids), tensor veli palatini, and tensor tympani
VI: abducens	Contraction of lateral rectus muscle
VII: facial	1. Parasympathetic—lacrimal, submandibular, and sublingual glands 2. Mm of facial expression, stapedius, stylohyoid, and the posterior belly of the digastric muscle 3. Taste—anterior two-thirds of tongue 4. Sensation—skin of external ear
VIII: vestibulocochlear	Hearing and sense of balance
IX: glossopharyngeal	1. Parasympathetic—parotid gland 2. Motor—stylopharyngeus mm 3. Taste—posterior one-third tongue 4. Sensation—parotid gland, carotid body and sinus, pharynx, and middle ear 5. Cutaneous sensation—external ear canal
X: vagus	1. Parasympathetic—trachea, bronchi, heart, GI tract 2. Contraction of laryngeal, pharyngeal, and esophageal striated mm 3. Taste—epiglottis and palate 4. Sensation—trachea, GI tract 5. Cutaneous sensation—external ear

XI: accessory	Movement of sternocleidomastoid and trapezius muscles
XII: hypoglossal	Contraction of muscles of tongue

Which three cranial nerves are purely sensory nerves?	1. CN I 2. CN II 3. CN VIII
Which five cranial nerves are purely motor nerves?	1. CN III 2. CN IV 3. CN VI 4. CN XI 5. CN XII
Which four cranial nerves have both motor and sensory components?	1. CN V 2. CN VII 3. CN IX 4. CN X
Which two cranial nerves are rostral to the midbrain?	1. CN I 2. CN II
Which two cranial nerve nuclei are located in the midbrain?	1. CN III 2. CN IV
Which four cranial nerves have at least a portion of their nuclei in the pons?	1. CN V 2. CN VI 3. CN VII 4. CN VIII
Which seven cranial nerves have at least a portion of their nuclei in the medulla?	1. CN V 2. CN VI 3. CN VII 4. CN VIII 5. CN IX 6. CN X 7. CN XII
Name the only cranial nerve that crosses the midline and exits the brainstem posterior to the ventricular system:	CN IV—exits the brainstem posteriorly and crosses the midline after exiting the caudal midbrain
What nucleus serves as the origin of preganglionic parasympathetic fibers projecting to the ciliary ganglion?	Edinger-Westphal nucleus of CN III
What visceral sensory nucleus, located in the medulla, is a relay center for taste, sensory input from the carotid sinus, carotid body, and the vagus nerve?	Nucleus Solitarius

What visceral motor nucleus, located in the medulla, is involved in coordinating swallowing and speech?

Nucleus aMbiguus

Which are the afferent and efferent limbs of the corneal reflex?

CN V$_1$ and CN VII

Which are the afferent and efferent limbs of the pupillary light reflex?

CN II and CN III

Which are the afferent and efferent limbs of the gag reflex?

CN IX and CN X

Name the site of a lesion, within the visual tract, capable of causing each of the following deficits:

    Ipsilateral blindness

Transection of the optic nerve

    Binasal hemianopia

Bilateral lateral compression of optic chiasm

    Bitemporal hemianopia

Midsagittal transection or midline pressure on the optic chiasm (often caused by a pituitary tumor)

    Right hemianopia *without* macular sparing

Transection of the left optic radiation

    Right upper quadrantanopia

Transection of the lower division of the left optic radiation

    Right lower quadrantanopia

Transection of the upper division of the left optic radiation

    Right hemianopia *with* macular sparing

Destruction of the left visual cortex

What are five key structures of the pupillary light reflex pathway?

1. Ganglion cells of the retina
2. Pretectal nucleus of the midbrain
3. Edinger-Westphal nucleus
4. Ciliary ganglion
5. Postganglionic parasympathetic fibers of CN III

What are four key structures of the pupillary dilation pathway?

1. Paraventricular nucleus of the hypothalamus
2. Ciliospinal center of Budge at the level of T1 to T2
3. Superior cervical ganglion
4. Postganglionic sympathetic fibers traveling along the internal carotid artery and its branches to the eye

What part of the cortex is responsible for voluntary eye movements?

Frontal eye field (Brodmann area 8)

What side will a patient's eyes deviate toward if there is a lesion of the right frontal eye field?

Right side ("Look toward the lesion of frontal eye fields")

What structure connects the nucleus of CN VI and the nucleus of CN III?

Medial longitudinal fasciculus (MLF)

What type of lesion will result in medial rectus palsy (inability to adduct the eye) on attempted lateral gaze but normal adduction on accommodation?

Intranuclear ophthalmoplegia (a lesion of the MLF)

What classic idiopathic lesion is characterized by ptosis, miosis, and anhydrosis?

Horner syndrome

Name the condition characterized by a pupil that will accommodate but cannot react to light:

Argyll-Robertson pupil (associated with tertiary syphilis, lupus, and diabetes mellitus)

Name the condition caused by a lesion in the afferent fibers of the light reflex pathway:

Marcus Gunn pupil

What are the primary sensory receptors of the auditory pathway?

Inner hair cells of the organ of Corti

Where does the auditory pathway terminate?

Bilateral input from both auditory tracts terminates in primary auditory cortex in superior temporal gyrus (Brodmann areas 41 and 42)

What type of cells are responsible for relaying auditory stimuli from the organ of Corti to the cochlear nuclei?

Bipolar cells of the spiral or cochlearganglion

What thalamic nucleus plays a key role in relay of impulses from the cochlear nuclei to higher cortical centers?

Medial geniculate body of the thalamus

What pontine nucleus plays a key role in sound localization?

Superior olivary nucleus

What are key structures of the hearing pathway?

Cochlear → cochlear nucleus → decussating fibers in Trapezoid body → superior olivary nucleus → lateral lemniscus → inferior colliculi → medial geniculate nucleus → primary auditory cortex

Conduction deafness is caused by a lesion of which components of the auditory system?

External auditory canal, tympanic membrane, or the middle ear

Sensorineural deafness is caused by a lesion of which components of the auditory system?

Cochlea, cochlear nerve, or the cochlear nuclei

Patients with presbycusis have trouble hearing what types of sounds?

High-frequency sounds

Which cells of the vestibular system respond to angular acceleration and deceleration?

The hair cells of the three semicircular canals

What structures of the vestibular system respond to linear acceleration and deceleration?

The hair cells of the utricle

What type of cells are responsible for relaying vestibular stimuli from the hair cells to the vestibular nuclei?

Bipolar cells of the vestibular ganglion

What structures provide input to the vestibular nuclei?

Hair cells of the semicircular canal, hair cells of the utricle, and the flocculonodular lobe of the cerebellum

What structures receive signals from the vestibular nuclei?

The thalamus, spinal cord, cerebellum, and CNs III, IV, and VI

Cerebellum, Thalamus, Hypothalamus

What are the three primary functions of the cerebellum?

1. Maintenance of posture and equilibrium
2. Control of muscle tone
3. Coordination of voluntary muscle activity

What type of tremor may result from a cerebellar lesion?

Intention tremor

A positive Romberg sign (loss of balance when the eyes are closed) suggests a lesion to which tract of the CNS?

Dentothalamic tract (the main cerebellar pathway) or dorsal column (tabes dorsalis in neurosyphilis)

Name the thalamic nucleus/nuclei responsible for the relay of impulses for each modality listed below:

Vision

Lateral geniculate nucleus ("Lateral to Look")

Hearing	Medial geniculate nucleus ("Medial for Music")
Proprioception, pain, pressure, touch, vibration	Lateral portion of ventral posteriornucleus (VPL, "Posterior for Proprioception, Pain")
Facial sensation	Medial portion of ventral posterior nucleus (VML)
Motor	Ventral anterior/lateral nuclei
Limbic function	Dorsomedial, anterior nuclei
Name the largest thalamic nucleus:	Pulvinar
What is the function of the pulvinar?	Integration of visual, auditory, and somesthetic input
Which portion of the internal capsule contains fibers of the corticobulbar tract?	The genu
Which portion of the internal capsule contains fibers of the corticospinal, spinothalamic, visual, and auditory tracts?	The posterior limb
Which arteries supply the posterior limb of the internal capsule?	Perforating branches of the anteriorchoroidal artery and lenticulostriate arteries
Name the major hypothalamic nucleus (or nuclei) responsible for each function listed below:	
Regulation of the release of gonadotropic hormones	Medial preoptic nucleus (which contains the sexually dimorphic nucleus)
Regulation of circadian rhythms	Suprachiasmatic nucleus
Regulation of body temperature	Anterior nucleus (lesion results in hyperthermia) and posterior nucleus (lesion results in poikilothermia)
Regulation of water balance, synthesis of antidiuretic hormone, oxytocin, and corticotropin-releasing factor	Paraventricular and supraoptic nuclei
Regulation of appetite	VentroMedial nucleus (lesion resulting from eating Very Much [hyperphagia, obesity]) and lateral hypothalamic nucleus (lesions cause anorexia and starvation)

Regulation of hypothalamus	Arcuate or infundibular nucleus
Regulation of emotional expression	Mammillary nucleus (a component of the limbic system)
What are the major structures of the Papez circuit?	Septal area, mammillary body, anteriornucleus of thalamus, cingulate gyrus, entorhinal cortex, and hippocampal formation
What is the most epileptogenic part of the cerebrum?	The hippocampus
What system within the CNS plays a central role in the initiation and coordination of somatic motor activity?	The striatal or extrapyramidal motor system
What are the major components of the striatal motor system?	Neocortex, basal ganglia (striatum [caudate + putamen], globus pallidus, subthalamic nucleus, substantia nigra), and thalamus

Neurotransmitters

Name the NT described below:

Major NT of the PNS	ACh
NT which is increased in the CNS of patients with schizophrenia	Dopamine
Major NT of the parasympathetic nervous system	ACh
NT believed to cause panic attacks when released suddenly by the locus coeruleus	NE
Major NT of the preganglionic sympathetic nervous system	ACh
NT highly concentrated in the substantia nigra that plays a key role in pain transmission	Substance P
Major NT of the postganglionic sympathetic neurons supplying sweat glands and certain blood vessels	ACh
NT which is depleted from the basal nucleus of Meynert in Alzheimer disease	ACh

NT which is depleted from the substantia nigra in patients with Parkinson disease	Dopamine
NT that causes renal vasodilation	Dopamine
Two NTs believed to be depleted in depression	1. NE 2. Serotonin
Powerful analgesic NT found exclusively in the hypothalamus	β-Endorphin
Opiate peptides which play a role in pain suppression	Enkephalins
NT that regulates release of GH and TSH; markedly ↓ Alzheimer disease	Somatostatin
Major inhibitory NT of the cortex	GABA
Major inhibitory NT of the spinal cord	Glycine
Major excitatory NT of the brain	Glutamate
Gaseous, vasoactive NT involved in memory	Nitrous oxide
NT important in the initiation of sleep	Melatonin
NT which inhibits the reticular activating center, thereby increasing total sleep time	ACh
Which two amino acids can serve as a precursor for the synthesis of catecholamines?	1. Phenylalanine 2. Tyrosine

Cerebral Cortex

What are the six layers of neocortex?	1. Layer I: molecular layer 2. Layer II: external granular layer 3. Layer III: external pyramidal layer 4. Layer IV: internal granular layer 5. Layer V: internal pyramidal layer 6. Layer VI: multiform layer

Name the site of a lesion, within the cortex, capable of causing each of the following deficits:

Right-sided flaccid hemiparalysis — Left primary motor area (Brodmann area 4)

Left-sided pronator drift — Right primary motor area (Brodmann area 4)

Loss of abstract thought and self-restraint — Bilateral loss of frontal lobes anterior to the frontal eye fields

Slowed speech without any impairment of language comprehension — Broca speech area (Brodmann areas 44, 45; always in the dominant hemisphere, usually left)

Loss of right-sided tactile sensation and proprioception — Left somesthetic area (Brodmann areas 3, 1, 2)

Cortical deafness — Bilateral destruction of the auditory areas (Brodmann areas 41, 42); unilateral destruction of the auditory area causes a slight ↓ in hearing.

Inability to understand spoken language and verbalize coherent thoughts — Wernicke speech area (Brodmann area 22) in the dominant hemisphere, usually left

Ipsilateral anosmia (inability to smell) — Primary olfactory area (Brodmann area 34)

Alexia and agraphia (inability to read and write) — Angular gyrus (Brodmann area 39)

Loss of ability to transfer information from short-term to long-term memory — Bilateral destruction of the hippocampal cortex

Psychic blindness, hyperphagia, docility, and hypersexuality (Klüver-Bucy syndrome) — Bilateral destruction of the anterior temporal lobes (amygdala)

Loss of ability to recognize faces — Inferomedial right occipitotemporal area

Loss of vision in the right visual field with macular sparing — Destruction of the left primary visual area (Brodmann area 17)

Name the term used to describe a deficit in the ability to draw a geometric figure: Construction apraxia

Name the term used to describe a "magnetic gait," commonly seen in normal-pressure hydrocephalus: Gait apraxia

What part of the nervous system is involved in maintaining wakefulness? Reticular activating system and bilateral cortex

PATHOLOGY OF THE NERVOUS SYSTEM

Congenital Disorders

Name the type of neural tube defect
with the following features:

Failure of posterior vertebral arch closure (not evident on clinical examination)	Spina bifida occulta
Failure of posterior vertebral arch closure accompanied by herniation of the meninges	Spina bifida cystica
Herniation of the meninges outside of the spinal canal	Meningocele
Herniation of nervous tissue and meninges outside of the spinal canal	Myelomeningocele
Complete cerebral agenesis due to lack of closure of the anterior neuropore	Anencephaly
Diverticulum of malformed CNS tissue	Encephalocele

What factor is used to screen pregnant mothers for neural tube defects? α-Fetoprotein

What is the most common cause of mental retardation? Fetal alcohol syndrome, often associated with cardiac and facial anomalies

What are two common chromosomal genetic causes of mental retardation?
1. Trisomy 21
2. Fragile X

Name the condition characterized by an excess of CSF in the cranial cavity: Hydrocephalus

What type of hydrocephalus is characterized by obstruction in the flow of CSF through the ventricular system and subarachnoid space? Noncommunicating hydrocephalus

What type of hydrocephalus is characterized by free flow of CSF but abnormal CSF absorption? Communicating hydrocephalus

What congenital malformation of the CNS is characterized by herniation of the cerebellar tonsils and medulla through the foramen magnum (which may result in obstruction of CSF circulation)? Arnold-Chiari malformation (type 1)

What congenital malformation of the CNS is associated with syringomyelia (central cavitation of the spinal cord)?	Arnold-Chiari malformation (type 2)
What congenital malformation of the CNS is characterized by cystic dilation of fourth ventricle, agenesis of vermis, and associated with hydrocephalus?	Dandy-Walker malformation
What complication of premature babies usually results in hypoxic/ischemic injuries of brain?	Subependymal germinal matrix bleed

Stroke

Describe the artery that has been occluded in each of the following stroke syndromes:

Paresis and sensory loss of contralateral lower extremity	ACA
Hemiparesis, contralateral hemisensory loss, homonymous hemianopsia, aphasia	MCA supplying the dominant hemisphere, usually left hemisphere
Loss of consciousness, hemisensory loss, homonymous hemianopsia with macular sparing	PCA
Amaurosis fugax	Ophthalmic artery
Vertigo, cranial nerve palsies, impaired level of consciousness, dysarthria	Vertebrobasilar artery
Sensory neglect and apraxia	MCA supplying the nondominant hemisphere, usually right hemisphere
Urinary incontinence, suck and grasp reflexes	Middle or ACA supplying the frontal lobe
Ipsilateral loss of pain and temperature for face, contralateral pain and temperature for body	PICA—Wallenberg syndrome (lateral medulla)

What are the most frequent sites of thrombotic occlusion in the cerebral vasculature?	Carotid bifurcation, MCA, and basilar artery
What is the most frequent site of embolic occlusion in the cerebral vasculature?	MCA

Which cardiac arrhythmia is associated with embolic stroke?	Atrial fibrillation
What type of stroke, associated with HTN, causes the formation of small, cystic, moon-shaped pits?	Lacunar infarctions
Where do lacunar strokes usually occur?	Basal ganglia, thalamus, internal capsule, white matter, pons, cerebellum
Name the term used to describe small aneurysms of the cerebral vasculature, caused by long-standing HTN, that may result in intracerebral hemorrhage:	Charcot-Bouchard aneurysms
What are the most common locations for Charcot-Bouchard aneurysms?	Thalamus and basal ganglia
Within the cerebral vasculature, what are the most common sites of berry aneurysm formation?	At the bifurcations of the circle of Willis
What is the most common complication of berry aneurysms?	Rupture causing subarachnoid hemorrhage
What are three disorders that predispose to the formation of berry aneurysms?	1. Polycystic kidney disease 2. Ehlers-Danlos syndrome 3. Marfan syndrome
Which cranial nerve palsy is associated with internal carotid or posterior communicating artery aneurysms?	CN III palsy causing papillary dilation
Name the term used to describe paroxysmal, self-limiting episodes of neurologic deficit, commonly including transient aphasia.	Transient ischemic attack
Which syndrome is characterized by loss of all motor function except that of CN III and IV?	Locked-in syndrome (usually a result of infarction or tumor at the base of the pons)

Seizures

Name the type of seizure associated with the following clinical findings:	
Loss of consciousness followed by loss of postural control, a tonic phase of muscle contraction and clonic limb jerking	Tonic-clonic seizure

A child who appears to be daydreaming in class and is found to have a 3-second spike-and-wave pattern on EEG	Absence seizure
Sudden, brief muscle contractions	Myoclonic epilepsy
Motor, sensory, visual, psychic, or autonomic phenomena with preserved level of consciousness	Simple partial seizure
Seizure begins with behavioral arrest, which is followed by auditory or visual hallucination, automatisms, and finally by postictal confusion	Complex partial seizure
What disorder is characterized by paroxysmal episodes of sharp, shooting facial pain in the distribution of one or more branches of CN V?	Trigeminal neuralgia
What is the drug of choice for trigeminal neuralgia?	Carbamazepine
What is the triad of cerebellar dysfunction?	1. Loss of balance (disequilibrium) 2. Hypotonia 3. Loss of coordinated muscle activity (dyssynergia)
Name the terms used to describe traumatic injury to the cortex at the site of impact and opposite the side of impact:	Coup injury (at the site of impact); contrecoup injury (opposite the site of impact)

Intracranial Hemorrhage

Name the type of intracranial hemorrhage associated with the following features:

Bloody or xanthrochromic CSF on lumbar puncture	Subarachnoid hemorrhage
Hematoma following the contour of a cerebral hemisphere on computed tomography (CT) scan	Subdural hematoma
Laceration of bridging cerebral veins	Subdural hematoma
Laceration of middle meningeal artery due to fracture of the temporal bone	Epidural hematoma
Lucid interval followed by rapid decline in mental status	Epidural hematoma

Most common type of intracranial hemorrhage resulting from trauma	Subdural hematoma
Ruptured berry aneurysm or arteriovenous malformation	Subarachnoid hemorrhage
Seen in patients with long-standing, poorly controlled HTN	Intraparenchymal hemorrhage
Lens-shaped hematoma on CT scan	Epidural hematoma
Crescentic hematoma on CT scan	Subdural hematoma
Seen more commonly in alcoholics and the elderly	Subdural hematoma
What is the most common cause of subarachnoid hemorrhage?	Trauma

Meningitis/Encephalitis

Name the type of meningitis associated with the following CSF findings:

Greater than 1000 polymorphonuclear mononuclear leukocytes, ↓ glucose, increased protein	Bacterial meningitis
Increased lymphocytes, minor elevation in protein, normal CSF pressure	Viral meningitis
Increased lymphocytes, minor elevation in protein, elevated CSF pressure	Fungal meningitis

Perivascular cuffing, inclusion bodies, and glial nodules may be seen in what cerebral infection?	Viral meningoencephalitis
Name the three most common bacteria causing neonatal meningitis:	1. Group B Streptococcus 2. *Escherichia coli* 3. Listeria
Name the parasite spread from cats to humans that causes periventricular calcifications and congenital disorders in offspring of infected mothers:	*Toxoplasma gondii*
Name the fungal meningitis most commonly associated with diabetics in DKA:	Mucormycosis

Bullet-shaped intracytoplasmic inclusions, Negri bodies are characteristic of which CNS viral infection?	Rabies
Hemorrhagic necrosis of temporal lobes is most commonly associated with which viral encephalitis?	HSV-1
Which infectious disease is characterized by neuronal vacuolization leading to small cysts in the gray matter of the brain *without* an associated inflammatory response?	Spongiform encephalopathy
Which disease is characterized by progressive ataxia, dementia, and spongiform gray matter changes?	Creutzfeldt-Jacob disease

Demyelinating Disorders

Name the demyelinating disorder associated with the following clinical and pathologic features:

Most common demyelinating disorder	Multiple sclerosis
Associated with JC virus infection in AIDS patients	Progressive multifocal leukoencephalopathy
Periventricular calcification; spinal lesions typically in the white matter of the cervical cord	Multiple sclerosis
Postviral autoimmune syndrome causing demyelination of peripheral nerves, especially motor fibers	Guillain-Barré syndrome
Triad of intention tremor, scanning speech, and nystagmus	Multiple sclerosis
May present with intranuclear ophthalmoplegia (MLF syndrome) or sudden visual loss due to optic neuritis	Multiple sclerosis
Ascending paralysis, facial diplegia, and autonomic dysfunction	Guillain-Barré syndrome
Oligoclonal bands in the CSF	Multiple sclerosis

Albuminocytologic dissociation (↑ CSF protein with normal cell count)	Guillain-Barré syndrome
↑ CSF protein, normal glucose, ↑ lymphocytes	Multiple sclerosis

Leukodystrophies and Neurocutaneous Syndromes

Name the type of leukodystrophy associated with the following features:

Globoid bodies in white matter	Krabbe disease
Deficiency of β-galactocerebrosidase	Krabbe disease
Deficiency of arylsulfatase A	Metachromatic leukodystrophy
Nervous tissue demonstrates loss of myelin and appears yellowish brown, build up of cerebroside in myelin sheath	Metachromatic leukodystrophy
Peroxisomal deficiency, demyelination starts in occipital lobe and moves anteriorly	Adrenoleukodystrophy (X-linked)

Name the type of neurocutaneous syndromes associated with the following features:

Cutaneous and plexiform neurofibromas, Lisch nodules on iris, café au lait spots, axillary freckling	Neurofibromatosis (NF1)
Bilateral schwanomas, meningioma, ependyoma	NF2
Capillary hemagiomas, hemagioblastomas in cerebellum and retina, increased incidence of renal cell carcinoma	von Hippel-Lindau
Nasolabial subcutaneous angiofibroma, epilepsy, subependymal nodules, ungual fibroma, shagreen patch, ash leaf spots	Tuberous sclerosis
What is the inheritance pattern of neurocutaneous syndromes?	Autosomal dominant (AD)
What is the inheritance pattern of leukodystrophies?	Autosomal recessive (AR)

Neurodegenerative Disorders

What are the two most common causes of dementia in the elderly? — Alzheimer dementia and multi-infarct dementia

Name the neurodegenerative disorder associated with the following clinical and pathologic features:

Hirano bodies, neurofibrillary tangles, senile plaques (accumulations of β-amyloid protein) — Alzheimer dementia

Stepwise dementia in a patient with focal neurologic deficits — Multi-infarct dementia

Thiamine deficiency from alcohol abuse causing ophthalmoplegia, ataxia, nystagmus — Wernicke encephalopathy

Long-term alcohol abuse causing retrograde and anterograde amnesia, confabulation, and shrunken, petechial hemorrhage in mammillary bodies — Korsakoff psychosis

Progressive dementia with predominantly frontal and temporal gliosis and neuronal loss — Pick disease

Degeneration of the caudate nucleus — Huntington disease

Lewy bodies and depigmentation of the substantia nigra — Parkinson disease

Parkinsonian symptoms with autonomic dysfunction, including orthostatic hypotension — Shy-Drager syndrome

Resting tremor, cogwheel rigidity, akinesia, postural instability — Parkinson disease

Can be caused by MPTP use — Parkinson disease

Slowly progressive ataxia, dysarthria associated with kyphoscoliosis, diabetes, arrythmias, and myocarditis due to triplet repeat GAA on chromosome 9 — Friedreich ataxia

Autosomal dominant (AD) inheritance and anticipation (worsening of disease in future generations) due to increasing number of CAG repeats on chromosome 4 — Huntington disease

UMN and LMN signs due to loss of myelinated fibers of the corticospinal tract	Amyotrophic lateral sclerosis (ALS)
Viral infection → inflammatory response in anterior horn of the spinal cord → LMN loss	Poliomyelitis
Childhood ataxia associated with telangiectasias of the skin and conjunctiva associated with *ATM* gene mutation	Ataxia-telangiectasia
Floppy baby (hypotonia) due to LMN degeneration, tongue fasciculation	Werdnig-Hoffman disease
Which protein gives rise to the amyloid fibrils of Alzheimer disease?	A-β
Which is the conformation of A-β protein in neuritic plaques?	β-Pleated sheet
The A-β protein is derived from processing of which larger molecule?	Amyloid precursor protein (APP)

Brain Tumors

Where are the majority of adults versus children CNS tumors found?	Supratentorial for adults, infratentorial for children
Name the brain tumor associated with each of the following clinical or pathologic findings:	
Most common pediatric intracranial tumor	Juvenile pilocytic astrocytoma
Most common pituitary tumor	Pituitary adenoma
Most common pituitary adenoma	Prolactinoma
Most common pediatric supratentorial tumor	Craniopharyngioma
Most common primary brain tumor	Glioblastoma multiforme
Most common intracranial tumor	Metastases
Malignant pediatric tumor which metastases through CSF pathways	Medulloblastoma
Malignant pediatric tumor found exclusively in the posterior fossa	Medulloblastoma
Vascular tumor of cerebellum and retina in patients with von Hippel-Lindau syndrome	Hemangioblastoma

Abundant capillaries and vacuolated foam cells	Hemangioblastoma
Type of tumor that is found bilaterally in patients with neurofibromatosis II	Vestibular schwannoma
Tumor of the dorsal root that may grow in a dumbbell configuration through a vertebral foramen	Schwannoma
Tumor which originates from the vestibular division of CN VIII	Schwannoma
Tumor which grows in a mixture of Antoni A or Antoni B patterns	Schwannoma
Small round blue cell tumor	Medulloblastoma
Bipolar cells, Rosenthal fibers, and microcysts	Juvenile pilocytic astrocytoma
Verocay bodies	Schwannoma
Tumor derived from Rathke pouch	Craniopharyngioma
Two tumors often presenting with bitemporal hemianopia	Pituitary adenoma and craniopharyngioma
Tumor characterized by concentric whorls and calcified psammoma bodies	Meningioma
Tumor arising from ependymal lining of ventricular system	Ependymoma
Tumor commonly arising in the pineal region causing obstructive hydrocephalus by compromising the aqueduct of Sylvius	Germinoma
EBV positive B-cell tumor of the CNS in AIDS patients	CNS lymphoma
Tumor of the foramen of Monro causing obstructive hydrocephalus	Colloid cyst of the third ventricle
Benign tumor characterized by calcifications and cells with fried-egg appearance or perinuclear halos	Oligodendroma
Tumor characterized by highly malignant cells bordering necrotic areas	Glioblastoma multiforme
Benign tumor derived from arachnoid cap cells with well-delineated margins	Meningioma

Disorders of the Spinal Cord

Name a disease of the spinal cord
associated with each of the following
neurologic findings:

Loss of all spinal modalities except tactile discrimination, vibratory sensation, and proprioception	Ventral spinal artery occlusion
Impaired tactile discrimination, vibratory sensation, and proprioception	Tabes dorsalis
Loss of pain and temperature sensation in a cape-like distribution and flaccid paralysis of the intrinsic muscles of the hand	Syringomyelia
Impaired tactile discrimination, vibratory sensation and proprioception, UMN signs, and ataxia	Vitamin B_{12} deficiency

Miscellaneous

What complication affecting the brainstem can be caused by rapid correction of hyponatremia?	Central pontine myelinolysis
Describe how transtentorial herniation causes contralateral hemiparesis.	Compresses the right crus cerebri → corticospinal and corticobulbar fibers are compromised (Kernohan notch)
Describe how transtentorial herniation causes pupillary dilation.	Tension on CN III causes pupillary dilation.
Name a life-threatening complication of transforaminal or tonsillar herniation:	Compression of the medullary respiratory center → respiratory insufficiency
What is the term used to describe brainstem hemorrhages caused by transtentorial and transforaminal herniation?	Duret hemorrhages
What is the systemic response to increased intracranial pressure (Cushing triad)?	1. HTN 2. Bradycardia 3. Irregular respirations

What is the most common reversible cause of dementia in the elderly?

Normal pressure hydrocephalus

Normal pressure hydrocephalus is a common complication of what type of intracranial pathology?

Subarachnoid hemorrhage

What is the triad of normal-pressure hydrocephalus?

1. Ataxic, magnetic gait (Wobbly)
2. Dementia and/or short-term memory loss (Weird)
3. Urinary incontinence (Wet)

What diuretic is commonly used to manage increased intracranial pressure?

Mannitol (provides osmotic diuresis)

What is the protein change associated with prion diseases?

Conformational change in PrPc (α-helix isoform) to PrPsc (β-pleated sheet isoform)

PHARMACOLOGY OF THE NERVOUS SYSTEM

Antiepileptics

For each of the following drugs, name:

1. The mechanism of action (MOA)
2. Indication(s) (IND)
3. Significant side effects or important toxicity (TOX) (if any)

Carbamazepine

MOA: Na^+ channel blocker

IND: Tonic-clonic, partial, and Jacksonian seizures

TOX: ↑ LFT, agranulocytosis, a plastic anemia

Ethosuximide

MOA: May block T-type Ca^{2+} channels in thalamus

IND: Absence seizures

TOX: GI upset, Stevens-Johnson syndrome

Diazepam

MOA: Facilitates GABA action by ↑ frequency of Cl channel opening

IND: Status epilepticus

TOX: Sedation

Lamotrigine

MOA: Blocks Na^+ channels

IND: Adjuvant antiepileptic agent

TOX: Life-threatening rash and Stevens-Johnson syndrome

Phenytoin

MOA: Na^+ channel blocker

IND: Tonic-clonic, partial, and status

TOX: Nystagmus, ataxia, gingivalhyperplasia, hirsutism, megalobasticanemia, teratogenic

Phenobarbital

MOA: Facilitates GABA action by ↑ duration of Cl channel opening

IND: Tonic-clonic seizures

TOX: Induces P-450, drowsiness

Valproic acid

MOA: Unknown—may facilitate GABA action

IND: Myoclonic seizures

TOX: Hepatotoxicity, GI toxicity, inhibits P-450, thrombocytopenia

Name the drug(s) of choice for each of the following types of epilepsy:

Simple and complex partial

Phenytoin, carbamazepine

Absence

Ethosuximide

Febrile

Phenobarbital

Myoclonic

Valproic acid, clonazepam

Status epilepticus

Phenytoin, diazepam

Tonic-clonic

Phenytoin, carbamazepine

Antiparkinsonian Agents

For each of the following drugs, name:

1. **The mechanism of action (MOA)**
2. **Indication(s) (IND)**
3. **Significant side effects or important toxicity (TOX) (if any)**

Amantidine

MOA: May enhance dopamine release

IND: Helpful for rigidity and bradykinesia

TOX: Acute psychosis (rare)

Benztropine

MOA: Antimuscarinic

IND: Adjuvant therapy

TOX: Similar to atropine

Bromocriptine	**MOA:** Dopamine receptor agonist
	IND: Used with levodopa
	TOX: Hypotension, confusion, hallucinations, nausea
Levodopa	**MOA:** Dopamine precursor converted to dopamine in CNS
	IND: Combined with carbidopa, levodopa is the most efficacious regimen for Parkinson disease
	TOX: Nausea, tachycardia, hypotension, hallucinations, dyskinesias
Carbidopa	**MOA:** Inhibition of dopamine decarboxylase → ↑ levodopa availability in CNS
	IND: Used with levodopa
	TOX: spasms of the eyelid, irregular heartbeat, confusion, agitation, hallucinations
Selegiline	**MOA:** Inhibition of MAOb → ↑ dopamine levels in CNS
	IND: Used as adjuvant to levodopa
	TOX: HTN

Anesthetics

For each of the following drugs, provide:

1. The mechanism of action (MOA)
2. Indication(s) (IND)
3. Significant side effects or important toxicity (TOX) (if any)

Halothane	**MOA:** CNS depression
	IND: Prototype general anesthetic; potent anesthetic but weak analgesic
	TOX: Arrhythmias, ↓ cardiac output, hypotension, hepatotoxicity
Nitrous oxide	**MOA:** CNS depression
	IND: Weak general anesthetic, strong analgesic
	TOX: Anoxia, vitamin B_{12} deficiency (with chronic use)

Thiopental	**MOA:** Prolongs inhibitory postsynaptic potentials by ↑ GABA levels (similar to phenobarbital)
	IND: Surgical anesthesia
	TOX: Laryngospasm
Benzodiazepines (diazepam, midazolam)	**MOA:** Facilitates GABA action by ↑ frequency of Cl⁻ channel opening
	IND: Sedative, hypnotic, anxiolytic
	TOX: Sedation
Ketamine	**MOA:** PCP analog
	IND: General anesthetic
	TOX: Postoperative hallucinations, amnesia, respiratory depression
Propofol	**MOA:** CNS depression
	IND: General anesthetic—rapid onset and clearance
	TOX: Cannot be given to patients with egg or soybean allergies
Local anesthetics (procaine, cocaine, tetracaine, lidocaine, bupivacaine)	**MOA:** Block Na^+ channels
	IND: Anesthetic for minor procedures, spinal blocks
	TOX: Arrhythmias, HTN; cardiotoxicity (bupivacaine), seizures
Succinylcholine	**MOA:** Depolarizing neuromuscular blocker
	IND: Rapid sequence induction
	TOX: Malignant hyperthermia when given with halogenated inhaled anesthetic; contraindicated in patients with glaucoma because of ↑ intraocular pressure (IOP)
Tubocurarine	**MOA:** Nondepolarizing neuromuscular blocker
	IND: Adjuvant to general anesthesia
	TOX: Hypotension
Why is epinephrine commonly combined with local anesthetics?	To prolong the duration of the anesthetic effect by causing local vasoconstriction
What types of fibers are affected most by local anesthetic agents?	Pain > temperature > touch > pressure; small unmyelinated fibers most affected; large, myelinated fibers least affected

Which drug is used to reverse
the effects of the nondepolarizing
muscle blockers?

Neostigmine

Which drug is used to treat malignant
hyperthermia?

Dantrolene

Analgesics

For each of the following drugs, provide:

1. The mechanism of action (MOA)
2. Indication(s) (IND)
3. Significant side effects and unique
   toxicity (TOX) (if any)

   Acetaminophen

   MOA: COX inhibitor

   IND: Pain, fever (but not used as anti-
   inflammatory)

   TOX: Overdose causes hepatic
   necrosis

   Aspirin

   MOA: Irreversible inhibition of COX-1
   and COX-2

   IND: Analgesic, antipyretic, anti-
   inflammatory, antiplatelet drug

   TOX: GI ulcers, platelet dysfunction,
   hypersensitivity reactions,
   bronchoconstriction, tinnitus, Reye
   syndrome in children

   Celecoxib

   MOA: COX-2 inhibitor

   IND: Osteoarthritis, rheumatoid arthritis

   TOX: Similar to aspirin but less GI
   toxicity

   Gabapentin

   MOA: Structural analog of GABA

   IND: Neuropathic pain

   TOX: Sedation, movement disorders

   Indomethacin

   MOA: Reversible inhibition of COX-1
   and COX-2

   IND: Acute gout, neonatal patent
   ductus arteriosus

   TOX: GI upset, headache

   Meperidine

   MOA: μ opioid receptor agonist

   IND: Analgesic

   TOX: Seizures; side effects similar
   to morphine

Morphine

MOA: μ opioid receptor agonist; opioid receptor binding activates G proteins and adenylyl cyclase.

IND: Analgesic, cough suppressant.

TOX: Constipation, emesis, sedation, respiratory depression, miosis, urinary retention.

Note: these symptoms are typical for heroin overdose.

Nalbuphine

MOA: Opioid mixed agonist-antagonist analgesic that activates κ and weakly blocks μ receptors

IND: Analgesic with less abuse potential

Naloxone

MOA: μ opioid receptor antagonist

IND: Used to reverse the effects of opioid agonists

TOX: CNS depression

What two types of opioid receptors mediate analgesia, respiratory depression, and physical dependence?

1. μ
2. δ

What type of opioid receptors mediate spinal analgesia and the sedative effects of opioids?

κ

CHAPTER 5

Cardiovascular

EMBRYOLOGY

What are the five dilatations of the primitive heart tube?

1. Truncus arteriosus
2. Bulbus cordis
3. Primitive ventricle
4. Primitive atrium
5. Sinus venosus

Name the structures in the mature heart that are derived from the following embryonic structures:

Truncus arteriosus

Ascending aorta and pulmonary trunk

Bulbus cordis

Smooth parts of left (aortic vestibule) and right (conus arteriosus) ventricle

Primitive ventricle

Trabeculated parts of left and right ventricle

Primitive atria

Trabeculated parts of left and right atria

Left horn of sinus venosus

Coronary sinus

Right horn of sinus venosus

Smooth part of right atrium (sinus venarum)

Transient common pulmonary vein

Smooth part of left atrium

Right common cardinal vein and right anterior cardinal vein

Superior vena cava

Which embryonic layer gives rise to most of the cardiovascular system?

Mesoderm

What structure divides the truncus arteriosus and bulbus cordis?

Aorticopulmonary septum

Name the structure between the atria that develops from the walls of the septum primum and septum secundum:

Foramen ovale

Name the three physiologic shunts in the fetal circulation and the structures they shunt between:	1. Foramen ovale (right to left atrium) 2. Ductus arteriosus (pulmonary artery to aortic arch) 3. Ductus venosus (umbilical vein to IVC)

ANATOMY

What are the two anatomic divisions of the pericardium?	1. Serous pericardium (made of visceral epicardial layer and parietal layer) 2. Fibrous pericardium
Which nerve lies between the fibrous paricardium and mediastinal pleura?	Phrenic nerve (runs with pericardiophrenic vessels)

Name the chamber associated with each heart surface:

Sternocostal surface	Right ventricle
Posterior surface (base)	Left atrium
Diaphragmatic surface	Right and left ventricles
Pulmonary surface and apex	Left ventricle

Name the structures that compose each heart border:

Right border	Right atrium
Left border	Left ventricle, left auricle
Inferior border	Right ventricle
Superior border	Right and left auricles, great vessels

Name the major artery that commonly supplies each of the following structures:

Right atrium and right ventricle	Right coronary artery (RCA)
Sinoatrial (SA) and atrioventricular (AV) nodes	RCA
Left atrium and left ventricle	Left coronary artery (LCA)
Interventricular septum 1. Anterior 2/3 2. Posterior 1/3	1. Left anterior descending (LAD) 2. Posterior interventricular artery
Which artery determines dominance of cardiac blood supply?	Posterior interventricular artery

What are the most common sites for coronary occlusion?	Left anterior descending (LAD) > RCA > circumflex
Trace the general pathway of venous drainage from myocardium.	Great, middle, and small cardiac veins → coronary sinus → right atrium
Trace the conduction pathway of a cardiac impulse.	SA node → AV node → bundle of His → right and left bundle branches → Purkinje fibers
Which nerve supplies parasympathetic input to heart?	Vagus nerve
Which syndrome is characterized by arm claudication, syncope, vertigo, nausea, and a supraclavicular bruit?	Subclavian steal syndrome (occlusion in subclavian artery proximal to take vertebral artery take-off → "stealing" of blood from vertebral artery to distal subclavian artery)
Describe the best location for auscultation of the following cardiac valves:	
Tricuspid valve	Left sternal border, fifth intercostal space
Pulmonary valve	Left sternal border, second intercostal space
Mitral valve	Apex of heart, fifth intercostal space
Aortic valve	Right sternal border, second intercostal space

PHYSIOLOGY

Cardiac Electrophysiology

Name the electrical event in the heart associated with each feature of a normal electrocardiogram:	
P wave	Atrial depolarization
PR interval	Atrial depolarization and conduction delay through AV node
QRS complex	Depolarization of the ventricles
T wave	Ventricular repolarization
Which ion primarily dictates the resting membrane potential of a myocyte?	Potassium. Membrane has high K^+ permeability through K^+ channels.

Which membrane protein maintains the ion gradient?	Sodium-potassium ATPase
What is the effect of potassium efflux from a myocardial cell?	Hyperpolarization
What is the effect of potassium influx into a myocardial cell?	Depolarization

Describe the electrochemical events that cause the following phases of the cardiac myocyte action potential:

Phase 0 (the upstroke)	Influx of Na^+ into cell
Phase 1 (initial repolarization)	Efflux of K^+ out of cell and $\downarrow Na^+$ influx
Phase 2 (the plateau)	Influx of Ca^{2+} into cell, efflux of K^+ out of cell
Phase 3 (repolarization)	Efflux of K^+ out of cell
Phase 4 (resting membrane potential)	Equilibrium potential, balance between K^+ leak current and Na^+/K^+ ATPase

What unique electrochemical feature of SA node allows it to act as a pacemaker for the heart?	Phase 4 depolarization causing **automaticity**
What ion and channel are responsible for automaticity?	Na^+ conductance via I_f channel.

Describe the electrochemical events that cause the following phases of the SA nodal action potential:

Phase 0 (the upstroke)	Influx of Ca^{2+} into cell
Phase 3 (repolarization)	Efflux of K^+ out of cell
Phase 4 (slow depolarization)	Increasing Na^+ influx into cell

What phase 4 characteristic determines heart rate?	Slope which represents rate of depolarization
Name the component of the cardiac conduction system where phase 4 depolarization is *fastest*:	SA node
Name the component of the cardiac conduction system where phase 4 depolarization is *slowest*:	Bundle of His and Purkinje fibers

Define conduction velocity.	The rate at which an impulse spreads throughout cardiac tissue
What determines conduction velocity?	Rate of depolarization (phase 0 upstroke)
Where is conduction velocity *fastest*?	The Purkinje system
Where is conduction velocity *slowest*?	The AV node
What is the significance of the conduction delay at the AV node?	The delay in conduction allows for ventricular filling

Cardiac Contractility and Output

Describe the function of each myocardial cellular component:

Sarcomere	Contractile unit
Intercalated disks	Cell adhesion
Gap junction	Electrochemical communication between myocardial fibers
T tubules	Carry action potentials into the cell interior
Sarcoplasmic reticulum	Storage and release of calcium

Which ion determines the magnitude of tension in a contracting myocardial cell?	Amount of intracellular calcium

Describe the effect of each of the following on contractility:

Increased heart rate	Increased contractility
Catecholamines	Increased contractility
Digoxin	Increased contractility
Acetylcholine (ACh)	Decreased contractility

What is the Frank-Starling relationship?	The greater the end-diastolic volume (preload), the greater is the stroke volume.
How does contractility affect cardiac output?	Cardiac output increases as contractility increases.
Name the four factors that determine myocardial oxygen consumption:	1. Afterload 2. Size of heart (wall tension) 3. Contractility 4. Heart rate

Provide formulas for each of the following:

Stroke volume

End-diastolic volume – end-systolic volume =

Cardiac output

Stroke volume × heart rate =

Ejection fraction

Stroke volume/end-diastolic volume =

Stroke work

Aortic pressure × stroke volume

Cardiac output based on Fick principle

O_2 consumption/(arterial O_2 – venous O_2)

Heart Sounds

Name the event associated with each heart sound:

S_1

Closure of the AV (tricuspid, mitral) valves

S_2

Closure of semilunar (aortic, pulmonary) valves

S_3

Flow of blood from atria into ventricles during diastole (often seen with large ventricular volumes, ie, CHF; often benign in youth and trained athletes)

S_4

Flow of blood from atria into ventricles during atrial systole (often present in patient with stiffened ventricle)

Maintenance of Blood Pressure

What is the site of highest resistance in the cardiovascular system?

Arterioles

Which vascular bed has the largest cross-sectional and surface areas?

Capillaries

Which vascular bed contains the largest volume of blood at any given time?

Veins

Define the following terms:

Systolic blood pressure

Highest arterial blood pressure during a cardiac cycle

Diastolic blood pressure

Lowest arterial blood pressure during a cardiac cycle

Pulse pressure

Difference between systolic and diastolic blood pressure

What is the most important determinant of pulse pressure?	Stroke volume
What is the effect of aging on pulse pressure?	Aging widens pulse pressure due to ↓ capacitance of blood vessels
How is left atrial pressure estimated clinically?	Pulmonary capillary wedge pressure
Where are the carotid baroreceptors located?	Bifurcation of common carotid arteries
What is the function of the carotid baroreceptors?	Minute to minute regulation of blood pressure
Which nerve carries information from baroreceptors to the vasomotor center in the brainstem?	Cranial nerve IX
Describe the phases of the Valsalva maneuver and changes occurring with BP and heart rate.	Phase 1: forceful expiration against closed glottis (↑ BP with ↑ intrathoracic pressure, ↓ HR with baroreflex)
	Phase 2: accommodation (↓ BP with reduced venous return, ↑ HR with baroreflex)
	Phase 3: breathe in (↓ BP with ↓ intrathoracic pressure, ↑ HR with baroreflex)
	Phase 4: recovery (↑ BP with normal venous return, marked ↓ HR with baroreflex overshoot)
Name two ways that the vasomotor center responds to decreased mean arterial pressure:	1. ↓ Parasympathetic output 2. ↑ Sympathetic output
Name the hormone(s) responsible for each of the following functions:	
Long-term regulation of blood pressure	Renin-angiotensin-aldosterone system
Stimulation of aldosterone secretion and arterial vasoconstriction	Angiotensin II
Water retention and direct arteriolar vasoconstriction causing an increase in blood pressure	Vasopressin
Inhibition of renin release, stimulation of salt and water excretion, and vascular smooth muscle relaxation	Atrial natriuretic peptide

Name three stimuli for renin secretion:

1. ↓ Renal blood pressure
2. ↓ Na^+ delivery to macula densa of JGA
3. ↑ Sympathetic tone

What is the effect of cerebral ischemia on blood pressure and heart rate?

Cushing reflex: blood pressure ↑ and heart rate ↓

What is the mechanism of increased blood pressure in cerebral ischemia?

Chemoreceptors in the vasomotor center stimulate increased sympathetic outflow

What is the mechanism of decreased heart rate in cerebral ischemia?

Baroreceptor reflex to increase in BP leads to increased parasympathetic outflow to heart

Where are the carotid chemoreceptors located?

Bifurcation of common carotid arteries and the aortic arch at carotid body

What do chemoreceptors sense?

Oxygen, CO_2, pH, and temperature

What is the Starling equation?

$J_v = K_f [(P_c - P_i) - (\pi_c - \pi_i)]$

Describe the effect of each of the following on capillary filtration:

Increased capillary hydrostatic pressure

Increased fluid filtration

Increased interstitial hydrostatic pressure

Decreased fluid filtration

Increased capillary oncotic pressure

Decreased fluid filtration

Increased interstitial oncotic pressure

Increased fluid filtration

Define autoregulation.

The capacity of an organ to maintain constant blood flow despite changes in mean arterial pressure

Define active hyperemia.

The capacity of an organ to increase blood flow in response to metabolic demands

Name the primary mechanism of blood flow regulation in the following tissues:

Coronary arteries

Local metabolic control

Cerebral vasculature

Local metabolic control

Muscle

Local metabolic control

Skin

Sympathetic control

Pulmonary

Local metabolic control

Name five key metabolites which cause vasodilation:

1. Lactate
2. K^+
3. Adenosine
4. CO_2
5. H^+

Name the primary vasoactive metabolite in the following tissues:

Coronary arteries O_2, adenosine

Cerebral vasculature CO_2 (most important), H^+

Muscle   Lactate, K^+, adenosine

Pulmonary O_2

CARDIOVASCULAR PATHOLOGY AND PATHOPHYSIOLOGY

Murmurs

Name the valvular defect causing each murmur described below:

Harsh midsystolic murmur in the left second intercostal space at the left sternal border

Pulmonic stenosis

Harsh midsystolic murmur in the right second intercostal space at the right sternal border, radiating to the neck (carotid arteries) and apex

Aortic stenosis

Harsh midsystolic murmur at the left third and fourth interspaces radiating down the left sternal border; murmur louder with decreased preload (ie, on Valsalva); S_4 and biphasic apical impulse often present

Hypertrophic cardiomyopathy

Blowing holosystolic murmur at apex radiating to the left axilla with increased apical impulse

Mitral regurgitation

Blowing holosystolic murmur at the lower left sternal border radiating to the right of the sternum; may ↑ with inspiration

Tricuspid regurgitation

Soft, late systolic murmur at the left sternal border or apex, accompanied by midsystolic click

Mitral valve prolapse

Harsh holosystolic murmur at the lower left sternal border, accompanied by a thrill	Ventricular septal defect (VSD)
Blowing, high-pitched diastolic murmur at the left second to fourth interspaces radiating to the apex	Aortic regurgitation
Low-pitched diastolic murmur at the apex that gets louder prior to S_1; an opening snap is often present just after S_2	Mitral stenosis
Systolic flow murmur at left upper sternal border; fixed splitting of S_2	Atrial septal defect (ASD)

What congenital valvular defect is associated with aortic stenosis?

Bicuspid aortic valve

What are two common manifestations of aortic stenosis?

Angina and syncope

Which disorder results from myxomatous degeneration of the mitral valve?

Mitral valve prolapse

Patients with mitral valve prolapse are at increased risk of which infection?

Infective endocarditis

Heart Failure

What are the most common causes of left-sided heart failure?

Ischemic heart disease, HTN, mitral and aortic valvular disease, myocardial disease (cardiomyopathy, myocarditis)

Name four key mechanisms of compensation in congestive heart failure (CHF):

1. Hypertrophy
2. Ventricular compensation
3. Blood volume expansion
4. Tachycardia

Name two major clinical signs/ symptoms of left-sided heart failure:

1. Pulmonary congestion
2. Pulmonary edema causing dyspnea and orthopnea

Name three consequences of suboptimal renal perfusion:

1. RAA axis activation leading to salt and water retention
2. Ischemic acute tubular necrosis (ATN)
3. Prerenal azotemia

What is the consequence of impaired cerebral perfusion in CHF?	Hypoxic encephalopathy
What is the most common cause of right-sided heart failure?	Left-sided heart failure
Name two major pulmonary causes of right-sided heart failure:	1. Interstitial fibrosis 2. Pulmonary HTN
Name four key clinical signs of right-sided heart failure:	1. Portal, systemic, peripheral congestion, and edema 2. Hepatomegaly 3. Congestive splenomegaly 4. Renal congestion
Describe the phases of pathologic change in the liver that result from chronic right-sided heart failure.	Nutmeg appearance → centrilobular necrosis → central hemorrhagic necrosis → cardiac sclerosis (cirrhosis)
What is the most common cause of acute right-sided heart failure in a patient with a deep venous thrombosis?	Massive pulmonary embolus
What EKG findings may be seen with acute right-sided heart stress?	$S_1Q_3T_3$: S wave in lead 1, Q wave in lead 3, T-wave inversion in lead 3

Ischemic Heart Disease

Name four important manifestations of ischemic heart disease:	1. Angina 2. Myocardial infarction (MI) 3. Lethal arrhythmia causing sudden cardiac death 4. Chronic CHF
What are the two major etiologies of myocardial ischemia?	1. ↓ Coronary perfusion 2. ↑ Myocardial O_2 demand
What conditions compound the consequences of impaired myocardial perfusion?	Anemia, advanced lung disease, cigarette smoking, congenital heart disease
Name the type of angina:	
Pain precipitated by exertion, relieved by rest/vasodilators	Stable angina
Paroxysmal chest pain at rest in patient with or without coronary risk factors	Prinzmetal angina
Severe substernal pain/pressure at rest	Unstable angina

Describe the underlying pathology for each type of angina:

    Stable angina

        Greater than 75% occlusion of coronary artery

    Prinzmetal angina

        Coronary vasospasm

    Unstable angina

        Plaque disruption with resulting occlusive thrombosis within a coronary artery

Describe the associations between myocardial ischemia, injury, and infarction.

1. Ischemia—insufficient blood supply to the myocardium, occurs first
2. Injury—results when the ischemic process is prolonged
3. Infarction—describes necrosis or death of myocardial cells

Name the type of myocardial damage described below:

    Full-thickness infarction caused by complete occlusion of a coronary artery

        Transmural infarction

    Infarction of the inner half (or less) of the ventricular wall supplied by a partially occluded coronary artery

        Subendocardial infarction

    T-wave inversion on ECG

        Transmural ischemia

    ST depression on ECG

        Subendocardial injury

    ST elevation on ECG

        Transmural injury

    Q waves present on ECG

        Transmural infarction

What is the initial event in the development of a transmural infarction?

Acute plaque disruption

What are the most common symptoms of a myocardial infarct?

Crushing retrosternal chest pain or pressure, dyspnea, pain radiating into left arm or neck, diaphoresis, nausea

What type of necrosis is seen in myocardium within 24 hours of infarction?

Coagulative necrosis

What type of inflammatory cells are seen in the myocardium within 24 hours of infarction?

Neutrophils

What is the most common type of inflammatory cell seen in myocardium from the 2nd to 10th day after an infarction?

Macrophages

When is the risk of myocardial rupture greatest and why?

At 4 to 7 days. Tissue is weakest following phagocytosis of debris by macrophages and prior to growth of granulation tissue.

How many days does it take to form granulation tissue in a region of infarcted myocardium?

7 to 10 days

How many weeks does it take to form contracted scar tissue in a region of infarcted myocardium?

7 weeks

What is the diagnostic test of choice in a patient with suspected MI?

ECG

What two classic ECG changes are seen during an MI?

1. Q waves
2. ST elevation

When does CK-MB begin to rise, peak, and return to normal?

Rise: 3 to 8 hours

Peak: 10 to 24 hours

Return to normal: 2 to 3 days

When does troponin I begin to rise, peak, and return to normal?

Rise: 3 to 8 hours

Peak: 24 to 48 hours

Return to normal: 5 to 10 days

What are the advantages and disadvantages of the CK-MB serum cardiac marker?

Allows diagnosis of re-infarction as levels quickly return to normal; may be falsely elevated with skeletal muscle injury

What are the advantages of the Troponin test?

Very specific to cardiac injury; allows diagnosis of late presenting MI

What are the two most common complications of MI?

1. Cardiac arrhythmia
2. CHF

List five less common but severe complications of MI:

1. Cardiogenic shock
2. Ventricular aneurysm or rupture
3. Papillary muscle rupture
4. Mural thrombosis with resulting peripheral embolism
5. Dressler syndrome

Cardiomyopathy

How does the left ventricle respond to long-standing HTN?

Concentric hypertrophy

What are the three types of cardiomyopathy?

1. Dilated or congestive
2. Hypertrophic
3. Restrictive

What are the most common nongenetic etiologies of dilated cardiomyopathy?

"ABCDE"

Alcohol abuse

Beriberi (thiamine deficiency)

Coxsackie B myocarditis, **C**ocaine, **C**hagas disease

Doxorubicin toxicity

pr**E**gnancy

Name the type of cardiomyopathy associated with the following clinical and pathologic features:

30% to 40% of cases are genetic

Dilated

100% of cases are genetic

Hypertrophic

Associated with alcoholism and thiamine deficiency

Dilated

Associated with coxsackie virus B and with *Trypanosoma cruzi*

Dilated

Associated with doxorubicin

Dilated

Associated with eosinophilia

Restrictive (Loeffler endocarditis)

Associated with pregnancy

Dilated

Asymmetric septal hypertrophy, banana-shaped left ventricle without dilatation

Hypertrophic

Can be caused by sarcoidosis, amyloidosis, scleroderma, hereditary hemochromatosis, endocardial fibroelastosis, radiation-induced fibrosis

Restrictive

Cardiomyopathy most commonly caused by endomyocardial fibrosis

Restrictive

Causes sudden death in young, otherwise healthy athletes

Hypertrophic

Commonly inherited in an autosomal-dominant (AD) fashion

Hypertrophic

Four-chamber hypertrophy and dilation	Dilated
Left ventricular outflow obstruction	Hypertrophic
Myocyte tangles, disorientation	Hypertrophic
Symptoms relieved by squatting	Hypertrophic

Pericarditis and Cardiac Tumors

Name the type of pericarditis based on the following exudates descriptions:	
Clear, straw colored, minimal inflammation, decreased fibrin	Serous pericarditis
Fibrin rich	Fibrinous pericarditis
Bloody	Hemorrhagic pericarditis
What are the most common etiologies of serous pericarditis?	Uremia, systemic lupus erythematosus (SLE), rheumatic fever
What are the most common etiologies of fibrinous pericarditis?	Uremia, SLE, rheumatic fever, coxsackie viral infection, MI, trauma
What are the most common etiologies of hemorrhagic pericarditis?	Trauma, malignancy, tuberculosis
What ECG and BP findings are seen in pericarditis?	ECG: diffuse ST elevations in all leads BP: pulsus paradoxus
What is the most common cardiac tumor of adults?	Metastases (eg, melanoma)
What is the most common primary cardiac tumor of adults?	Left-sided atrial myxoma
What is the most common primary cardiac tumor in children?	Rhabdomyoma, commonly associated with tuberous sclerosis

Congenital Heart Disease

| Name the congenital heart defect associated with each of the following statements: | |
| Three most common causes of R->L shunting | 1. Atrial septal defect (ASD)
2. VSD
3. Patent ductus arteriosus (PDA) |

Two most common defects	1. VSD 2. PDA
Five defects causing cyanosis at birth	"5 T's": 1. Tetralogy of Fallot 2. Transposition of the great vessels 3. Truncus arteriosus 4. Total anomalous pulmonary venous return 5. Tricuspid atresia
Continuous machinery-like murmur	PDA
Pulmonic stenosis, right ventricular hypertrophy, overriding aorta, VSD ("PROVe")	Tetralogy of Fallot
Boot-shaped cardiac silhouette	Tetralogy of Fallot
Defect causing lower body cyanosis	Preductal coarctation
Defect causing upper extremity HTN and diminished lower extremity pulses	Postductal coarctation (stenosis distal to the ductus arteriosus)
Associated with Turner syndrome	Coarctation of the aorta
Associated with Down syndrome	ASDs, VSDs, and AV valve abnormalities (due to endocardial cushion abnormalities)
Associated with Rubella	Patent ductus arteriosus
Associated with 22q11 syndrome	Truncus arteriosus, Tetralogy of Fallot
Common cyanotic congenital heart defect in children born to diabetic mothers	Transposition of the great vessels
Aorta arises from *right* ventricle and pulmonary trunk arises from *left* ventricle	Transposition of the great vessels
Valvular defect associated with increased risk of infective endocarditis and calcification	Bicuspid aortic valve
What is the consequence of leaving a left-to-right shunting untreated?	Right → left shunting
What type of infection are patients with VSD at an increased risk for?	Infective endocarditis
What drug is used to induce closure of a PDA?	Indomethacin

What drug is used to prevent closure of a PDA?	Prostaglandins
What is the most common genetic cause of congenital heart disease?	Trisomy 21

Cardiac Infectious Disorders

What type of infection is responsible for causing rheumatic fever?	Group A streptococcal pharyngitis
How does streptococcal pharyngitis cause rheumatic heart disease?	Antistreptococcal antibodies cross-react with a cardiac antigen
What serologic test is elevated in rheumatic heart disease:	Antistreptolysin antibodies (ASO)
Name the five major Jones criteria for rheumatic heart disease:	1. Joints: migratory polyarthritis 2. ♥ (o) = pancarditis 3. Nodules: subcutaneous nodules 4. Erythema marginatum 5. Syndeham chorea
Name five minor Jones criteria for rheumatic heart disease:	1. Fever 2. Arthralgia 3. Elevated ESR/CRP 4. Leukocytosis 5. Heart block on ECG
What term is used to describe the foci of pink collagen surrounded by lymphocytes and Anitschkow cells (macrophages) that are pathognomonic for rheumatic heart disease?	Aschoff bodies
Which valve is most commonly affected in rheumatic heart disease?	Mitral valve
What is the most commonly observed valvular deformity in rheumatic heart disease?	Fishmouth or buttonhole stenosis of the mitral valve
What are the three major categories of endocarditis?	1. Infective 2. Nonbacterial thrombotic or marantic 3. Libman-Sacks
What is the most common valve affected by bacterial endocarditis?	Mitral valve

What is the most common valve affected by bacterial endocarditis in IV drug users?	Tricuspid valve

Name the type of endocarditis described in each of the following vignettes:

25-year-old (y/o) IV drug user with rapid onset of high fever, rigors, malaise, and tricuspid regurgitation	Acute infective endocarditis
60-y/o woman with mitral valve prolapse, who has recently undergone dental extraction, presents with low-grade fever and flu-like symptoms	Subacute infective endocarditis
65-y/o man with metastatic colon cancer and new murmur consistent with mitral regurgitation	Nonbacterial thrombotic endocarditis
30-y/o woman with SLE	Libman-Sacks endocarditis
Which organism most often causes acute infective endocarditis?	*Staphylococcus aureus*
Which organism most often causes subacute infective endocarditis?	*Streptococcus viridians*
What are the clinical signs of bacterial endocarditis?	Fever Roth spots Osler nodes Murmur Janeway lesions Anemia Nail bed hemorrhages Emboli

Define the following eponyms used to describe signs of bacterial endocarditis:

Osler nodes	Tender, raised lesions on finger and toe pads
Janeway lesions	Small, erythematous lesions on palms and soles
Roth spots	Erythematous spots with white centers on retina
What are some sequelae to bacterial endocarditis?	Valvular injury, renal injury (glomerulonephritis), septic emboli to brain, kidneys causing infarction or abscess

Atherosclerosis

What are the major risk factors for coronoary heart disease?	Age (men > 45, women > 55 or with premature menopause)
	Family history of premature heart attacks (MI or sudden cardiac death in men < 55, women < 65)
	Cigarette smoking
	Hypertension (HTN)
	HDL < 40, HDL > 60 negates one risk factor
What are the two main histopathologic components of an atheroma?	Superficial fibrous cap overlying a necrotic core
What are the components of the fibrous cap?	Smooth muscle cells, macrophages, foam cells, lymphocytes, collagen, and elastin.
What is the pathologic precursor to atheroma?	Fatty streak
What is the term for ulcerated, calcified, hemorrhagic atheromas that predispose to thrombosis?	Complicated plaques
What is the underlying pathologic basis for the initiation of atherosclerosis?	Endothelial injury
What may produce this endothelial injury?	Hypercholesterolemia, mechanical injury, HTN, immune mechanisms, toxins, etc.
How are foam cells created?	Macrophages that ingest oxidized LDL that has accumulated in the vessel wall become foam cells.
Which lipids are most commonly found in an atheromatous plaque?	Cholesterol and cholesterol esters (LDL)
What is the function of smooth muscle cells in an atheroma?	Smooth muscle cells when activated by growth factors proliferate and migrate into intima. They then secrete extracellular matrix glycoproteins.
What are the major cell types associated with the formation of an atheroma?	Macrophages (foam cells), T lymphocytes (attracted to zone of injury), smooth muscle cells, and endothelial cells

What are the most common locations for atherosclerotic disease?	Abdominal aorta, coronary arteries, popliteal arteries, and carotid arteries
What are the four major clinical manifestations of atherosclerosis?	1. Arterial insufficiency (ie, stroke, MI, peripheral vascular disease, ischemic bowel disease) 2. Thrombus formation due to plaque rupture 3. Atheroembolism 4. Aneurysm, dissection, or rupture of a major vessel

Arteriolosclerosis

Name the type of arteriolosclerosis associated with the following clinical and pathologic features:

Hyaline deposits causing thickening of arteriolar walls	Hyaline arteriolosclerosis
Onion skin arteriolar thickening	Hyperplastic arteriolosclerosis
Deposition of calcium in the medial coat of arteries of the lower extremities	Monckeberg arteriosclerosis
Pipestem arteries with ringlike calcifications	Monckeberg arteriosclerosis
Two types of arteriolosclerosis that occur in patients with long-term HTN	1. Hyaline arteriolosclerosis 2. Hyperplastic arteriolosclerosis

Hypertension

HTN is the most important risk factor in which two vascular diseases?	1. Coronary artery disease 2. Cerebrovascular disease
What percentage of hypertensive patients have essential HTN?	90% to 95%
What are two common renal causes of secondary HTN?	1. Renal artery stenosis 2. Renal parenchymal disorders
What are some common endocrine causes of secondary HTN?	1. Pheochromocytoma 2. Conn syndrome (primary aldosteronism) 3. Hyperthyroidism 4. Oral contraceptive use 5. Cushing syndrome 6. Acromegaly

Name two common cardiac complications of long-standing HTN:	1. Left ventricular hypertrophy 2. Left-sided heart failure (a result of secondary to left ventricular hypertrophy)
Define hypertensive urgency and emergency.	Urgency: blood pressure > 200/120 without symptoms Emergency: blood pressure > 200/120 with symptoms or evidence of end organ damage

List the possible effects of malignant HTN on each organ system below:

Heart	Acute LV failure, MI
Aorta	Dissection
Lungs	Pulmonary edema
Kidneys	Acute renal failure
Eyes	Papilledema, fundal hemorrhages, blurred vision
Brain	Headache, encephalopathy, seizure, hemorrhagic cerebrovascular accident (CVA)
What is the most common cause of death in patients with untreated HTN	Coronary artery disease

Aneurysms and Dissection

What is the most common site for atherosclerotic aneurysm?	Abdominal aorta, below renal arteries and above iliac bifurcation
What is the most common site for syphilitic aneurysm?	Thoracic aorta (often ascending)
What is the mechanism of syphilitic aneurysms?	Obliteration of the arteries supplying the aorta (endarteritis obliterans), leading to necrosis of the media

Name the type of aneurysm referred to in the following clinical vignettes:

55-y/o man, who is a smoker with HTN, diabetes, and coronary artery disease, is found to have a pulsatile midline abdominal mass.	Atherosclerotic, abdominal aortic aneurysm

35-y/o with a family history of polycystic kidney disease presents with the worst headache of his life.	Berry Aneursym rupture leading to subarachnoid hemorrhage
40-y/o prostitute with angina and shortness of breath (SOB) is found to have wide pulse pressure and a high-pitched blowing diastolic murmur.	Syphilitic/luetic, dilation of aortic root leads to aortic regurgitation
What are the most common etiologies for the development of aortic dissection?	HTN and connective tissue disorders (such as Marfan syndrome)
Name two characteristic histopathologic findings in the aorta in a patient with Marfan syndrome:	1. Elastic tissue fragmentation 2. Cystic medial degeneration
What is the genetic defect in Marfan disease?	Defect in fibrillin-1 which forms a scaffold for elastic fibers.
What is the classic clinical presentation of aortic dissection?	Sudden onset of severe tearing pain radiating to the back and descending as the dissection progresses
What is the underlying mechanism in the development of varicose veins?	Venous dilation or deformation leading to venous valvular incompetence
State two complications of varicose veins:	1. Varicose ulceration 2. Stasis dermatitis

Vasculitides

Name the type of vasculitis associated with the following clinical and pathologic features:	
Presence of C-ANCA	Wegener granulomatosis
Presence of P-ANCA	Microscopic PolyANgiitis, PolyArteritis Nodosa (PAN), and Churg-Strauss syndrome
Most common vasculitis in the United States	Temporal or giant cell arteritis
Fibrous thickening of origins of the great vessels leading to absent pulses	Takayasu arteritis
Well-demarcated, segmental fibrinoid necrosis of the arterial wall and diffuse neutrophilic infiltrates in medium-sized arteries	PAN

Commonly affecting the coronary arteries and may result in coronary aneurysm	Kawasaki disease
Segmental inflammation/thrombosis of arteries and adjacent veins, nerves, and connective tissue; results in painful ischemic disease and associated with smoking	Buerger disease (Thromboangiitis obliterans)
Vascular and mesangial deposition of IgA complexes with abdominal pain, palpable purpura especially on buttocks, glomerulonephritis, and arthritis	Henoch-Schonlein purpura
Which vessels are most commonly involved in temporal arteritis?	External carotid artery and its branches
What is the triad of Wegener granulomatosis?	1. Focal necrotizing vasculitis of upper airways and lungs 2. Necrotizing granulomas of upper and lower respiratory tract 3. Necrotizing glomerulitis
What are the six clinical signs of acute arterial occlusion?	"Six P's": 1. Pain 2. Pallor 3. Poikilothermia 4. Paresthesia 5. Paralysis 6. Pulselessness
Name the type of vasculitis associated with each of the following clinical vignettes:	
70-y/o white man with constitutional symptoms, headache, jaw claudication, acute onset of blindness; W/U: ↑ ESR	Temporal (giant cell) arteritis
30-y/o Korean woman with constitutional symptoms, arthritis; physical examination (PE): loss of carotid and radial pulses	Takayasu arteritis
35-y/o hepatitis B positive man with fever, HTN; W/U: neutrophilia, P-ANCA ⊕	PAN

12-y/o girl recovering from a viral infection presents with exertional chest pain; PE: febrile, conjunctival injection, cervical lymphadenopathy, strawberry tongue, diffuse erythematous rash, edema of hands and feet	Kawasaki disease
40-y/o man with asthma; PE: palpable purpura, diffuse wheezes; CBC: eosinophilia; transbronchial biopsy: upper airway granulomas and elevated P-ANCA and ESR	Churg-Strauss syndrome
8-y/o boy presents with abdominal pain, hematuria, and recent history of URI; PE: palpable purpura, heme ⊕ stools; W/U: vascular biopsy shows perivascular granulocytes, IgA deposition	Henoch-Schonlein purpura
55-y/o man presents with chronic cough, rhinorrhea, ulcerations of nasal septum; W/U: RBC casts in urine and C-ANCA ⊕	Wegener granulomatosis
21-y/o woman smoker with pallor and cyanosis of fingertips after exposure to cold	Raynaud disease

Vascular Tumors

Name the vascular disorder associated with the following clinical or pathologic features:

Most common tumor of infancy	Port-wine stain birthmark
Cutaneous vascular tumor commonly seen in patients with end-stage liver disease (hyperestrinism)	Spider telangiectasia
AD condition is characterized by a localized dilation of venules and capillaries in skin and mucous membrane leading to epistaxis and GI bleeding	Hereditary hemorrhagic telangiectasia (Rendu-Osler-Weber) syndrome
AD condition is characterized by the presence of multiple cavernous hemangiomas of skin, liver, pancreas, and spleen and hemangioblastomas of cerebellum with ↑ risk of renal cell carcinoma	von Hippel-Lindau disease

Vascular tumor associated with thorium contrast material and polyvinyl chloride	Hemangiosarcoma
Vascular tumor commonly seen in men of eastern European descent and in those infected with HIV consisting of red or purple cutaneous plaques on the lower extremities	Kaposi sarcoma
Vascular tumor caused by human herpesvirus (HHV) 8 or HIV	Kaposi sarcoma
Syndrome is characterized by cyanosis and edema of upper extremities, head, and neck in a patient with bronchogenic carcinoma	Superior vena cava syndrome

PHARMACOLOGY

Antianginal Agents

What are the three classes of antianginal drugs?	1. Organic nitrates 2. β-Blockers 3. Calcium channel blockers
How do nitrates cause vasodilation?	Nitrates are metabolized to nitric oxide (NO) → NO causes ↑ in cyclic guanosine monophosphate (cGMP) in endothelial cells → vasodilation
Describe how nitrates reduce angina.	1. Vasodilation causes venous pooling, which reduces preload and consequently myocardial oxygen consumption. 2. Coronary vasodilation improves oxygen delivery to the myocardium.
What is the most common side effect of nitrates?	Headache
Describe how each of the following drugs reduces angina:	
β-Blockers	By ↓ contractility and heart rate
Nifedipine	Coronary arteriaolar vasodilation
Verapamil	Decreased heart rate and contractility, slowed conduction (especially through AV node)

What is the antianginal drug of choice for Prinzmetal angina?   Diltiazem

What antianginal drug is contraindicated in patients with asthma and COPD?   β-Blockers

Inotropic Support

Name the only oral inotropic agent: Digoxin

Describe the three-step mechanism by which digitalis potentiates myocardial contractility.
1. Inhibition of Na^+/K^+ ATPase.
2. Buildup of intracellular Na^+.
3. High intracellular Na^+ impairs Na^+-Ca^{2+} antiport, causing increased intracellular Ca^{2+}.

What is the unique side effect of digoxin on the heart?   Dysrhythmia

Which agent can be used to counteract the cardiac toxicity of digoxin? By what mechanism? K^+ supplementation. Digoxin binds near K^+ site on Na^+/K^+ ATPase. When K^+ is low, digoxin has better access and vice versa.

What are the unique neurotoxicities of digoxin?   Headache, nausea, altered color perception, blurred vision, tinnitus

For which arrhythmia is digoxin commonly used?   Atrial fibrillation

What is the β-agonist of choice for inotropic support in heart failure?   Dobutamine

Which antiarrhythmic is useful for abolishing torsades de pointes and digoxin toxicity? Mg^{2+}

By which mechanism do β-agonists and phosphodiesterase inhibitors potentiate myocardial contractility?   These agents increase cAMP which promotes increased intracellular Ca^{2+}.

Antiarrhythmics

For each class of antiarrhythmic agent, state the mechanism of action. (Note: many of these agents have multiple mechanisms of action.):

IA Na^+ channel blocker, some K^+ blockade

IB Na^+ channel blocker

IC	Na^+ channel blocker
II	β-Blocker
III	K^+ channel blocker
IV	Ca^{2+} channel blocker

For each class of antiarrhythmic agent, describe how the myocyte action potential is affected:

IA	Slows phase 0 depolarization, slows phase 3 repolarization
IB	Shortens phase 3 repolarization
IC	Slows phase 0 depolarization
II	Suppresses phase 4 depolarization
III	Prolongs phase 3 depolarization
IV	Shortens duration of action potential

For each class of antiarrhythmic agent, name several commonly used agents:

IA	Quinidine, amiodarone, procainamide, disopyramide
IB	MeLT: Mexilitine, Lidocaine, Tocainamide
IC	Flecainide, encainide, propafenone
II	Propranolol, esmolol, metoprolol, atenolol
III	Sotalol, ibutilide, bretylium, amiodarone
IV	Verapamil, diltiazem

For each subtype of class I antiarrhythmics, describe binding affinity for Na channels and the effect on APD

IA	Intermediate binding affinity to Na^+ channels, also blocks K^+ channels; prolongs AP duration
IB	Rapid rate of binding and release; shortens AP duration
IC	Tight binding and slow release; minimal change in AP duration

For each antiarrhythmic agent, name the unique toxicity/toxicities:

Quinidine — Cinchonism—headache, tinnitus, thrombocytopenia, torsades de pointes

Procainamide — Reversible drug-induced lupus

Lidocaine — CNS depression, cardiac depression, local anesthetic

Flecainide — Proarrhythmic

Propranolol — Sedation and fatigue, erectile dysfunction, exacerbation of asthma and COPD, masks effects of hypoglycemia

Bretylium — Severe postural hypotension

Amiodarone — Interstitial pulmonary fibrosis, thyroid dysfunction, hepatotoxicity, tremor, ataxia, neuropathy, bluish discoloration of skin, corneal deposits

What is the drug of choice for abolishing acute supraventricular tachycardia (SVT)? — Adenosine

Antihypertensives

For each of the following drugs, provide:

1. **The mechanism of action (MOA)**
2. **Indication(s) (IND)**
3. **Significant side effects and unique toxicity (TOX) (if any)**

β-Blockers

MOA: β-blockade ↓ cAMP

IND: intravenous agent for the short-term management of HTN

TOX: impotence, asthma, mask signs of hypoglycemia, CV effects (bradycardia, CHF, AV block), sedation

Prazosin, terazosin, doxazosin

MOA: α-blocker

IND: essential HTN, benign prostatic hypertrophy

TOX: first-dose hypotension

Phentolamine

MOA: reversible α-blocker

IND: diagnosis of pheochromocytoma

Phenoxybenzamine

MOA: irreversible α-blocker

IND: diagnosis of pheochromocytoma

Nifedipine

MOA: dihydropyridine Ca^{2+} blockers, selective for vascular smooth muscle

IND: essential HTN

TOX: bradycardia, hypotension, metabolic acidosis

Diltiazem, verapamil

MOA: nondihydropyridine Ca^{2+} blockers, verapimil is cardioselective, diltiazem has intermediate affinity for heart and vascular smooth muscle

IND: essential HTN

TOX: mild LFT abnormality, sexual dysfunction

Clonidine

MOA: centrally acting α_2-agonist that decreases sympathetic outflow

IND: mild-to-moderate HTN

TOX: dry mouth, rebound hypotension with sudden withdrawal

α-Methyldopa

MOA: converted to α-methyl norepinephrine (NE) to act centrally as an α-agonist and decrease sympathetic outflow

IND: pregnant patients with HTN

TOX: positive Coombs test, drowsiness

Hydralazine

MOA: causes arteriolar vasodilation by increasing cGMP in vascular smooth muscle

IND: essential HTN

TOX: drug-induced lupus, angina

Minoxidil

MOA: causes arteriolar vasodilation by causing K^+ channels to open on vascular smooth muscle hyperpolarizing the membrane and decreasing voltage-gated Ca^{2+} current

IND: HTN, alopecia

TOX: hypertrichosis, pericardial effusion

Nitroprusside

MOA: metabolism of nitroprusside releases NO which causes vasodilation via cGMP.

IND: malignant HTN.

TOX: cyanide toxicity (avoided if drug is mixed just prior to administration).

For each condition listed below, select the best antihypertensive agent(s):

Angina pectoris	β-Blockers, Ca^{2+} channel blockers
Diabetes	Angiotensin-converting enzyme inhibitors (ACEi), Ca^{2+} blockers, β-blockers
Hyperlipidemia	ACEi, Ca^{2+} blocker
SVT	β-Blockers
CHF	Diuretics, ACEi, β-blockers
History of MI	β-blockers, ACEi
Chronic renal failure	Diuretics, Ca^{2+} blockers
Anxiety	β-Blockers
Benign prostatic hyperplasia	α_1-Selective antagonist
Pheochromocytoma	Phenoxybenzamine, phentolamine
Hypertrophic obstructive cardiomyopathy	β-Blockers
Asthma, COPD	Diuretics, Ca^{2+} blockers
Hyperthyroidism	β-Blockers
Moderate bradycardia	β-Blockers with intrinsic sympathomimetic activity: pindolol and acebutol
Pregnancy	α-Methyldopa
Migraine headaches	β-Blockers

For each condition listed below, list the antihypertensive agent that should be avoided:

CHF	Verapamil
Asthma, COPD	β-Blockers

What class of diuretics is especially useful in black and elderly patients?	Thiazide diuretics
What class of diuretics is useful in patients who have not responded to thiazides?	Loop diuretics
What class of antihypertensives is useful in patients who cannot tolerate the side effects of ACEi?	Angiotensin receptor blockers (ARBs)

What classes of antihypertensive agents are absolutely contraindicated in pregnant patients?

ACEi and ARBs

List three agents useful in the management of malignant HTN:

1. Sodium nitroprusside
2. Hydralazine
3. Labetalol

Lipid-Lowering Agents

Cholestyramine

MOA: bile acid–binding resin, ↓ bile acid stores, ↑ catabolism of plasma LDL

IND: adjuvant therapy for patients with familial hypercholesterolemia, ↓ LDL

TOX: constipation, GI discomfort, may interfere with intestinal absorption of other drugs, LFT changes, myalgias

Statins

MOA: hydroxymethylglutaryl-CoA (HMG-CoA) reductase inhibitors, rate-limiting step of XOL synthesis

IND: hypercholesterolemia: to ↓ LDL

TOX: hepatotoxicity, rhabdomyolysis

Niacin

MOA: reduces release of fatty acids from adipose; ↓ LDL synthesis in liver

IND: hypercholesterolemia: to ↑ HDL and ↓ LDL

TOX: flushing, pruritus (both reversible with aspirin), hepatotoxicity, GI upset, paresthesias

Gemfibrozil, clofibrate

MOA: stimulate lipoprotein lipase to increase catabolism of VLDL and triglycerides (↓ VLDL, ↓ TGs)

IND: hypercholesterolemia; dramatically ↓ TGs, ↑ HDL

TOX: myositis, hepatoxicity

Autonomics

Direct cholinergic agonists

ACh

MOA: physiologic cholinergic agonist

IND: no clinical use; ACh decreases heart rate, cardiac output, and blood pressure

TOX (for all direct cholinergic agonists):
1. Diarrhea
2. Diaphoresis
3. Miosis
4. Nausea
5. Urinary urgency

Bethanechol

MOA: binds primarily at muscarinic receptors; stimulates bowel and bladder smooth muscle contraction

IND: postoperative ileus and urinary retention

Pilocarpine

MOA: direct cholinergic agonist that activates ciliary muscle of the eye and pupillary sphincter

IND: glaucoma

Indirect cholinergic agonists (anticholinesterases)

Neostigmine, physostigmine

MOA: inhibitor of acetylcholinesterase → accumulation of ACh at synapses

IND: postoperative ileus, urinary retention, myasthenia gravis, reversal of neuromuscular blockade; atropine overdose (physostigmine)

TOX: generalized convulsions (rare)

Edrophonium, pyridostigmine

MOA: inhibitor of acetylcholinesterase

IND: diagnosis (edrophonium) and treatment (pyridostigmine) of myasthenia gravis

Echothiophate

MOA: irreversible inhibitor of acetylcholinesterase

IND: treatment of organophosphate overdose, galucoma

List the toxicities of acetylcholinesterase poisoning (caused by parathion or organophosphates):

"DUMBELS"
Diarrhea
Urination
Miosis
Bronchoconstriction
Excitation of skeletal muscles
Lacrimation
Sweating and **S**alivation

Atropine

MOA: nonselective muscarinic antagonist

IND: pupillary dilation, reduction of gastric acid secretion, reduction of GI motility, reduction of airway and salivatory secretions, organophosphate/ cholinergic poisoning

TOX: "Dry as a bone, Red as a beet, Blind as a bat, Mad as a hatter, Hot as a hare."

Dry as a bone: ↓ perspiration, lacrimation, salivation

Red as a beet: dry, red skin

Blind as a bat: blurry vision

Mad as a hatter: hallucinations, delirium

Hot as a hare: hyperthermia

Describe how atropine acts on the following organs or systems:

Eyes

Pupillary dilation (bella donna alkaloid), mydriasis, cycloplegia

Airways

Blocks bronchial secretion, bronchodilation

Salivary glands

Blocks salivary secretion

Heart

Bradycardia initially; tachycardia ultimately

Scopolamine

MOA: nonselective muscarinic antagonist

IND: motion sickness

Ipratropium

MOA: nonselective muscarinic antagonist

IND: bronchodilator used for asthma or COPD

Benztropine

MOA: centrally acting antimuscarinic agent

IND: adjuvant therapy for Parkinson disease

Hexamethonium

MOA: competitive nicotinic ganglion blocker

IND: used for HTN in the past

Succinylcholine

MOA: depolarizing neuromuscular blocker (nicotinic antagonist)

IND: neuromuscular blockade during general anesthesia

TOX: malignant hyperthermia when combined with halogenated anesthetic agents in susceptible patients (treat with dantrolene)

Tubocurarine, atracurium, vecuronium

MOA: nondepolarizing neuromuscular blocker

IND: neuromuscular blockade during general anesthesia; atracurium and vecuronium are degraded in the plasma and therefore preferred in patients with renal failure

TOX: may cause histamine release resulting in bronchospasm, skin wheals, and hypotension

Pralidoxime

MOA: cholinesterase regenerator

IND: used for organophosphate poisoning

State the MOA for each of the following agents:

Hemicholinium

Inhibits reuptake of choline in cholinergic neurons (rate-limiting step in ACh synthesis)

Botulinum

Inhibits release of ACh in cholinergic neurons

Reserpine

Inhibits VMAT transporter of dopamine into storage vesicles in adrenergic neurons

Guanethidine

Inhibits release of NE from adrenergic neurons

Amphetamine

Stimulates release of NE from adrenergic neurons (indirect-acting amines)

Cocaine, tricyclic antidepressants

Inhibit reuptake of NE from synapse

Direct adrenergic agonists

Epinephrine

MOA: agonist at α_1, α_2, β_1, β_2 receptors

IND: acute, refractory asthma (bronchodilator), open angle glaucoma, anaphylactic shock, used with local anesthetic to $\uparrow$ duration of action (local vasoconstriction)

TOX: CNS disturbance, HTN, arrhythmia, pulmonary edema

**Describe the effect of epinephrine
on each of the following organs
or tissues:**

Myocardium	Positive inotropic and chronotropic effects (β_1)
Blood vessels	Overall $\uparrow$ blood pressure (vasoconstriction of cutaneous mucous membrane and visceral vasculature; vasodilation of liver and skeletal muscle vasculature) ($\alpha_1 > \beta_2$)
Lungs	Bronchodilation (β_2)
Liver	Increased glycogenolysis, increased insulin release (β_2)
Adipose tissue	Increased lipolysis (α_2, β_1, β_2, β_3)
Pupils	Mydriasis (α_1 radial dilator muscle contraction); accommodation for far vision (β_2 ciliary muscle relaxation)
Skin	Piloerection(α_1)
Norepinephrine	**MOA:** Selective adrenergic agonist. Strong α-agonist that also stimulates β_1 receptors. NE produces only minimal stimulation of β_2 receptors.
	IND: Useful in maintaining blood pressure in shock.
Compare the effects of NE and epinephrine (EPI) at the different adrenergic receptors.	α_1 EPI $\geq$ NE α_2 EPI $\geq$ NE β_1 EPI = NE β_2 EPI >> NE *creates difference
Phenylephrine	**MOA:** direct adrenergic agonist; stimulates $\alpha_1 > \alpha_2$
	IND: nasal decongestant
	TOX: causes HTN
Clonidine	**MOA:** direct adrenergic agonist; stimulates $\alpha_2 > \alpha_1$
	IND: HTN (especially in pregnant patients), nicotine, heroin, and cocaine withdrawal
	TOX: rebound HTN, dry mouth, drowsiness
Isoproterenol	**MOA:** direct adrenergic agonist; stimulates β_1 and β_2 receptors equally
	IND: Bronchodilator used in asthma

Dobutamine	**MOA:** direct adrenergic agonist; stimulates $\beta_1 > \beta_2$
	IND: positive inotropic agent used to improve cardiac output in heart failure
Albuterol, terbutaline	**MOA:** direct adrenergic agonist; stimulates $\beta_2 > \beta_1$
	IND: bronchodilator used in asthma; slows preterm labor by inhibiting uterine contraction (terbutaline)
	TOX: tremor, tachycardia
Dopamine	**MOA:** direct adrenergic agonist; stimulates D_1 and D_2 receptors equally
	IND: maintenance of blood pressure in shock
What is the toxicity of most adrenergic agonists?	1. CNS disturbance—fear, anxiety, tension, headache 2. HTN 3. Arrhythmias 4. Pulmonary edema

Indirect adrenergic agonists

Amphetamine	**MOA:** stimulates release of NE from adrenergic neurons
	IND: attention deficit hyperactivity disorder, narcolepsy, appetite control
	TOX: psychosis, anxiety
Tyramine	**MOA:** stimulates release of NE from adrenergic neurons
	IND: no clinical indications; found in fermented foods
	TOX: severe vasopressor effects in combination with MAOIs
Ephedrine	**MOA:** stimulates release of NE from synaptic vesicles in adrenergic neurons
	IND: nasal decongestant, enhances athletic performance
	TOX: causes HTN
Cocaine	**MOA:** inhibition of catecholamine reuptake
	IND: local anesthetic
	TOX: arrhythmias, MI, seizures

Adrenergic antagonists

Phenoxybenzamine

MOA: irreversible adrenergic antagonist; blocks $\alpha_1 > \alpha_2$

IND: HTN 2° to pheochromocytoma

TOX: nasal congestion, postural hypotension, compensatory tachycardia

Phentolamine

MOA: reversible adrenergic antagonist; blocks α_1 and α_2 receptors equally

IND: diagnosis of pheochromocytoma; management of intraoperative HTN

Prazosin, terazosin

MOA: adrenergic antagonist; selectively blocks α_1 receptors

IND: treatment of HTN and benign prostatic hypertrophy

TOX: orthostatic hypotension

Propranolol

MOA: adrenergic antagonist, blocks both β_1 and β_2 receptors

IND: HTN, angina prophylaxis, antiarrhythmic, anxiety, thyroid storm, migraine prophylaxis

TOX: bronchoconstriction, arrhythmias, sexual dysfunction, CNS sedation, and fatigue

Describe the effect of propranolol on each of the following tissues:

Heart	Decreased cardiac output
Blood vessels	Reflex peripheral vasoconstriction
Kidneys	Increased Na^+ retention
Lungs	Bronchoconstriction

Metoprolol, atenolol, esmolol

MOA: adrenergic antagonist; selectively blocks β_1 receptors

IND: HTN, angina prophylaxis, MI, superventricular tachycardia (esmolol)

TOX: Hypotension, bradycardia, hyperglycemia, ventricular dysrhythmias

List two β-blockers with intrinsic sympathomimetic activity:

1. Acebutolol
2. Pindolol

Which β-blocker also blocks α_1 receptors?

Labetalol

What are the six common side effects of β-blockers?

1. Bronchoconstriction/asthma attack
2. Arrhythmia
3. Sexual dysfunction
4. Fasting hypoglycemia, masking of hypoglycemic signs
5. CNS sedation, fatigue
6. Hypotension

Describe the effect of dopamine on each of the following organs or tissues:

Myocardium

Positive inotropic and chronotropic effects

Blood vessels

Vasoconstriction →↑ BP

Kidneys

Increases renal blood flow at low and moderate doses

CHAPTER 6

Pulmonary

EMBRYOLOGY

From what structure does the lung bud arise?	Foregut
From which embryonic layer is the lining of the respiratory tract derived?	Endoderm
From which embryonic layer is the muscle and connective tissue of the respiratory tract derived?	Mesoderm
What is the consequence of incomplete separation of the lung bud from the esophagus?	Tracheoesophageal fistula (TEF)
What is the most typical type of TEF?	Esophageal atresia (ends in blind pouch)
What other constellation of developmental abnormalities should you look for with TEF?	**VATER** syndrome: **V**ertebral, **A**nal, **T**racheal, **E**sophageal, **R**adial/**R**enal
At what gestational age is a human capable of respiration?	25 weeks
In what period do the majority of alveoli develop?	Postpartum
What histology is typical of cells lining the conducting airway?	Pseudocolumnar ciliated cells
Which cells produce surfactant?	Type II pneumocytes
List the structures the diaphragm is derived from:	"**S**everal **P**arts **B**uild **D**iaphragm"— **S**eptum transversum, **P**leuroperitoneal folds, **B**ody wall, **D**orsal mesentery of esophagus

| Which disorder results from abnormal development of the diaphragm? | Diaphragmatic or hiatal hernia |
| Where can pain from the diaphragm refer? | To the shoulder |

ANATOMY

Which nerve provides motor innervation to the diaphragm?	Phrenic nerve ("C3, C4, C5 keep the diaphragm alive")
Which muscles are involved in respiration?	Diaphragm (most important), external intercostals, sternocleidomastoids, anterior and medial scalene
What area of the left lung is most similar to the right middle lobe?	Lingula (technically part of the left upper lobe)
Which lobe does foreign body aspiration most commonly affect when supine?	Superior segment of right lower lobe (because right main stem bronchus is wider, more vertical, and the superior segment ostium is posteriorly located)
The bifurcation of the trachea occurs at the level of which vertebral body?	Intervertebral disk T4 to T5
What four structures make up a bronchopulmonary segment?	1. Segmental bronchus 2. Branch of the pulmonary artery 3. Branch of the bronchial artery 4. Tributaries of the pulmonary vein
Which syndrome can result from a malignant tumor in the region of the superior pulmonary sulcus?	Pancoast syndrome (lower trunk brachial plexopathy and Horner syndrome)

PHYSIOLOGY

Lung Volumes and Capacities

Name the lung volume defined below:

| Expired volume with each normal breath | Tidal volume (TV) |
| Volume that can be inspired beyond the TV | Inspiratory reserve volume (IRV) |

Volume that can be expired beyond the TV	Expiratory reserve volume (ERV)
Volume that remains in the lungs after maximal expiration	Residual volume (RV)

Name the lung capacity defined below:

TV + IRV	Inspiratory capacity (IC)
ERV + RV	Functional residual capacity (FRC)
TV + IRV + ERV	Vital capacity (VC)
Volume which can be forcibly expired in 1 second after maximal inspiration	Forced expiratory volume (FEV_1)
Total volume which can be forcibly expired	Forced VC (FVC)
TV + IRV + ERV + RV	Total lung capacity (TLC)
What is the formula for minute ventilation?	TV × respiratory rate (breaths per minute)

Lung Compliance and Resistance

What is the relationship between compliance and elasticity?	Compliance and elasticity are inversely related.
Name four common causes of decreased lung compliance:	1. Pulmonary fibrosis 2. Atelectasis 3. Acute respiratory distress syndrome 4. Neonatal respiratory distress syndrome
What is a common smoking-related cause of increased lung compliance?	Emphysema, normal aging lungs
What is the effect of surfactant on alveolar surface tension and lung compliance?	Surfactant decreases surface tension to allow small alveoli to stay open and increases compliance.
What is the law of Laplace?	Pressure = 2 × surface tension/radius. The larger the radius of the vessel/ airway, the more stable and less likely it is to collapse.
What is the relationship between airflow and resistance?	Airflow is inversely proportional to airway resistance.
What is the relationship between airway radius and resistance?	Resistance is inversely proportional to the fourth power of the radius (Poiseuille law).

For each factor below, state whether airway resistance will be increased or decreased:

Bronchoconstriction	Increased
Parasympathetic stimulation	Increased
Sympathetic stimulation	Decreased
High lung volumes	Decreased
Low lung volumes	Increased

Hemoglobin

For each of the factors below, determine whether the hemoglobin dissociation curve will be shifted to the left or to the right?

Increased P_{CO_2}	Right
Increased pH	Left
Decreased temperature	Left
Increased 2,3-bisphosphoglycerate (2,3-BPG) concentration	Right
Fetal hemoglobin	Left
Carbon monoxide poisoning	Left

Note: ↑ in any factor (except pH) results in right shift.

What is the mnemonic for right shift?

CADET face **RIGHT** (CO_2, Acid/Altitude, **D**PG (2,3-DPG), **E**xercise, **T**emperature

Which quaternary conformation of Hb has the highest affinity for oxygen?

The R (relaxed form)

How does hemoglobin's affinity for O_2 compare to that of CO?

The affinity of CO is 200 times as great as that of O_2.

What are the signs and symptoms of carbon monoxide toxicity?

Headache, nausea/vomiting, loss of consciousness, confusion

What are the three ways in which CO_2 is transported from the tissues to the lungs?

1. As HCO_3^- in erythrocytes
2. Bound to hemoglobin (carbaminohemoglobin)
3. Dissolved in blood

Which enzyme catalyzes the conversion of CO_2 into HCO_3^-?

Carbonic anhydrase

Which protein is the main buffer within erythrocytes?

Deoxyhemoglobin

Acclimatization to High Altitude

For each of the values below, determine how they are affected by high altitude *acutely*:

Ventilation

Increased

PAO_2, PaO_2

Decreased (due to decreased partial pressure of atmospheric O_2)

$PACO_2$, $PaCO_2$

Decreased (due to hyperventilation)

Systemic arterial pH

Increased

Hemoglobin saturation

Decreased

Hemoglobin concentration

No change

For each of the values below, determine how they are affected by high altitude *chronically*:

Ventilation

Increased

PAO_2, PaO_2

Decreased (due to decreased partial pressure of atmospheric O_2)

$PACO_2$, $PaCO_2$

Decreased (due to hyperventilation)

Systemic arterial pH

Increased (but closer to normal due to renal excretion of bicarbonate)

Hemoglobin saturation

Decreased

Hemoglobin concentration

Increased (polycythemia due to increased erythropoietin production)

Lung Zones

Choose the zone or region of the lungs that fits each description below:

Alveolar pressure > arterial pressure > venous pressure

Zone 1

Arterial pressure > alveolar pressure > venous pressure

Zone 2

Arterial pressure > venous pressure > alveolar pressure	Zone 3
$V/Q \approx 3 \rightarrow$ wasted ventilation	Apex
$V/Q \approx 0.6 \rightarrow$ wasted perfusion	Base

What is the effect of hypoxia on pulmonary blood vessels?

Vasoconstriction. **Note:** hypoxia causes vasodilation in all other vascular beds.

What is the quotient of V/Q in a lung where the pulmonary artery is completely occluded (shunt-unventilated blood)?

0

What is the quotient of V/Q in complete airway obstruction (physiologic dead space)?

∞

Neurologic Regulation of Respiration

Describe the function of each of the following neural structures in the control of respiration:

Medullary respiratory center	Determines the rhythm of breathing by controlling inspiration and expiration
Pontine apneustic center	Stimulates inspiration
Cerebral cortex	Voluntary control of respiration
Lung stretch receptors in bronchial smooth muscle	Reflexive slowing of respiratory frequency (Hering-Breuer reflex)
Irritant receptors in airway epithelial cells	Initiate coughing
Juxtacapillary (J) receptors in alveolar walls	Cause rapid shallow breathing in congestive heart failure
Joint and muscle receptors	Stimulate respiration at the initiation of exercise
Medullary chemoreceptors	Increase breathing rate in response to low pH
Peripheral chemoreceptors in the carotid and aortic bodies	Increase breathing rate in response to low arterial P_{O_2}, low pH, and high P_{CO_2}

PATHOLOGY

Pulmonary Edema, ARDS, and Neonatal RDS

Which syndrome is characterized by diffuse alveolar damage, pulmonary edema, and respiratory failure?

Adult respiratory distress syndrome (ARDS)

What type of material is seen in the alveoli of a patient in the acute phase of ARDS?

Hyaline membranes formed by a fibrinous exudate and necrotic cellular debris

What are some of the causes of ARDS?

Shock of any etiology, fat embolism, gram-negative sepsis, severe bacteria/viral infections, near-drowning, aspiration of GI contents, acute pancreatitis, heroin overdose, oxygen toxicity, cytotoxic drugs

What is the most common cause of respiratory failure in the newborn and also of death in premature infants < 28 weeks gestational age?

Neonatal respiratory distress syndrome (hyaline membrane disease)

What is the typical clinical presentation of neonatal respiratory distress syndrome?

Preterm infants with initially normal respirations followed by cyanosis, tachypnea, and signs of respiratory distress

What is the pathogenesis of neonatal respiratory distress syndrome?

Deficiency of pulmonary surfactant leading to increased surface tension

What type of cells produce pulmonary surfactant?

Type II pneumocytes

What is the predominant chemical in pulmonary surfactant?

Dipalmitoyl phosphatidylcholine (lecithin)

What is the diagnostic test of choice to judge fetal lung maturity?

Amniotic fluid lecithin: sphingomyelin ratio (a ratio of 2:1 implies adequate surfactant is present)

What are the three strongest risk factors for neonatal respiratory distress syndrome?

1. Prematurity
2. Maternal diabetes
3. Delivery by caesarean section

What is the classic pathologic finding in the alveoli of an infant with neonatal respiratory distress syndrome?

Intra-alveolar hyaline membranes

Infants surviving an initial bout of neonatal respiratory distress syndrome are at risk for which five complications?	1. Bronchopulmonary dysplasia (resulting in part from oxygen therapy) 2. Retinopathy of prematurity (resulting from oxygen therapy) 3. Patent ductus arteriosus 4. Intraventricular cerebral hemorrhage 5. Necrotizing enterocolitis
What medications can you give to prevent neonatal respiratory distress syndrome?	Glucocorticoids given to the mother can accelerate fetal lung maturation and reduce the risk of neonatal respiratory distress syndrome.

Pulmonary Embolism

What are the most common clinical presentations of PE?	Tachycardia, tachypnea, dyspnea, pleuritic chest pain, or hemoptysis
What is the etiology of 95% of pulmonary emboli?	Dislodged deep venous thromboses (DVT) from the deep veins of the thigh or pelvis
What factors favor the development of a DVT?	Virchow triad: (1) stasis, (2) hypercoagulability, (3) endothelial damage
How do you diagnose a PE radiographically?	V/Q scan or CT angiogram (1st line), pulmonary angiography (gold standard)
What type of tumors commonly cause a DVT by inducing a hypercoagulable state?	Adenocarcinomas
What is the most common genetic disease that predisposes to the development of DVT?	Factor V Leiden
What type of embolism can develop uniquely in a peripartum woman?	Amniotic fluid embolism
For what type of embolism is a patient with a long bone fracture at risk?	Fat emboli from bone marrow, pulmonary thromboembilsm due to trauma and stasis
What type of infarction results from a PE?	Hemorrhagic infarction (appears as wedge-shaped opacity on chest x-ray [CXR])

What therapy is indicated for high-risk patients during the workup of PE and for patients diagnosed with PE?

Full treatment doses of heparin (unfractionated or low molecular weight)

What is used for long-term prophylaxis for patients at risk of developing DVT?

Warfarin

What is an alternative to warfarin for outpatient DVT prophylaxis?

Subcutaneous heparin (low molecular weight or unfractionated)

Obstructive Lung Disease

What are the most common disease categories causing pulmonary hypertension?

1. Chronic obstructive pulmonary disease (COPD)
2. Left-sided heart disease
3. Recurrent PE
4. Autoimmune disorders

How is the heart affected by long-standing pulmonary hypertension?

Pulmonary hypertension causes right ventricular hypertrophy and dilatation.

What is the reversal of a left-to-right shunt to a right-to-left shunt due to long-standing pulmonary hypertension?

Eisenmenger syndrome

What is the most common cause of COPD?

Cigarette smoking

What is the effect of COPD on hematocrit (Hct)?

Chronic hypoxia leads $\rightarrow \uparrow$ Hct

What is the effect of COPD on FEV_1/FVC?

$\downarrow FEV_1/FVC < 0.8$

Name the obstructive pulmonary disorder described by the following pathologic features:

Smooth muscle and goblet cell hyperplasia; mucus-plugged airways containing Curschmann spirals, eosinophils, and Charcot-Leyden crystals

Bronchial asthma

Hyperplasia of bronchial submucosal glands, hypersecretion of mucus, squamous metaplasia or dysplasia of bronchial epithelium

Chronic bronchitis

Permanent airway dilation and scarring; inflammation and necrosis of bronchial walls and alveolar fibrosis

Bronchiectasis

Alveolar enlargement due to alveolar wall destruction; ↓ lung elasticity

Pulmonary emphysema

Diagnosed clinically by productive cough for > 3 consecutive months for 2+ years

Chronic bronchitis

Name the chronic disorder characterized by increased airway reactivity, resulting in paroxysmal bronchial contraction:

Bronchial asthma

Name the two types of bronchial asthma:

1. Atopic or immune asthma
2. Nonatopic or nonimmune asthma

What type of hypersensitivity response is seen in atopic asthma?

Type I hypersensitivity response mediated by IgE and mast cells, eosinophils, and basophils

What other conditions are typically seen in association with atopic asthma?

Allergic rhinitis, eczema

Name several common triggers of atopic asthma:

Dust, pollen, food, and animal dander

Name several triggers of nonatopic asthma:

Respiratory tract infection, cold, chemical irritants, exercise

What are the two common presenting features of bronchial asthma?

1. Dyspnea
2. Wheezing

Which four conditions are commonly associated with bronchiectasis?

1. Bronchial obstruction from tumor or foreign body
2. Cystic fibrosis (CF)
3. Kartagener syndrome
4. Necrotizing pneumonia

What are the three common presenting features of bronchiectasis?

1. Abundant, copious, often foul-smelling sputum
2. Chronic cough
3. Hemoptysis

What are the components of an acinus of the lungs?

Alveoli, air ducts, respiratory bronchioles, terminal bronchioles

Name the type of emphysema described below:

Enlargement of bronchioles, typically in the upper lobes and apices (most often associated with smoking)

Centriacinar emphysema

Destruction and dilation of entire acinus, typically in the lower lobes; associated with α_1-antitrypsin deficiency

Panacinar emphysema

Destruction of the distal acinus occurring typically near the pleura and areas of fibrosis that may cause pneumothorax

Paraseptal emphysema

Irregular involvement of the acinus that may be related to inflammatory processes of the lungs

Irregular emphysema

How does smoking cause emphysema?

Smoke particles recruit inflammatory cells, promote the release and enhance the activity of elastase, and inhibit the activity of α_1-antitrypsin.

What is the role of α_1-antitrypsin deficiency in the development of emphysema?

The lack of this protease inhibitor results in the digestion of the elastin in alveolar walls by elastase.

What is the effect of emphysema on the anteroposterior diameter of the chest and the TLC?

Both are increased.

Restrictive Lung Disease

What general category of pulmonary disease is characterized by dyspnea, decreased lung volumes, and decreased compliance?

Restrictive lung disease

What is the effect of restrictive lung disease on FEV_1/FVC?

$\downarrow FEV_1/FVC \geq 0.8$

What are the two categories of restrictive lung disease?

1. *Pulmonary*: interstitial lung disease or pneumonitis, resulting in poor lung expansion
2. *Extrapulmonary*: extrapulmonary disease associated with disorders of the chest wall, pleura, or respiratory muscles

What are the common causes of pulmonary restrictive lung disease?	Idiopathic, connective tissue disease, drug-related, sarcoidosis (all → *poor lung expansion*)
What are the common causes of extrapulmonary restrictive lung disease?	Neuromuscular disease (polio), obesity, pleural disease, and scoliosis (all → *poor breathing mechanics*)

Name the specific type of restrictive lung disease described below:

65-year-old (y/o) hay farmer with recent exposure to moldy hay presents with chronic dry cough, chest tightness; physical examination (PE): bilateral diffuse rales; bronchoscopy: interstitial inflammation; bronchioalveolar lavage: lymphocyte and mast cell predominance	Hypersensitivity pneumonitis
35-y/o man presents with intermittent hemoptysis and hematuria; W/U demonstrates alveolar hemorrhage and acute glomerulonephritis	Goodpasture syndrome
40-y/o with progressive hypoxemia and cor pulmonale; lung biopsy demonstrates chronic inflammation of the alveolar wall in a pattern consistent with honeycomb lung; bronchioalveolar lavage: mild eosinophilia	Idiopathic pulmonary fibrosis
58-y/o former shipbuilder presents with the insidious onset of dyspnea; transbronchial biopsy demonstrates interstitial pulmonary fibrosis, ferruginous bodies; chest CT scan demonstrates pleural effusion and dense pleural fibrocalcific plaques	Asbestosis
55-y/o miner (nonsmoker) presents with dyspnea and dry cough; pulmonary function tests (PFTs) show both obstructive and restrictive pattern; chest x-ray (CXR): hilar lymphadenopathy with eggshell calcifications	Silicosis

60-y/o male with 100 pack-year history of (h/o) smoking presents with pleuritic chest pain, hemoptysis, and dyspnea; PE: dullness to percussion and absent breath sounds in the right lower lung field

Pleural effusion (secondary to malignancy)

50-y/o former heavy smoker presents with multiple lung and rib lesions; biopsy: cells (similar to the Langerhans cells of the skin) containing tennis racket–shaped Birbeck granules

Eosinophilic granuloma

30-y/o black female presents with DOE, fever, arthralgia; PE: iritis, erythema nodosum; W/U: eosinophilia, ↑ serum ACE levels; PFT: restrictive pattern; CXR: bilateral hilar lymphadenopathy interstitial infiltrates; lymph node biopsy: noncaseating granulomas

Sarcoidosis

Which typically asymptomatic disorder causes visible black deposits in the lungs of coal workers?

Anthracosis

Which three medications are known to commonly cause interstitial lung disease?

Bleomycin, methotrexate, and amiodarone

Pulmonary Infections

What infection is characterized by fever > 39°C, chills, cough productive of blood-tinged, purulent sputum, pleuritic pain, hypoxia, and lobar infiltrate on CXR?

Acute pneumonia

What infection is characterized by fever < 39°C, nonproductive cough, GI upset, and diffuse patchy infiltrates on CXR?

Atypical pneumonia

Name the most common organism(s) associated with the pulmonary infection described below:

Community-acquired acute pneumonia

Streptococcus pneumoniae

Commonly follow a viral respiratory infection	*Staphylococcus aureus* and *Haemophilus influenzae*
Interstitial pneumonia	*Mycoplasma pneumoniae* (most common), *Chlamydia pneumoniae*
Fungal pneumonia in an AIDS patient	*Pneumocystis jiroveci* (previously *Pneumocystis carinii*)
Typical pneumonia in neonate	*Streptococcus agalactiae* (group B streptococcus)
Typical pneumonia in an alcoholic after aspiration	*Klebsiella pneumoniae*
Atypical pneumonia in patient with positive cold agglutinin test	*Mycoplasma pneumoniae*
Atypical pneumonia in a neonate with trachoma	*Chlamydia trachomatis*
Atypical pneumonia in a dairy worker	*Coxiella burnetti*
Atypical pneumonia in a rabbit hunter	*Francisella tularensis*
Pneumonia in a bird owner with splenomegaly and bradycardia	*Chlamydia psittaci*
Hospitalized patient with lobar pneumonia	*Streptococcus pneumoniae* > *S. aureus*
Pneumonia in an IV drug user	*Streptococcus pneumoniae*, *K. pneumoniae*, and *S. aureus*
Pneumonia in a patient recovering from viral upper respiratory infection	*Staphylococcus aureus*, *H. influenzae*
Atypical pneumonia in a spelunker from the Ohio river valley	*Histoplasma capsulatum*
Atypical pneumonia in a patient from the southwestern United States	*Coccidioides immitis*
Associated with spread by inhalation of contaminated water droplets from air conditioners	*Legionella pneumophila*

Name the most common causative pathogen(s) of pneumonia for each age group below:

Neonates	Group B streptococci, *Escherichia coli*, *Listeria*
Children (6 weeks-18 years)	RSV and other viruses, *M. pneumoniae*, *C. pneumoniae*, *S. pneumoniae*

Adults (18-40 years old)	*Mycoplasma pneumoniae, C. pneumoniae, S. pneumoniae*
Adults (45-65 years old)	*Streptococcus pneumoniae, H. influenzae,* anaerobes, viruses, *M. pneumoniae*
Adults (> 65 years old)	*Streptococcus pneumoniae,* viruses, anaerobes, *H. influenzae,* gram-negative rods

Name four common complications of lobar pneumonia:	1. Abscess formation (especially *S. aureus* and anaerobes) 2. Empyema or spread of infection to the pleural cavity 3. Organization of exudate to form scar tissue 4. Sepsis
What type of pulmonary infection is characterized by localized suppurative necrosis of lung tissue?	Lung abscess
Name several bacterial pathogens capable of causing lung abscess:	*Staphylococcus aureus,* aerobic and anaerobic streptococci, gram-negative bacilli, and anaerobic oral flora

Cystic Fibrosis

What is the most common lethal genetic disease in Caucasians?	CF
What is the mode of inheritance of CF?	Autosomal recessive (chromosome 7)
Which membrane protein is defective in CF?	The cystic fibrosis transmembrane conductance regulator (CFTR), a chloride channel protein
What is the function of CFTR?	Regulation of sodium, chloride, and bicarbonate transport across the plasma membrane
What is the most common genetic lesion causing CF?	Deletion of three nucleotides encoding phenylalanine 508 in the CFTR; ΔF508 prevents the normal expression of CFTR
Describe how the ΔF508 mutation prevents normal expression of CFTR:	Altered membrane folding precludes glycosylation and transport to the plasma membrane.
What is the end result of the ΔF508 mutation of the *CFTR* gene?	Complete loss of CFTR in the plasma membrane

How does a defect in the CFTR affect exocrine glands?

Altered CFTR activity causes the accumulation of hyperviscid mucus that blocks the secretions of exocrine glands.

What tests are used to diagnose CF in infants?

Sweat chloride test, measurement of nasal potential difference, genotyping (definitive)

How does CF typically present in an infant?

Failure to thrive, meconium ileus, mother complains child "tastes salty"

Describe the effect of CF on each of the following organs:

Lungs

Recurrent pulmonary infections, bronchiesctasis; $\uparrow$ RV and TLC in chronic disease; $\downarrow$ FEV_1/FVC in acute exacerbation; pulmonary hemorrhage may occur

Pancreas

Variable defects in pancreatic exocrine function; may cause pancreatic insufficiency and diabetes mellitus

Intestines

Mucus plugs $\rightarrow$ small bowel obstruction; meconium ileus in some infants

Liver

Plugging of bile cannaliculi $\rightarrow$ cirrhosis

Epididymis and ductus deferens

Bilateral absence of the vas deferens

Salivary glands

Ductal dilation; squamous metaplasia of ductal epithelium and glandular atrophy

Which organisms are commonly responsible for pulmonary infections in CF?

Pseudomonas aeruginosa, S. aureus, and *Pseudomonas cepacia*

What is a common nutritional deficiency in CF?

Deficiency of the fat-soluble vitamins (vitamins A, D, E, and K)

What type of heart disease is common in patients with CF?

Cor pulmonale

Lung Cancer

What is the most common cause of cancer deaths in the United States for both men and women?

Lung cancer

What is the most common type of malignant tumor in the lungs?

Metastasis

What are the most common primary lung tumors?	Adenocarcinoma is slightly more common than squamous cell carcinoma
Name the type(s) of primary lung cancer associated with the following features:	
Central location	Squamous cell and small (oat) cell carcinomas
Peripheral location	Adenocarcinoma, large cell carcinoma, bronchioalveolar carcinoma
Dysplasia and carcinoma in situ precede development of this tumor	Squamous cell carcinoma
Strongest link to smoking	Squamous cell and small (oat) cell carcinomas
Least linked to smoking, frequently seen in nonsmoking women	Bronchioalveolar carcinoma
Most aggressive tumor	Small (oat) cell carcinoma
Associated with production of PTH-related peptide, hypercalcemia	Squamous cell carcinoma
Associated with production of ADH (SIADH) and ACTH (Cushing syndrome)	Small (oat) cell carcinoma
Carcinoembryonic antigen (CEA) positive	Adenocarcinoma
Secretion of 5-hydroxytryptamine (5-HT, serotonin)	Carcinoid
Oat-like, dark blue cells	Small (oat) cell carcinoma
Tumor cells lining alveolar walls	Bronchioalveolar adenocarcinoma
Giant pleomorphic cells, poor prognosis, and high likelihood of cerebral metastasis	Large cell carcinoma
Tumor at apex of lung causes Horner syndrome or lower brachial plexopathy	Pancoast tumor
Rare pleural tumor is found in patients with a h/o exposure to asbestos	Malignant mesothelioma
Most common cancer in patients with h/o exposure to asbestos	Lung cancer

OTHER PATHOLOGY

Immotile cilia secondary to a dynein
arm defect, associated with situs
inversus, infertility, bronchiectasis

Kartagener syndrome

Causes stridor, toxic presentation,
may be life threatening, thumbprint
sign on x-ray, caused by *H. influenzae*

Acute epiglotittis

Causes stridor, nontoxic presentation,
steeple sign on x-ray, caused by
parainfluenza virus

Laryngotracheobronchitis, croup

PHARMACOLOGY

For each of the following drugs, provide:

1. The mechanism of action (MOA)
2. Indication(s) (IND)
3. Significant side effects
   and unique toxicity (TOX) (if any)

Albuterol

MOA: β_2-agonist → bronchodilator,
short acting

IND: asthma

TOX: tachycardia, arrhythmias, tremor,
hyperglycemia

Inhaled corticosteroids
(beclomethasone, fluticasone,
triamcinolone)

MOA: anti-inflammatory; inhibits
smooth muscle hyperreactivity

IND: moderate-to-severe asthma

TOX: oropharyngeal thrush, dysphonia

Cromolyn

MOA: anti-inflammatory; inhibits
histamine release from mast cells

IND: prophylaxis for asthmatic attack

TOX: laryngeal edema (very rare)

Ipratropium

MOA: bronchodilator; cholinergic
antagonist

IND: COPD.

TOX: Rare—minor systemic manifestations
of anticholinergic effect

Leukotriene inhibitors (zileuton,
zafirlukast, montelukast)

MOA: inhibits leukotriene synthesis
(zileuton) or blocks leukotriene
receptors (zafirlukast, montelukast)

IND: prophylaxis for asthmatic attack

TOX: elevation of liver enzymes

Theophylline

MOA: bronchodilator; exact mechanism unknown

IND: asthma

TOX: seizures and arrhythmias

What is the drug of choice for mild asthma?

Inhaled albuterol as needed

Which three classes of bronchodilators are useful in the management of asthma and COPD?

1. Anticholinergic agents (eg, ipratropium)
2. β-Agonists (eg, albuterol)
3. Theophylline (much less useful)

What is the drug of choice in an asthmatic requiring daily albuterol use?

Inhaled glucocorticoids

Describe how glucocorticoids act on airways to control asthma:

Glucocorticoids reduce inflammation and decrease the reactivity of airways to irritants such as cold, cigarette smoke, allergens, and exercise.

What type of therapy may be required in patients with daily asthma attacks?

Systemic steroid therapy; usually with oral prednisone or IV methylprednisolone

Name three agents used in the treatment of allergic rhinitis:

1. Antihistamines (eg, diphenhydramine, loratadine, terfenadine)
2. α-Agonist aerosols (eg, phenylephrine)
3. Corticosteroid nasal sprays (eg, beclomethasone, fluticasone, triamcinolone)

Which class of bronchodilators is useful in patients who cannot tolerate β-agonists?

Anticholinergic agents (eg, ipratropium)

CHAPTER 7

Gastroenterology

EMBRYOLOGY

What portion of the GI tract is derived from the embryonic foregut?

From the intra-abdominal esophagus → pancreas (distal to sphincter of Oddi)

What portion of the GI tract is derived from the embryonic midgut?

From the second part of the duodenum → proximal two-thirds of the colon (at the splenic flexure)

What portion of the GI tract is derived from the embryonic hindgut?

From the distal one-third of the colon → rectum (proximal to the pectinate line)

What GI structures are derived from the embryonic ectoderm?

Oropharynx (anterior two-thirds of tongue, lips, parotids, tooth enamel), anus, and rectum (distal to the pectinate line)

Name the embryonic layer supplied by the following arteries:

Celiac trunk — Foregut

Inferior mesenteric artery — Hindgut

Superior mesenteric artery — Midgut

What embryonic structure gives rise to the anterior two-thirds of the tongue?

First branchial arch

What embryonic structure gives rise to the posterior one-third of the tongue?

Third and fourth branchial arches

What disorder results from failure of fusion of the maxillary and medial nasal processes?

Cleft lip

What disorder results from failure of fusion of the nasal septum, lateral palatine processes, and/or median palatine process?

Cleft palate

What is Meckel diverticulum?	Persistence of the vitelline duct or yolk stalk that may contain ectopic tissue. **Remember: "The rule of 2's": 2** in long, **2**% of population, **2** ft from ileocecal valve, presents within **2** years of life, can contain **2** types of epithelia (gastric, pancreatic).
What primordial embryonic structures give rise to the pancreas?	Ventral bud → pancreatic head, uncinate process, main duct
	Dorsal bud → everything else (body, tail, isthmus, accessory duct)
What congenital defect is caused by abnormal fusion of the ventral and dorsal buds of the pancreas?	Annular pancreas (leads to ring around duodenum and obstruction)
What congenital defect results from failure of migration of neural crest cells, causing an absence of parasympathetic ganglion cells in the distal colon?	Hirschsprung (congenital aganglionic) megacolon
What congenital defect results from incomplete canalization of the bile ducts during development and presents shortly after birth with clay-colored stools and jaundice?	Biliary atresia

ANATOMY

What are the four main layers of the wall of the digestive tract?	1. Mucosa
	2. Submucosa
	3. Muscularis
	4. Serosa
Name the enteric plexus associated with the following descriptions:	
Located between mucosa and inner layer of smooth muscle in GI tract wall	Submucosal (Meissner) plexus
Located between inner (circular) and outer (longitudinal) layer of smooth muscle in GI tract wall	Myenteric (Auerbach) plexus
Coordinates motility along the entire gut wall	Myenteric plexus = Motility
Controls local secretions, absorption, and blood flow	Submucosal plexus = Secretions

Name the lymphoid tissue found in lamina propria and submucosa of small intestine:	Peyer patches
What is the major function of the Peyer patch?	Detect antigens → secrete IgA into lumen
In the liver, which zone of the portal acinus contains the highest O_2 concentration and nutrients?	Zone 1
Which zone of the portal acinus contains the lowest O_2 concentration and nutrients?	Zone 3
Name the three major branches of the abdominal aorta and their approximate vertebral level:	1. Celiac trunk (T12) 2. Superior mesenteric artery (L1) 3. Inferior mesenteric artery (L3)
What structure provides collateral venous drainage to the superior vena cava (SVC) when there is obstruction of the inferior vena cava (IVC)?	Azygous vein
Name the four key sites for portal-systemic shunt and the veins involved:	1. Esophagus (left gastric → esophageal) 2. Umbilicus (paraumbilical → superficial/inferior epigastric) 3. Rectum (superior rectal → middle/inferior rectal) 4. Posterior abdominal wall (colic → lumbar)
Which two vessels merge to form the portal vein?	Splenic (inferior mesenteric vein has already joined the splenic vein) and superior mesenteric veins
What important neural structure traverses the parotid gland?	Facial nerve (CN VII)
Which syndromes may result from reinnervation of the CN VII after Bell palsy or surgical severance of nerve?	Frey syndrome (sweating occurs along with salivation), crocodile tears syndrome (tearing occurs along with salivation)
What are the muscles of mastication?	Three open: masseter, temporalis, and medial pterygoid; one close: lateral pterygoid
What types of muscle are found in the esophagus?	Proximal one-third = skeletal; distal one-third = smooth; middle one-third = both

What is the function of the pylorus?	Acts as muscular sphincter to regulate movement of food out of the stomach and prevents reflux of duodenal contents
Which blood vessel lies posterior to the first part of the duodenum?	Gastroduodenal artery (a concern in cases of posterior perforation due to ulcers)
The common bile duct and main pancreatic duct empty into what portion of the duodenum?	Second (descending) part
The common bile duct and pancreatic duct drain into the duodenum through what structure?	Hepatopancreatic ampulla (of Vater)
What structure controls the release of bile into the duodenum?	Sphincter of Oddi
Which two ducts combine to form the common bile duct?	1. Common hepatic 2. Cystic duct
What structures make up the porta hepatis?	Hepatic artery, portal vein, common bile duct
What structure keeps the cystic duct open at all times for bile to flow freely in both directions?	Spiral valve (of Heister)
What is the "bare area" of the liver?	A portion of the diaphragmatic surface of the liver that is devoid of peritoneum
What divides the left and right lobes of the liver?	Interlobar fissure (an invisible line running from the gallbladder to the IVC)
What structure supports the duodenum at the duodenojejunal flexure?	Suspensory ligament (of Treitz)
Name the intestinal structures (duodenum, ileum, jejunum, or colon) associated with each of the following characteristics:	
Long, finger-shaped villi	Jejunum
Intestinal glands (crypts) and < 3 cm luminal diameter	Ileum
No villi, large crypts, and 6 to 9 cm luminal diameter	Colon
Large, numerous, plicae circularis	Jejunum

Accounts for the terminal three-fifths of the small intestine	Ileum
Contains fatty tags (appendices epiploicae)	Colon
Contains prominent Peyer patches	Ileum
Contains long vasa recta	Jejunum

What term is used to describe the three longitudinal bands of smooth muscle in the colon?

Teniae coli

What is the name for the wall sacculations in the colon that are separated by the plicae semilunaries?

Haustra

What anatomic feature divides the upper and lower anal canal?

Pectinate line

What muscle holds the rectum in a 90° flexure?

Puborectalis muscle

Describe the arterial supply, venous drainage, and innervation of internal hemorrhoids:

Vasculature = superior rectal artery/vein (drains to portal circulation); visceral innervation → not painful

Describe the arterial supply, venous drainage, and innervation of external hemorrhoids:

Vasculature = inferior rectal artery/vein (drains to systemic circulation via IVC); somatic innervation → painful

What type of muscle is found in the internal anal sphincter?

Smooth muscle (under involuntary control via autonomic innervation)

What type of muscle is found in the external anal sphincter?

Striated muscle (under voluntary control via the pudendal nerve)

What are the boundaries of Hesselbach triangle?

Inferior epigastric artery, inguinal ligament, lateral border of rectus abdominus muscle

Name the types of hernia:

Peritoneum protrudes through Hesselbach triangle, medial to the inferior epigastric artery

Direct hernia

Retroperitoneal structures to enter the thorax because of defective development of pleuroperitonial membrane

Diaphragmatic hernia

Peritoneum protrudes through both the internal (deep) and external (superficial) inguinal rings	Indirect hernia
Stomach herniates upward through the esophageal hiatus of the diaphragm	Hiatal hernia
Occurs in infants as a result of failure of processus vaginalis to close	Indirect hernia
Protrudes below the inguinal ligaments and lateral to the pubic tubercle; more common in females	Femoral hernia

PHYSIOLOGY

Saliva

Which three glands produce saliva?	1. Parotid 2. Submandibular 3. Sublingual
Name three important functions of saliva:	1. Protection of dental health by buffering oral bacterial acids 2. Digestion (starches by α-amylase); triglycerides (TGs) by lingual lipase 3. Lubrication of food with mucins
What determines the relative composition of salivary contents?	Flow rate
How is the regulation of saliva production unique?	It is stimulated by *both* parasympathetic and sympathetic activity.

GI Hormones and Secretions

Name the source of the following
GI secretory products:

Intrinsic factor (IF)	Parietal cells (stomach)
Pepsinogen	Chief cells (stomach)
Histamine	Mast cells (stomach)
Gastric acid (H⁺)	Parietal cells (stomach)
Gastrin	Antral G cells and duodenum
Bicarbonate	Surface mucosal cells (of stomach and duodenum)

Secretin	S cells (duodenum)
Somatostatin	D cells (duodenum)
Cholecystokinin (CCK)	I cells (duodenum) and jejunum
Gastric inhibitory peptide (GIP)	Duodenum and jejunum

For each of the following substances, state the factors that regulate its secretion:

Gastric acid (H⁺)	↑ By histamine, acetylcholine (ACh), gastrin; ↓ by prostaglandin, somatostatin, GIP
Pepsinogen	↑ By vagal stimulation (ACh) and low pH
Gastrin	↑ By small peptides and amino acids (AAs) (Phe and Trp = most potent), gastric distention, and vagus (via gastrin-releasing peptide[GRP]); ↓ by pH < 3.0 and secretin
Bicarbonate in pancreatic secretions	↑ By secretin (potentiated by CCK and vagal input)
Secretin	Acid (H⁺ and fatty acids [FAs]) in the duodenum
Somatostatin	↑ By acid; ↓ by vagus
CCK	↑ By FAs, AAs, and small peptides
GIP	↑ By FAs, AAs, and oral glucose

List the most important functions of the following GI secretions:

IF	Binds vitamin B₁₂ for uptake in terminal ileum
Gastric acid (H⁺)	Converts pepsinogen to pepsin and sterilizes chyme. **Note:** inadequate acid production →↑ risk of *Salmonella* infections
Pepsinogen	Digests protein
Gastrin	↑ Secretion of IF, HCl, and pepsinogen; stimulates gastric motility and growth of gastric mucosa
Bicarbonate	Neutralizes acid → prevents autodigestion
Secretin	↑ Pancreatic HCO₃⁻ secretion; ↓ gastric acid secretion

Somatostatin	$\downarrow H^+$ and pepsinogen secretion, $\downarrow$ pancreatic and SI secretions, $\downarrow$ gallbladder contraction, $\downarrow$ release of both insulin and glucagon
CCK	$\uparrow$ Gallbladder contraction, $\uparrow$ pancreatic enzyme secretion, $\downarrow$ gastric emptying
GIP	$\uparrow$ Insulin (especially in response to oral glucose); $\downarrow H^+$ secretion
Which enzyme in the parietal cell catalyzes the production of H^+ and HCO_3^- from CO_2 and H_2O?	Carbonic anhydrase
How is H^+ secreted into the lumen of the stomach?	H^+/K^+ ATPase pumps H^+ out of cells and Cl^- diffuses concurrently to maintain electrical neutrality forming HCl.
Which chemical potentiates the actions of ACh and gastrin in stimulating H^+ secretion?	Histamine. (This is why H^+ receptor blockers are so effective in treating ulcers.)
Which prototypical drug blocks the effects of histamine at the level of the parietal cell?	Cimetidine (an H receptor blocker)
Why does not atropine block vagally mediated gastrin secretion?	Vagal stimulation of acid production is independent of ACh. (It is mediated by GRP.)
Which GI hormone is released by the small intestine in response to fats, proteins, and carbohydrates?	GIP

GI Motility

What are the two main divisions of the enteric nervous system?	1. Extrinsic (parasympathetic and sympathetic nervous systems) 2. Intrinsic (enteric nervous systems)
Parasympathetic innervation of the GI tract occurs via which nerves and has what general effect?	Vagus and pelvic $\rightarrow$ usually stimulatory
Sympathetic innervation of the GI tract occurs via which nerves and has what general effect?	Fibers originate in spinal cord and synapse in the celiac and superior mesenteric ganglia $\rightarrow$ usually inhibitory.
What term is used to describe the vasovagal reflex that accomodates for food entering the stomach?	Receptive relaxation

What reflex mediates colonic motility in response to food in the stomach?	Gastrocolic reflex

What are the two components of the gastrocolic reflex?	1. Fast: mediated by the autonomic nervous system 2. Slow: mediated by CCK and gastrin

What two centers of the brain are integral to vomiting?	1. Chemoreceptor trigger zone (floor of the fourth ventricle) 2. The vomiting center of the medulla

What pacemaker cells in the GI tract regulate the basal rate of gut contraction?	Interstitial cells of Cajal (ICC)

What are the frequencies of ICC's pacemaker activities?	Stomach—3/min, duodenum—12/min, ileum—10/min, colon—3/min

Miscellaneous GI Physiology

What part of the pancreas is responsible for synthesizing and releasing zymogens?	Secretory acinar cells

Which two chemicals stimulate the release of zymogens?	1. ACh 2. CCK

Which hormone acts on the pancreatic ductal cells to increase mucus and HCO_3^- secretion?	Secretin

Name the pancreatic enzymes responsible for the following actions:

Starch digestion	α-Amylase (secreted in active form)
Protein digestion	Proteases (eg, trypsin, chymotrypsin, elastase, carboxypeptidases—secreted as proenzymes)
Fat digestion	Lipase, phospholipase A, colipase

Which enzyme catalyzes the conversion of trypsinogen into trypsin?	Enterokinase (a brush-border enzyme)

Why is the conversion of trypsin an important part of protein digestion?	Trypsin converts proenzymes to their active forms (including trypsinogen to form a positive-feedback loop)

What is the rate-limiting step in carbohydrate digestion?	Production of monosaccharides by oligosaccharide hydrolases (at brush border)

What are the five major components of bile?	1. Water (97%) 2. Bile salts 3. Phospholipids 4. Cholesterol 5. Bilirubin (BR)
What property of bile salts allows them to solubilize lipids into micelles for absorption?	They are amphipathic (contain *both* hydrophilic and hydrophobic regions).
Where is bile produced and stored?	It is produced continuously by hepatocytes and stored in gallbladder.
What is the role of intestinal bacteria in the synthesis of bile acids?	They convert primary (1°) bile acids to secondary (2°) bile acids.
Which membrane protein is essential for bile acids recirculation?	Na^+-bile cotransporter in terminal ileum
Why does ileal resection result in steatorrhea?	Lack of bile acid recirculation $\rightarrow$ depletion of the bile acid pool $\rightarrow$ impaired fat absorption
What types of carbohydrates can be absorbed?	Monosaccharides only (eg, glucose, galactose, fructose)
By what mechanism are carbohydrates absorbed?	Glucose/galactose: Na^+-dependent cotransport; fructose: facilitated diffusion
How are fats absorbed?	Lipase breaks triglycerides into glycerol and FAs. Short- and medium-chain FAs undergo passive diffusion; long-chain FAs form micelles with bile salts for passive diffusion.
What metabolites of protein can be absorbed by the GI tract and what type of transport molecules are involved in their absorption?	AAs, dipeptides, and tripeptides; Na^+-dependent cotransporters

PATHOLOGY

Nonneoplastic Disorders of the Upper GI Tract

Name the nonneoplastic disorder of the upper GI tract with the following pathologic and clinical features:

Common vesicular circumoral lesion with eosinophilic intranuclear inclusions	Herpes labialis (usually herpes simplex virus [HSV]-1)

Connective tissue disorder characterized by xerostomia, keratoconjunctivitis sicca, and autoantibodies to SS-A (Ro) and SS-B (La)	Sjögren syndrome
Esophageal dysmotility caused by inability of the lower esophageal sphincter to relax (due to loss of ganglion cells in the myenteric plexus)	Achalasia
Type of hiatal hernia in which the stomach and the cardioesophageal junction slide in and out of the thorax	Sliding (axial) hernia
Pharyngeal outpouching involving >1 layer of the esophageal wall; results in food accumulation and chronic halitosis	Zenker (pharyngoesophageal) diverticulum
Retching-induced laceration of gastroesophageal (GE) junction resulting in hematemesis and mediastinitis; ↑ incidence in alcoholics	Mallory-Weiss tear
Complete rupture of the esophagus (all layers), often due to severe retching	Boerhaave syndrome
May result from Chagas disease causing the loss of myenteric plexus in the esophagus	2° achalasia
Hyperplasia of gastric surface mucosal cells	Ménétrier disease
Postvagotomy, unimpeded passage of hypertonic food to SI → distention and diarrhea	Dumping syndrome

Neoplastic Disorders of the Upper GI Tract

Name the neoplastic disorder of the upper GI tract described by each of the following statements:

Most common salivary gland tumor; contains a mix of epithelial and mesenchymal elements	Pleomorphic adenoma (mixed tumor)

Irregular white mucosal patches in the mouth of an AIDS patient as a result of Epstein-Barr virus (EBV)	Oral hairy leukoplakia
Accounts for 95% of oral cancers	Squamous cell carcinoma
Benign salivary tumor containing cystic spaces lined by double-layered eosinophilic epithelium (oncocytes) embedded in dense lymphoid tissue	Warthin tumor (papillary cystadenoma lymphomatosum)
Most common esophageal carcinoma; usually in proximal two-thirds; associated with alcohol and tobacco use	Squamous cell carcinoma
Intestinal metaplasia of squamous epithelium in distal esophagus in response to prolonged injury (often due to GERD)	Barrett esophagus
Mucin-producing glandular tumor of the distal one-third of the esophagus	Adenocarcinoma
Infiltrating carcinoma, causing extensive thickening of stomach wall; "leather-bottle stomach"	Linitis plastica (signet ring carcinoma)
Gastric carcinoma that has metastasized to the ovary	Krukenberg tumor

Name six important risk factors for gastric carcinoma:

These ↑ your **"CHANSE"** for gastric cancer:

1. **C**hronic gastritis
2. *Helicobacter pylori* infection
3. **A** blood type
4. **N**itrosamines
5. **S**ex (men > 50 years old)
6. **E**ating habits (low-fiber diet)

Name six important risk factors for esophageal carcinoma:

"ABCDEF"

1. **A**chalasia
2. **B**arrett esophagus
3. **C**orrosive esophagitis
4. **D**iverticuli
5. **E**sophageal webs
6. **F**amilial

What is the name for metastatic spread of gastric cancer to the supraclavicular node?

Virchow node

Pediatric GI Disorders

Name the GI disorder commonly
diagnosed in the pediatric population
with the following findings:

    Difficulty with feeding starting from   Tracheoesophageal fistula
birth, excessive oral secretions,
inability to pass NG tube, no gas
in abdomen, early pneumonia

    Nonbilious projectile vomiting,   Pyloric stenosis
abdominal "olive" in epigastric
region

    Bilious vomiting, "double bubble,"   Duodenal atresia
associated with Trisomy 21

    Commonly occurs at ileocecal   Intussuseption
junction, most common cause of
small bowel obstruction in toddlers

    Failure to pass meconium in the first   Meconium ileus
48 hours of birth, abdominal
distention, associated with CF

Gastritis

Name the type of gastritis associated
with the following findings:

    Autoimmune disorder with   Type A (fundal) chronic gastritis
autoantibodies to parietal cells   (**Remember:** the 5 A's for type A)
and IF, achlorhydria, pernicious
anemia, and aging

    "Coffee-ground emesis" from   Acute (erosive) gastritis
mucosal inflammation

    Helicobacter pylori infection   Type B (antral) chronic gastritis (**B = bug**)

    Left shoulder pain   Perforation of ulcer → irritation of left
diaphragm

Peptic Ulcer Disease

Name the type of peptic ulcer (gastric
or duodenal) disease associated with
each of the following findings:

    Pain is greater with meals   Gastric ulcer (pain is **G**reater with
meals) → weight loss

    Pain decreases with meals   Duodenal ulcer (pain **D**ecreases with
meals) → weight gain

Almost 100% associated with *H. pylori* infection	Duodenal ulcer
Due to ↓ mucosal protection against gastric acid	Gastric ulcer
Associated with nonsteroidal anti-inflammatory drug (NSAID) use	Gastric ulcer
Hypertrophy of Brunner glands	Duodenal ulcer
Blood type O	Duodenal ulcer
Elevated gastrin levels	Duodenal ulcer
Due to ↑ gastric acid secretion and/or ↓ mucosal protection	Duodenal ulcer

Name four common complications of peptic ulcer disease:

1. Bleeding
2. Penetration
3. Perforation
4. Obstruction

Name a classic complication of posterior duodenal ulcers:

Massive hemorrhage from erosion of the gastroduodenal artery

Malabsorption

Name the malabsorption syndrome associated with each of the following pathologic and clinical findings:

Gluten sensitivity	Celiac disease (nontropical sprue)
Brush-border enzyme deficiency resulting in bacterial digestion of unabsorbed disaccharide, causing osmotic diarrhea	Disaccharidase deficiency (#1 = lactase deficiency)
Steatorrhea, weight loss, hyperpigmentation, polyarthritis, fever, and lymphadenopathy in an older, white male; infectious etiology	Whipple disease (caused by *Tropheryma whippelii*)
Increased risk of T-cell lymphoma, GI, and breast malignancy	Celiac disease
Autosomal recessive (AR) defect in chylomicron assembly resulting in an absence of chylomicrons, very low-density lipoproteins (VLDLs), or low-density lipoprotein (LDL) in blood	Abetalipoproteinemia

Flat, proximal intestinal mucosa with marked villous atrophy; lymphocytes and plasma cells in lamina propria	Celiac disease
Distinctive periodic acid–Schiff (PAS)-positive macrophages in intestinal mucosa	Whipple disease
Associated with HLA-DQ2 and HLA-DQ8	Celiac disease
Gram-positive actinomycetes	Whipple disease
Acanthocytes (*burr* cells) in blood	Abetalipoproteinemia

Diverticular Disease

What is the most common cause of painless bleeding from the lower GI tract?	Diverticulosis
What is the prevalence of diverticulosis in the US population older than age 60?	~50%
What part of the colon is most frequently affected by diverticulosis?	Sigmoid colon
Name the disorder characterized by diverticular inflammation causing left lower quadrant (LLQ) pain, anorexia, nausea, and vomiting:	Diverticulitis
Name four complications of diverticulitis:	1. Perforation 2. Peritonitis 3. Abscess 4. Obstruction
What part of the GI tract is most commonly affected by ischemic bowel disease?	"Watershed" areas (splenic flexure, rectosigmoid junction)
Define intussusception.	Telescoping of the intestines resulting in intestinal obstruction
Define volvulus.	Complete twisting of the bowel around its mesenteric base
Where does volvulus most commonly occur?	Sigmoid colon (more common in elderly)
Name the inflammatory bowel disease which is often characterized by overgrowth of exotoxin-producing bacteria:	Pseudomembranous colitis

Which organism is responsible for pseudomembranous colitis?	*Clostridium difficile*
What disorder is characterized by nausea, vomiting, anorexia, leukocytosis, and pain at McBurney point?	Appendicitis

Inflammatory Bowel Disease

Ulcerative colitis or Crohn's disease?

Pancolitis with crypt abscesses	Ulcerative colitis (UC)
Fistulas and fissures	Crohn's disease
Associated with ankylosing spondylitis	Both
Associated with sclerosing cholangitis	UC
Amyloidosis	Crohn's disease
Can lead to toxic megacolon	UC
Longitudinal ulcers	Crohn's disease
Punched-out aphthous ulcers	Crohn's disease
Increased risk of colorectal carcinoma	UC >>> Crohn's disease
Skip lesions	Crohn's disease
Can involve any portion of the GI tract (usually terminal ileum and colon)	Crohn's disease
"String sign" on x-ray (due to bowel wall thickening)	Crohn's disease
Associated with pyoderma gangreosum	Both
Transmural inflammation	Crohn's disease
Noncaseating granulomas	Crohn's disease
Cobblestone mucosa	Crohn's disease

Neoplastic Disorders of the Lower GI Tract

What is the most common histologic type of GI lymphomas?	95% are B cell (**MALT**omas).
What is the most common tumor of the appendix?	Carcinoid tumor
What type of cells give rise to carcinoid tumors?	Neuroendocrine cells

What substances are secreted from carcinoid tumors?

Serotonin, histamine, and prostaglandins

Which carcinoid tumors tend to be more aggressive?

Ileal, gastric, and colonic

Metastases to which organ result in carcinoid syndrome?

Liver

Name five clinical findings of carcinoid syndrome:

1. Vasomotor dysfunction
2. GI hypermotility
3. Bronchoconstriction
4. Hepatomegaly
5. Right-sided heart valve stenosis

What laboratory test is used in the diagnosis of carcinoid syndrome?

5-Hydroxyindoleacetic acid (5-HIAA) in urine

Name the types of neoplastic polyp:

Usually benign and pedunculated; most common

Tubular adenoma (75%)

Highly malignant; sessile tumor > 4 cm with fingerlike projections

Villous adenoma

Shares features of both other types of polyps

Tubulovillous adenoma

Name five major risk factors for colon cancer:

1. Presence of colonic villous adenomas
2. Inflammatory bowel disease
3. Low-fiber, high animal fat diet
4. Age (> 60)
5. Positive family/personal history

How does colorectal carcinoma classically present?

Left side lesions → blood in stool; right side lesions → anemia (from occult blood loss)

Where is the most common site for colorectal cancer?

Sigmoid colon

Name the autosomal dominant (AD) polyposis syndrome associated with each of the following findings:

Colonic polyps, osteomas, and soft tissue tumors; associated with abnormal dentition

Gardner syndrome

Hundreds of colonic polyps; malignant potential ~100%

Familial adenomatous polyposis (FAP)

Colonic polyps and CNS tumors; malignant potential ~100%

Turcot syndrome

Defect in DNA repair → many colonic lesions (especially proximal); malignant potential ~50%	Hereditary nonpolyposis colorectal carcinoma (HNPCC)
Benign, hamartomas of GI tract; melanotic pigmentation of hand, mouth, and genitalia; no malignant potential (but ↑ risk of other tumors)	Peutz-Jeghers syndrome

What are the three tumor syndromes in which the APC gene is mutated?

1. FAP
2. Gardner syndrome
3. Turcot syndrome

Pancreatitis and Pancreatic Cancer

Name nine causes of acute pancreatitis:

"GET SMASHeD"

1. **G**allstones (major cause)
2. **E**thanol (major cause)
3. **T**rauma
4. **S**teroids
5. **M**umps
6. **A**utoimmune disorder
7. **S**corpion sting
8. **H**yperlipidemia
9. **D**rugs (especially ddI)

Other causes: ischemia, infections, pancreatic cancer, and peptic ulcer disease

Name seven possible sequelae of acute pancreatitis:

1. Progression to chronic pancreatitis
2. Abscess
3. Pseudocyst
4. Hypocalcemia
5. Focal fibrosis and diffuse fat necrosis
6. Acute respiratory distress syndrome (ARDS)
7. Disseminated intravascular coagulation (DIC)

Name four common laboratory abnormalities in acute pancreatitis:

1. ↑ Serum amylase (within 24 hours)
2. ↑ Serum lipase (72-96 hours)
3. Hypocalcemia
4. Glycosuria

Name five causes of chronic pancreatitis:

"ABCCD"

1. **A**lcoholism (#1 in adults)
2. **B**iliary tract disease
3. **C**ystic fibrosis (#1 in kids)
4. **C**a^{2+} (hypercalcemia)
5. **D**ivisum (pancreas divisum)

Most pancreatic tumors are found in what region of the pancreas? — Two-thirds of pancreatic tumors are found in the pancreatic head.

What is a common clinical presentation of a mass in the pancreatic head? — Painless jaundice causing malabsorption and Courvoisier (enlarged, palpable) gallbladder

What is Trousseau syndrome? — Migratory thrombophlebitis associated with visceral cancer, commonly pancreatic adenocarcinoma

What are the two most commonly mutated genes causing pancreatic adenocarcinoma? —
1. *K-ras* (> 90% mutated)
2. *p53* (60%-80% mutated)

What is the prognosis for pancreatic adenocarcinoma? — Averages 6 months or less (very aggressive)

Disorders of Bilirubin Metabolism

What type of hyperbilirubinemia results from cholestasis? — Conjugated

Name the hereditary hyperbilirubinemia described in each of the following statements:

Mildly ↓ UDP-glucuronyl transferase; asymptomatic; associated with stress in 6% of people — Gilbert syndrome

AR defect causing ↓ canalicular excretion of BR conjugates → grossly black liver; asymptomatic — Dubin-Johnson syndrome

AR absence UDP-glucuronyl transferase → ↑ unconjugated BR → jaundice, kernicterus, early death — Crigler-Najjar syndrome, type I

AR defect causing asymptomatic, conjugated bilirubinemia — Rotor syndrome

Liver Disorders

What three pathologic characteristics define cirrhosis? —
1. Fibrosis
2. Nodular regeneration of hepatocytes
3. Disruption of parenchymal architecture

Name four common causes of micronodular cirrhosis:

1. Chronic alcoholism (think of a **micro**brewery)
2. Hereditary hemochromatosis
3. 1° biliary cirrhosis
4. Wilson disease (hepatolenticular degeneration

Name four common causes of macronodular cirrhosis:

1. Hepatitis B virus (HBV)
2. Hepatitis C virus (HCV)
3. α_1-Antitrypsin deficiency
4. Wilson disease

List the effects of hepatic failure on the following body systems:

Eye

Scleral icterus

Neurologic

Coma, hepatic encephalopathy (asterixis, hyperreflexia, behavioral changes)

Systemic

Peripheral edema, malnutrition

Skin

Jaundice, palmar erythema, spider angiomata, caput medusae

Reproductive

Testicular atrophy, gynecomastia, loss of pubic hair

Hematopoietic

Anemia, bleeding tendency ($\downarrow$ coagulation factors), splenomegaly

Renal

Hepatorenal syndrome (ARF 2° to hypoperfusion)

GI

Fetor hepaticus, ascites, esophageal varices, hemorrhoids

Name the liver disorder associated with each of the following findings:

Mallory bodies

Alcoholic hepatitis

Occlusion of IVC or hepatic veins with centrilobular congestion → congestive liver disease; associated with polycythemia, pregnancy, and hepatocellular carcinoma

Budd-Chiari syndrome

Obliteration of hepatic vein radicals following bone marrow transplant

Veno-occlusive disease

Copper deposition in liver, kidneys, brain, and cornea → asterixis, basal ganglia degeneration, dementia

Wilson disease (hepatolenticular degeneration)

AST:ALT ratio > 1.5	Alcoholic hepatitis
Lymphoid aggregates and interface hepatitis	Chronic hepatitis
May be incidental finding in young woman taking oral contraceptives	Hepatic adenoma
Sinusoidal hepatic dilations from use of anabolic steroids	Peliosis hepatis
Hemolysis, elevated LFTs, and low platelets in a pregnant woman	**HELLP** syndrome (hepatic disease of pregnancy)
Elevated α-fetoprotein (AFP)	Hepatocellular carcinoma

Name the etiology of cirrhosis associated with each of the following findings:

Panacinar emphysema	α_1-Antitrypsin deficiency
Decreased ceruloplasmin	Wilson disease (hepatolenticular degeneration)
Triad of bronze diabetes, skin pigmentation, and micronodular pigment cirrhosis	Hemochromatosis
Antimitochondrial antibodies	Primary biliary cirrhosis
Nutmeg liver	Congestive heart failure
Kayser-Fleischer rings	Wilson disease (hepatolenticular degeneration)
Micronodular fatty liver; portal hypertension, asterixis, jaundice, and gynecomastia	Chronic alcohol abuse
↑ Ferritin, transferrin, and total iron; ↓ total iron-binding capacity (TIBC)	Hereditary hemochromatosis. **Note:** total body iron is sometimes high enough to trigger metal detectors.

Name the major risk factors for hepatocellular carcinoma:	**"WATCH for ABC"**
	Wilson disease
	α_1-**A**nti**T**rypsin
	Carcinogens (eg, aflatoxin B_1, polyvinyl chloride)
	Hemochromatosis
	Alcoholic cirrhosis
	Hepatitis **B**
	Hepatitis **C**

Hepatocellular carcinoma tends to spread through which route?	Hematogenous
What is the most common type of malignancy in the liver?	Metastasis
Which primary tumors tend to metastasize to the liver?	Colon > Stomach > Pancreas > Breast > Lung (**Remember:** "Cancer Sometimes Penetrates Benign Liver!")

Name the hepatobiliary disorder associated with the following:

Strawberry gallbladder	Cholesterolosis
Associated with *Opisthorchis sinenis* (liver fluke) infection in Asia	Cholangiocarcinoma
Tumor arising at the junction of the left and right hepatic ducts	Klatskin tumor
Inflammation of the bile duct; commonly due to *Escherichia coli* infection	Ascending cholangitis

Disorders of the Gallbladder

What is Courvoisier law?	An enlarged, palpable gallbladder with jaundice is likely the result of an underlying malignancy (often in head of the pancreas) and not from a stone in the common duct (because gallbladder is typically too scarred from infection).
What is Charcot triad?	Spiking fevers with chills, jaundice, and right upper quadrant (RUQ) pain (biliary colic); strongly suggests cholangitis
What are the risk factors for cholelithiasis?	4 F's: Fertile, Fat, Forty-year-old Female
What is the most common type of gallstone?	Mixed stone (components of pigment and cholesterol stones)
Name six complications of cholelithiasis:	1. Biliary colic and common bile duct obstruction 2. Cholecystitis (acute or chronic) 3. Ascending cholangitis 4. Acute pancreatitis 5. Gallstone ileus 6. Malignancy (adenocarcinoma)

Viral Hepatitis

Name the hepatitis virus (viruses) associated with the following features:

Fecal-oral transmission	Hepatitis A virus (HAV)
Water-borne transmission	Hepatitis E virus (HEV)
Infection may lead to a carrier state	HBV, HCV, and hepatitis D virus (HDV, delta agent)
Defective virus requiring HBsAg as its envelope	HDV (delta agent)
Sexual, parenteral, and transplacental transmission	HBV, HCV, HDV
DNA hepadnavirus	HBV
High mortality rate in pregnant women	HEV
Associated with IV drug use	HCV
Long incubation (~3 months)	HBV
Increased risk of hepatocellular carcinoma	HBV, HCV
Immune globulin vaccine available	HAV, HBV (and HDV)
Short incubation (~2 weeks)	HAV

Name the hepatitis serologic marker described below:

Antigen found on surface of HBV; continued presence suggests carrier state	HBsAg
Antigen associated with core of HBV	HBcAg
Antigen in the HBV core that indicates transmissibility	HBeAg
Antibody suggesting low HBV transmissibility	HBeAb
Acts as a marker for HBV infection during the "window" period (acute phase)	IgM-HBcAb
Provides immunity to HBV	HBsAb

What is the "window" period of a hepatitis infection?	Period during acute infection when HBsAg has become undetectable, but HBsAb has not yet appeared

Infectious Diarrhea

Name six infectious causes of bloody diarrhea:	1. *Salmonella* 2. *Shigella* 3. *Campylobacter jejuni* 4. Enteroinvasive and enterohemorrhagic *E. coli* 5. *Yersinia enterocolitica* 6. *Entamoeba histolytica*

Name the diarrhea-causing organism associated with the following statements:

Most common cause of diarrhea in infants	Rotavirus
Ten to twelve loose, bloody, and mucous diarrhea stools per day due to ingestion of cysts	*Entamoeba histolytica*
Comma-shaped organisms causing rice-water stools	*Vibrio cholera*
Second to rotavirus as a cause of gastroenteritis in kids	Caliciviruses (Norwalk-like and Sapporo-like)
Bloody diarrhea; very low ID_{50} (small numbers of organisms can cause disease); nonmotile	*Shigella*
Usually transmitted from pet feces	*Yersinia enterocolitica*
Motile; lactose nonfermenter; causes bloody diarrhea	*Salmonella*
Comma- or s-shaped organisms causing bloody diarrhea; grows at 42°C	*Campylobacter jejuni*
Watery diarrhea with extensive fluid loss in AIDS patient	*Cryptosporidium*
Foul-smelling diarrhea after returning from a camping trip	*Giardia lamblia*
Watery diarrhea caused by antibiotic-induced suppression of colonic flora	*Clostridium difficile*

Name the organism responsible for food poisoning from the following items:

Reheated rice	*Bacillus cereus*
Reheated meat dishes	*Clostridium perfringens*
Improperly canned food	*Clostridium botulinum*

Contaminated seafood or raw oysters	*Vibrio parahaemolyticus* and *Vibrio vulnificus*
Meats, mayonnaise, custards	*Staphylococcus aureus.* **Note:** starts and ends quickly
Undercooked beef products	*Escherichia coli* O157:H7
Raw poultry, milk, eggs, and meat	*Salmonella*

PHARMACOLOGY

For each of the following drugs, provide:
1. The mechanism of action (MOA)
2. Indication(s) (IND)
3. Significant side effects and unique toxicity (TOX) (if any)

Omeprazole, pantoprazole, lansoprazole	**MOA:** Irreversibly inhibits H^+/K^+-ATPase in parietal cells (proton pump inhibitor) **IND:** Peptic ulcer disease, Zollinger-Ellison syndrome, erosive esophagitis **TOX:** Liver toxicity, pancreatitis, agranulocytosis (rare)
Cimetidine, ranitidine, famotidine, nizatidine	**MOA:** H_2 receptor antagonist in parietal cell **IND:** GE reflux disease **TOX:** Endocrine effects (gynecomastia—primarily caused by cimetidine, galactorrhea, ↓ sperm count), potent inhibitor of P-450, ↓ renal creatinine clearance
Misoprostol	**MOA:** PGE_1 analog →↑ secretion of gastric mucus and bicarbonate **IND:** Prophylaxis for NSAID-induced peptic ulcer disease (PUD); maintenance of a patent ductus arteriosus (PDA) **TOX:** Abortifacient
Aluminum sucrose sulfate (sucralfate)	**MOA:** Polymerizes in stomach → binds to injured tissue, forming a protective coating over ulcers (**Note:** requires an acidic environment) **IND:** Peptic ulcer disease **TOX:** Osteodystrophy, osteomalacia (mainly in pts with renal failure)

Ondansetron, granisetron	**MOA:** 5-HT$_3$ receptor antagonist
	IND: Postoperative nausea/vomiting, chemotherapy-induced emesis
	TOX: Headache, diarrhea
Meclizine	**MOA:** H$_1$ receptor antagonist
	IND: Motion sickness
	TOX: Teratogenic
Loperamide, diphenoxylate	**MOA:** Antimotility agents (meperidine analogs)
	IND: Diarrhea
	TOX: Toxic megacolon in kids (loperamide)
Metoclopramide	**MOA:** Stimulates ACh release →↑ upper GI motility
	IND: Nausea, ileus
	TOX: Sedation, diarrhea, and extrapyramidal symptoms (EPS) (especially in kids)
Lactulose	**MOA:** Osmotic laxative
	IND: Hyperammonemia, colonic lavage precolonoscopy
	TOX: Dehydration with overuse

What is "triple therapy" for peptic ulcer disease?	Proton pump inhibitor (PPi), bismuth salicylate, and two of the following antibiotics: metronidazole, amoxicillin, clarithromycin, or tetracycline
What is the most important approach to healing peptic ulcers?	Eradicating *H. pylori*
How long does proton pump inhibition last?	48 hours
Name two uses for bismuth subsalicylate:	1. *Helicobacter pylori* infection 2. Traveler diarrhea
What two weak bases that are used as antacids have minimal systemic absorption?	1. MgOH$_2$ 2. AlOH$_3$ (combined to make milk of magnesia)
For each of the following antacids list the toxicity/toxicities:	
Antacids	Hypokalemia, alter absorption of other drugs

Sodium bicarbonate	Systemic alkalinization
Aluminum hydroxide	Constipation
Magnesium hydroxide	Diarrhea

Name the therapy of choice for each of the following disorders:

Hereditary hemochromatosis	Repeated phlebotomy and deferoxamine
Wilson disease	Chelation therapy (with penicillamine)
Acute cholecystitis from gallstones	Cholecystectomy

CHAPTER 8

Reproduction and Endocrinology

EMBRYOLOGY

During embryogenesis, when is male/female phenotypic differentiation complete?	By week 20
Which gene determines phenotypic differentiation?	*Sry* gene (encodes for a protein called testis-determining factor [TDF])
Which cells secrete Müllerian-inhibiting factor (MIF) during fetal development?	Sertoli cells
What factors are required to direct the indifferent embryo into a male phenotype?	TDF, MIF, testosterone, and dihydrotestosterone (DHT)
In what structure, within the testes, does spermatogenesis occur?	Seminiferous tubules
What molecule is the primary (1°) source of energy for sperm?	Fructose
Give the number of chromosomes and amount of DNA found in each of the following cell types:	
Spermatogonia	46,2N
1° spermatocyte/oocyte	46,4N
Secondary (2°) spermatocyte/oocyte	23,2N
Spermatid/ovum	23,1N

What stage is each cell type halted in and when is the stage finally completed?

1° oocyte	Prophase I, just prior to ovulation
2° oocyte	Metaphase II, at fertilization

Name the structure of the mature sperm associated with each of the following statements:

Derived from the Golgi apparatus	Acrosomal cap
Contains mitochondria	Middle piece (neck)
Derived from one of the centrioles	Flagellum (tail)

Name the congenital disorder that results from each of the following aberrations:

Complete lack of fusion of paramesonephric ducts	Double uterus with double vagina
Partial fusion of the paramesonephric ducts	Bicornate uterus
Testes fail to descend into the scrotum	Cryptorchidism (bilateral → sterility)
Patency of processus vaginalis	If small → hydrocele; if large → congenital inguinal hernia
Failure of urethral folds to close	Hypospadias (penile urethra opens on inferior/ventral side)
Faulty positioning of genital tubercle	Epispadias (penile urethra opens on superior/dorsal side)

Name the embryonic structure that gives rise to each of the following tissues:

Thyroid gland	Thyroid diverticulum
Thymus, inferior parathyroids	Third branchial pouch
Superior parathyroids and the parafollicular "C" cells	Fourth branchial pouch (fourth is *superior* to third)
Chromaffin cells of adrenal medulla	Neural crest cells
Adrenal cortex	Mesoderm

What is the most common site for ectopic thyroid tissue and why?   The tongue; during development, the thyroid migrates caudally from the level of the developing tongue.

Which syndrome is caused by a failure of the development of the third and fourth pharyngeal pouches?

DiGeorge syndrome

Describe the clinical features of DiGeorge syndrome:

"CATCH 22"

Cardiac abnormalities (eg, tetralogy of Fallot, interrupted aortic arch)

Abnormal facies

Thymic aplasia/hypoplasia and **T**-cell deficiency

Cleft palate

Hypocalcemia → tetany Chromosome 22q11

ANATOMY

Name the five types of endocrine cells found in the pars distalis of the anterior pituitary:

1. Somatotrophs (~50%)
2. Mammotrophs
3. Thyrotrophs
4. Corticotrophs
5. Gonadotrophs

Where is antidiuretic hormone (ADH) primarily produced?

Supraoptic nucleus of hypothalamus

Where is oxytocin primarily produced?

Paraventricular nucleus of hypothalamus

What part of the pituitary stores and releases ADH and oxytocin?

Neurohypophysis (posterior pituitary)

Where is the hypophyseal portal system located?

Adenohypophysis (in the pars tuberalis)

What is the 1° arterial supply to the gonads?

Testicular/ovarian arteries (directly from abdominal aorta branches)

What is the 1° venous drainage of the gonads?

Left testicular/ovarian vein → left renal vein; right testicular/ovarian vein → inferior vena cava (IVC)

Which lymph nodes filter lymph from the gonads?

Deep lumbar/para-aortic nodes

Which lymph nodes filter lymph from the scrotum?

Superficial inguinal nodes

What are the two pathways for venous drainage from the prostate gland?

1. Prostatic venous plexus → internal iliac veins → IVC
2. Prostatic venous plexus → vertebral venous plexus → cranial dural sinuses

Describe the type of innervation for each phase of the male sexual response cycle:

Erection

Parasympathetic nerves (**Point**)

Emission

Sympathetic nerves (**Shoot**)

Ejaculation

Visceral autonomic and somatic nerves

Name the structure(s) contained in the following uterine ligaments:

Transverse cervical (cardinal) ligament

Uterine vessels

Suspensory ligament of ovaries

Ovarian vessels, lymphatics, autonomic nerves

Broad ligament

Round ligaments of the uterus, ovarian ligament, ureters, uterine tubes, and uterine vessels

What is the anatomic relationship of the ureter and the uterine artery?

Ureter lies posterior and inferior to uterine artery. **"Water (ureter) under the bridge (uterine artery)"**

What is the normal position of the uterus?

Anteverted (uterus to cervix) and anteflexed (cervix to vagina)

What is the landmark for a pudendal nerve block?

Ischial spine

Name the part of the fallopian tube described below:

Opens into the peritoneal cavity

Infundibulum

Site of fertilization

Ampulla

Opens into the uterine cavity

Intramural

Majority of the length of the tube

Isthmus

Describe the venous drainage of the adrenal glands.

Right adrenal vein → IVC; left adrenal vein → left renal vein

What type of nerves synapse in the adrenal medulla?

Preganglionic sympathetic (through splanchnic nerves)

| In the adrenal medulla, onto what cells do the preganglionic sympathetic nerves synapse? | Chromaffin cells → secrete catecholamines |

PHYSIOLOGY

Second Messengers

Name the second messenger mechanism used by each of the following hormones:

Hypothalamic hormones—gonadotropin-releasing hormone (GnRH), thyrotropin-releasing hormone (TRH), growth hormone–releasing hormone (GHRH), oxytocin, ADH (V_1 receptor)	Inositol triphosphate (IP_3)
Hypothalamic hormones—corticotropin-releasing hormone and ADH (V_2 receptor)	cAMP
Anterior pituitary hormones—luteinizing hormone (LH), follicle-stimulating hormone (FSH), adrenocorticotropic hormone (ACTH), thyroid-stimulating hormone (TSH)	Cyclic adenosine monophosphate (cAMP)
Growth hormone (GH)	Tyrosine kinase activation
Insulin	Tyrosine kinase activation
Melanocyte-stimulating hormone (MSH)	cAMP
Angiotensin II	IP_3
Calcitonin	cAMP
Glucagon	cAMP
Parathyroid hormone (PTH)	cAMP
Insulin-like growth factor (IGF)-1	Tyrosine kinase activation
Atrial natriuretic peptide (ANP)	Cyclic guanosine monophosphate (cGMP)
Nitric oxide	cGMP

Steroid Hormones

How do steroid hormones circulate in the body?

They are bound to specific globulin carrier proteins (which ↑ solubility and delivery to target organs).

How are the cellular effects of steroids mediated?

Steroids pass through the cell membrane, bind cytoplasmic receptors, and translocate to the nucleus where they influence gene expression.

Adrenal Glands

Name the three layers of the adrenal cortex and their major secretory products:

GFR (from outside to inside), "the deeper you go, the sweeter it gets: salt, sugar, sex"

1. Zona **G**lomerulosa—mineralocorticoids
2. Zona **F**asciculata—glucocorticoids
3. Zona **R**eticularis—andogrens

How does the secretion of glucocorticoids vary throughout the day?

Highest before waking and lowest at midnight

By what mechanism does ACTH increase steroid hormone synthesis?

Stimulates cholesterol desmolase

What is the effect of glucocorticoids on ACTH and cortisol secretion?

Potent glucocorticoids inhibit ACTH and cortisol secretion (a negative feedback mechanism).

What test is used to evaluate the response of the hypothalamic-pituitary axis to glucocorticoids?

Dexamethasone suppression test

Name four general actions of cortisol:

1. Stimulates gluconeogenesis (↑ protein catabolism and lipolysis)
2. Anti-inflammatory effects (block arachidonic acid pathway)
3. Acute exposure enhances immune response; chronic exposure suppresses immune response (inhibits interleukin [IL]-2 production)
4. Maintains vascular responsiveness to catecholamines

Name three specific actions of aldosterone:

1. ↑ Renal Na^+ reabsorption
2. ↑ Renal K^+ secretion
3. ↑ Renal H^+ secretion

Sex Hormones

What is the function of LH in male reproduction?	LH acts on Leydig cells → stimulates cholesterol desmolase → testosterone
What is the function of FSH in male reproduction?	FSH acts on Sertoli cells → spermatogenesis and secretion of inhibin (inhibits FSH)
How does testosterone regulate LH secretion?	Acts to ↓ release of GnRH from hypothalamus and to ↓ release of LH from adenohypophysis
Which enzyme is required to convert testosterone to its active form, DHT?	5-α-Reductase
Which enzyme catalyzes conversion of testosterone to estrogen?	Aromatase
Name three androgens (in order of decreasing potency) and where they are produced:	1. DHT (prostate, peripheral tissues) 2. Testosterone (testes, adrenals) 3. Androstenedione (adrenals)
Name five important functions of testosterone:	1. Sexual differentiation during development 2. 2° Sexual development, growth spurt, and fusion of epiphyseal plates 3. ↑ Libido 4. Anabolic effects 5. Spermatogenesis maintenance
What is the average age of menarche?	Between 11 and 14 years (in the United States)
How does GnRH release change during puberty?	Pulsatile release of GnRH begins and it upregulates its own receptors in the adenohypophysis.
What is the function of LH in female reproduction?	LH acts on theca cells → stimulates cholesterol desmolase → testosterone
What is the function of FSH in female reproduction?	FSH acts on granulosa cells → stimulates aromatase → estrogen
What happens to LH:FSH ratio during puberty?	LH >> FSH
Where is estrogen made?	Blood (via aromatase), ovaries (estradiol), placenta (estriol), and testes

What is the relative potency of the major estrogens?	Estradiol > estrone > estriol
Which estrogen is an indicator of fetal well-being?	Estriol ($\uparrow$ 1000× in pregnancy)
Where is progesterone produced?	Corpus luteum, adrenal cortex, placenta, and testes

Decide whether each of the following are characteristics of estrogen, progesterone, or both:

Development of genitalia	Estrogen
Growth of follicle	Estrogen
Proliferation of endometrium	Estrogen
Maintains endometrium	Progesterone
Maintains pregnancy	Both
Produces thick cervical mucus	Progesterone
Hepatic synthesis of transport proteins	Estrogen
$\downarrow$ Myometrial excitability	Progesterone
Development of breasts	Both
$\uparrow$ Body temperature	Progesterone
Spiral artery development	Progesterone
LH surge	Estrogen
Typical female fat distribution	Estrogen
Uterine smooth muscle relaxation (prevents contractions)	Progesterone
Decrease → endometrial sloughing	Progesterone
Pubertal development	Estrogen

What are the two main phases of the menstrual cycle and when do they occur?	1. Follicular phase (days 1-14) 2. Luteal phase (days 14-28)

Classify the following as characteristics of the follicular or luteal phase:

Graafian follicle matures	Follicular phase
Corpus luteum develops causing the release of estrogen and progesterone	Luteal phase (early)

Basal body temperature increases	Luteal phase
Oocyte progresses from meiosis I to meiosis II	Follicular phase
Endometrial glands grow → spiral arteries	Luteal phase
FSH and LH levels suppressed	Follicular phase
Endometrial proliferation	Follicular phase
Progesterone peaks	Luteal phase
Menses	Follicular phase (early)
When does ovulation occur?	14 days before menses (regardless of cycle length)
What changes in cervical mucus occur during ovulation?	Cervical mucus is thinnest and most penetrable during ovulation.
What endocrine change induces ovulation?	Estradiol burst at end of follicular phase causes a positive feedback effect, resulting in a surge of LH.
Which hormone prevents lactation during pregnancy?	High estrogen and progesterone block the effects of prolactin on the breast.
Where is hCG made and what is its function?	Syncytiotrophoblast of placenta produces hCG to maintain corpus luteum so it can produce progesterone during the first trimester until placenta can produce progesterone during the second and third trimester.
Name three scenarios in which hCG is elevated:	1. Pregnancy (in urine 10 days after fertilization) 2. Hydatidiform moles 3. Choriocarcinoma
hCG peaks at what gestational age?	Gestational week 9
What happens to estrogen and progesterone just prior to delivery?	Both increase throughout; near term estrogen:progesterone ratio increases.
What is the average age of menopause?	51 (tends to occur earlier in smokers)
Name four hormonal changes characteristic of menopause:	1. ↓ Estrogen 2. ↑↑ FSH 3. ↑ LH 4. ↑ GnRH

Name four clinical findings characteristic of menopause:	Menopause wreaks **"HAVOC"** on your body 1. **H**ot flashes 2. **A**trophy of **V**agina 3. **O**steoporosis 4. **C**oronary artery disease risk increases

Anterior Pituitary

Name the hormones produced by the anterior pituitary:	**"FLAT PiG"** plus melanotropin (MSH) FSH LH ACTH TSH Prolactin GH
Name four compounds derived from proopiomelanocortin (POMC):	1. ACTH 2. MSH 3. β-Lipotropin 4. β-Endorphin
Which hormones share a common α-subunit?	**T.S.H.** and **TSH** = **T**he **S**ex **H**ormones (LH, FSH, hCG) and **TSH**
Which glycoprotein subunit determines hormone specificity?	β-Subunit
How is GH regulated?	↑ By GHRH, sleep, stress, exercise, hypoglycemia, and puberty; ↓ by somatomedins, somatostatin, obesity, pregnancy, and hyperglycemia
Name four direct actions of GH (somatotropin):	1. ↓ Glucose uptake into cells (diabetogenic) 2. ↑ Lipolysis 3. ↑ Protein synthesis in muscle 4. ↑ Production of somatomedins (IGF)
Name three effects of IGF on growth:	1. ↑ Linear growth (pubertal growth spurt) 2. ↑ Lean body mass 3. ↑ Organ size
Which clinical syndrome results from GH hypersecretion before puberty?	Increased linear growth (gigantism)

Which clinical syndrome results from GH hypersecretion after puberty?	Acromegaly (may include glucose intolerance)
Name four functions of prolactin:	1. Stimulates milk production 2. Inhibits ovulation 3. Stimulates breast development (with estrogen) 4. Inhibits spermatogenesis
How is prolactin regulated?	↑ By estrogen (pregnancy), breast-feeding, sleep, stress, TRH, dopamine (DA) antagonists; ↓ by DA and DA agonists, somatostatin, and prolactin
What are the effects of excess prolactin?	Galactorrhea, ↓ libido, and failure to ovulate
How does prolactin inhibit ovulation?	Inhibits GnRH synthesis and release

Posterior Pituitary

Which hormones are released from the posterior pituitary and what are their functions?	Oxytocin—milk ejection and uterine contraction; vasopressin (ADH)— ↑ H_2O reabsorption in kidneys
How is the release of oxytocin regulated?	↑ By suckling, dilation of the cervix, and orgasm
How is the release of ADH regulated?	↑ By high serum osmolarity, volume contraction, pain, nausea, nicotine, opiates; ↓ by low serum osmolarity, ethyl alcohol, ANP, and α-agonists

Thyroid

Which cells are responsible for thyroid hormone synthesis?	Follicular cells
Thyroid hormones are synthesized from which two molecules?	1. Iodide (I^-) 2. Tyrosine
Which enzyme catalyzes the oxidation of I^- to I_2?	Thyroid peroxidase
What is the relative proportion of T_4:T_3 released into the bloodstream?	T_4 = 90%, T_3 = 10%
Which thyroid hormone has the greatest biological activity?	$T_3 \gg T_4$ (T_4 converted into T_3 by liver and kidneys)

Which protein produced by and used entirely within the thyroid is used to produce and store T_4 and T_3?	Thyroglobulin
Which carrier protein is necessary for delivery of thyroid hormone to the tissues?	Thyroxine-binding globulin (TBG)
How is thyroid hormone production regulated?	↑ By TRH and TSH; T_3 down-regulates TRH receptors in AP→↓ TSH
List four key functions of thyroid hormone:	Remember the **4 B's of T_3** 1. **B**rain maturation 2. **B**one and cartilage growth (synergistic with GH) 3. **β**-Agonist effects (↑ cardiac output [CO], heart rate [HR], stroke volume [SV]) 4. ↑ **B**MR (by ↑ Na^+/K^+ ATPase →↑ O_2 consumption)

Calcium Regulation

What is meant by a "negative Ca^{2+} balance?"	Intestinal Ca^{2+} absorption is less than Ca^{2+} excretion.
Which is the most important hormone in the regulation of Ca^{2+} levels and where is it made?	PTH is synthesized and secreted by the chief cells of the parathyroid gland.
What is the major stimulus for PTH secretion?	↓ Serum Ca^{2+} (also mildly ↓ Mg^{2+})
Which hormone is stimulated in response to ↑ PTH levels and ↓ serum Ca^{2+}?	Vitamin D (1,25-$(OH)_2^-$ cholecalciferol is active form.)
Which enzyme in the kidney catalyzes the activation of vitamin D?	1α-Hydroxylase
What factors increase 1α-hydroxylase activity?	↓ Serum Ca^{2+}, ↑ PTH, ↓ serum phosphate
What clinical syndrome results from vitamin D deficiency?	Kids → rickets; adults → osteomalacia
Which hormone is released in response to ↑ serum Ca^{2+} and where is it made?	Calcitonin is synthesized and secreted by the parafollicular "C" cells of the thyroid gland.

What is the effect of calcitonin on bones?	Blocks PTH-mediated resorption of bones

List the effects of PTH on each of the following organs:

Kidneys	$\downarrow$ Phosphate reabsorption (by $\uparrow$ urinary cAMP), $\uparrow$ Ca^{2+} reabsorption in distal convoluted tubule of kidneys
Intestines	$\uparrow$ Ca^{2+} absorption (by stimulating 1α-hydroxylase to activate vitamin D)
Bone	$\uparrow$ Resorption (brings Ca^{2+} and phosphate into extracellular fluid [ECF])

List the effects of vitamin D on each of the following organs:

Kidneys	$\uparrow$ Ca^{2+} and phosphate reabsorption
Intestines	$\uparrow$ Ca^{2+} and phosphate absorption
Bone	$\uparrow$ Resorption

Pancreas

Name the three major cell types in the pancreatic islets of Langerhans, their location, and function:	1. **Alpha** (outer rim) $\rightarrow$ glucagons 2. **Beta** (central rim of islet) $\rightarrow$ insulin 3. **Delta** (intermixed) $\rightarrow$ somatostatin (SS) and gastrin
List three major actions of glucagon on the liver and adipose tissue:	1. $\uparrow$ Glycogenolysis and gluconeogenesis 2. $\uparrow$ Lipolysis and ketoacid production 3. $\uparrow$ Urea production
List five major functions of insulin:	1. $\downarrow$ Blood glucose 2. $\uparrow$ Fat deposition ($\downarrow$ lipolysis) 3. $\downarrow$ Blood amino acids 4. $\downarrow$ Blood K^+ 5. $\uparrow$ Protein synthesis
What is the 2° structure of insulin?	An α-chain and a β-chain, joined by two disulfide bridges
What is C-peptide and why is it important?	A connecting peptide removed from proinsulin, packaged and secreted with insulin; serves as a useful monitor of β-cell function and exogenous insulin administration
What are some factors that $\uparrow$ insulin secretion?	$\uparrow$ Blood glucose (major), $\uparrow$ AAs, $\uparrow$ FAs, GH, cortisol, glucagon, ACh

How does glucose trigger insulin release?	Binds to GLUT-2 receptor on β-cells → closes K^+ channels → cell depolarization → opens Ca^{2+} channels → insulin secretion
Which drugs mimic the action of glucose on β-islet cells?	Sulfonylurea drugs
What is the effect of starvation and obesity on insulin receptor expression?	↑ In starvation; ↓ in obesity

PATHOLOGY

Male Reproductive System

Name the male genitourinary disease characterized by each of the following statements:

Intractable, painful erection; associated with venous thrombosis, trazodone, and sickle cell disease	Priapism
Inflammation of the glans associated with poor hygiene	Balanitis
Bent penis due to acquired fibrous tissue formation	Peyronie disease
Twisting of the testicular vasculature; may be spontaneous or the result of trauma	Torsion
Collection of serous fluid in the tunica vaginalis	Hydrocele
Palpable, "bag of worms" dilation of multiple veins of the pampiniform venous plexus of the spermatic cord	Varicocele
Acute purulent urethritis caused by gram-negative diplococci	Gonorrhea
Fever, chills, and dysuria; tender, boggy prostate; > 10 WBCs per high-power field on examination of prostatic secretions	Acute bacterial prostatitis

What are the possible sequelae of cryptorchidism?	5 to 10× ↑ risk of germ cell tumors (GCTs), atrophy, sterility, and inguinal hernias

What is the treatment for cryptorchidism?

Orchiopexy. **Note:** ↓ risk of sterility, but no ↓ risk of malignancy

What are the most common etiologies of orchitis?

Mumps virus (1 week postparotiditis)

Name the most likely organism(s) responsible for epididymitis in the following groups:

Pediatric patients

Gram-negative rods

Sexually active, < 35-year-old (y/o)

Neisseria gonorrhoeae, Clamydia trachomatis

Older men

Escherichia coli, Pseudomonas sp.

Name the penile neoplasm associated with each of the following:

Human papillomavirus (HPV) types 6 and 11

Condyloma acuminate

Single, grayish plaque on shaft/scrotum; associated with ↑ risk of visceral malignancy

Bowen disease

Premalignant, multiple wart-like, reddish lesions with HPV type 16 viral sequence

Bowenoid papulosis

HPV types 16, 18, 31, and 33

Squamous cell carcinoma of the penis

Single erythematous plaque representing carcinoma in situ of the penis, often on glans

Erythroplasia of Queyrat

What category of testicular tumors accounts for ~95% of all cases and has a peak incidence of 15- to 34-y/o?

GCTs

Name the testicular tumor associated with each of the following:

Malignant, painless enlargement of testis; most common GCT, radiosensitive

Seminoma

Malignant, chemosensitive GCT

Nonseminoma GCT

Malignant, painful GCT that has peak incidence in childhood; ↑ α-fetoprotein (AFP)

Yolk sac tumor (endodermal sinus tumor)

Malignant GCT made of 2+ embryonic layers and multiple tissue types; more common in kids	Teratoma
Malignant, aggressive GCT with > 1 neoplastic pattern	Mixed GCT
Benign, androgen-producing stromal tumor with intracytoplasmic Reinke crystals	Leydig cell tumor (interstitial)
Malignant, hemorrhagic tumor arising from trophoblastic cells; ↑ β-hCG	Choriocarcinoma
Most common testicular cancer in older men	Testicular lymphoma

Benign prostatic nodular hyperplasia or prostatic carcinoma?

Commonly affects peripheral zone	Prostatic carcinoma
Caused by age-related increase in DHT, testosterone, and estrogen	Nodular hyperplasia
Associated with bladder distention and urinary tract infections (UTIs)	Nodular hyperplasia
Enlarged, firm, nodular prostate on digital rectal examination (DRE)	Prostatic carcinoma
Commonly presents with nocturia and hesitancy	Nodular hyperplasia
Primarily affects central zone	Nodular hyperplasia
Primarily affects corpora amylacea	Nodular hyperplasia
↑ Total prostate-specific antigen (PSA), with ↓ fraction of free PSA	Prostatic carcinoma
↑ Total PSA, with proportionate ↑ in fraction of free PSA	Nodular hyperplasia

Hypermethylation of which gene is commonly associated with prostatic carcinoma?	GSTP1

What do the following findings suggest in a patient with prostatic carcinoma?

↑ Prostatic acid phosphatase	Capsule of the prostate has been penetrated.
↑ Alkaline phosphatase	Osteoblastic lesions from bony metastasis

Female Reproductive Pathology

Name the gynecologic infectious disorder characterized by each of the following features:

Clue cells in pap smear; ⊕ "whiff test"	Bacterial vaginosis (eg, *Gardnerella vaginitis*)
Thick, white discharge with vulvovaginal pruritis; most common form of vaginitis	Candidiasis
Fever, vomiting, diarrhea with desquamating rash; caused by exotoxins from *Staphylococcus aureus* associated with tampon use	Toxic shock syndrome
Soft, painful ulcerative lesion caused by *Haemophilus ducreyi*	Chancroid
Firm, painless chancre caused by a spirochete *Treponema pallidum*	1° syphilis
Small papule/ulcer associated with lymphadenopathy and caused by *C. trachomatis* serotypes L1, L2, or L3	Lymphogranuloma venereum
Donovan bodies on biopsy	Granuloma inguinale
Most common STD; frequent cause of pelvic inflammatory disease (PID) (though often asymptomatic); associated with Reiter syndrome	Chlamydial cervicitis (types D-K)
Sexually transmitted infection often associated with extragenital manifestations (eg, proctitis, arthritis, and neonatal conjunctivitis)	Gonorrhea
STD resulting in benign venereal warts caused by HPV types 6 and 11	Condyloma acuminatum
Painful vesicles/ulcers; cytologic evidence of multinuclear giant cells with viral inclusions	Herpes genitalis (most often HSV type 2)
STD caused by flagellated protozoan; #2 cause of vaginitis	Trichomoniasis
Commonly caused by *C. trachomatis* or *N. gonorrhoeae*; findings may include cervical motion tenderness, salpingitis, endometritis, or tubo-ovarian abscess	PID—at ↑ risk for ectopic pregnancy and infertility

Name the female reproductive disorder associated with each of the following features:

Triad of 2° amenorrhea, obesity, and hirsutism, ↑ testosterone, ↑ LH, ↓ FSH

Polycystic ovary (Stein-Leventhal) syndrome

Menstrual disorder associated with excessive bleeding during or between menstrual periods

Dysfunctional uterine bleeding

Cyclic pain and bleeding from proliferation of ectopic endometrial tissue

Endometriosis

Islands of endometrium found in the myometrium that may cause the uterus to grow to two to four times its normal size

Adenomyosis

Chocolate cysts

Endometriosis (in ovaries)

Name the tumor of the vulva or vagina associated with each of the following statements:

Eczematous lesion; biopsy shows large cells in epidermis with marginal clearing

Paget disease of vulva. **Note:** not always associated with underlying adenocarcinoma

Rare, malignant tumor of vagina associated with maternal use of diethylstilbesterol (DES) during pregnancy

Clear cell adenocarcinoma

Associated with HPV types 16, 18, 31, 33, and 45; #1 malignancy of vulva; ↑ in older women

Squamous cell carcinoma of vulva

"Bunch of grapes" protruding from vagina; usually in girls < 5-y/o, desmin positive

Sarcoma botryoides

Accounts for 95% of neoplasms of vagina; usually from extension of cervical cancer

Squamous cell carcinoma of vagina

Name the uterine tumor associated with each of the following statements:

Neoplastic changes in the endometrium occurring at squamocolumnar junction; associated with HPV infection

Cervical intraepithelial neoplasia (CIN)

Invasive carcinoma evolving from CIN	Squamous cell carcinoma of the cervix
Very common, benign, estrogen-sensitive smooth muscle tumor of the uterus; usually 20- to 40-y/o	Leiomyoma (fibroid)
Most common gynecologic malignancy; associated with prolonged estrogen exposure; usually 55- to 65-y/o	Endometrial carcinoma
Highly aggressive, bulky tumor with areas of necrosis; arises de novo; ↑ incidence in blacks	Leiomyosarcoma

What HPV types are commonly associated with a high risk of squamous cell carcinoma?

Types 16, 18, 31, 33

What are the HPV viral proteins associated with squamous cell carcinoma?

E6 and E7

What role do HPV viral proteins play in the development of invasive cervical carcinoma?

Proteins E6 and E7 bind to and inactivate gene products of *p53* and *Rb*, respectively.

What are the distinguishing histopathologic features of carcinoma in situ (CIN 3)?

Atypical changes extending through entire thickness of the epithelium

Name four factors associated with increased risk for invasive cervical carcinoma:

1. Early sexual activity
2. Multiple sex partners
3. ↓ Socioeconomic status
4. Cigarette smoking

What is the most effective screening tool for cervical cancer?

Routine pap smears

Name five factors that predispose to endometrial carcinoma:

1. Nulliparity
2. Obesity
3. Diabetes
4. Unopposed estrogen exposure (eg, estrogen-producing tumors, hormone replacement therapy [HRT])
5. Tamoxifen

How does endometrial carcinoma typically present?

Postmenopausal vaginal bleeding

Name the ovarian cyst associated with each of the following statements:

Distention of unruptured graafian follicle; may be associated with ↑ estrogen endometrial hyperplasia

Follicular cyst

Hemorrhage into persistent corpus luteum; menstrual irregularity

Corpus luteum cyst

Due to gonadotropin stimulation; often bilateral/multiple; associated with choriocarcinoma and moles

Theca-lutein cyst

Name the ovarian tumor associated with each of the following statements:

Malignant tumor of epithelial origin; two-thirds are bilateral; psammoma bodies

Serous cystadenocarcinoma

Benign adenoma; frequently bilaterally; lined with fallopian tubelike epithelium

Serous cystadenoma

Malignant GCT that is homologous to seminoma and may occur in childhood

Dysgerminoma

Malignant tumor of epithelial origin; can rupture and cause pseudomyxoma peritonei

Mucinous cystadenocarcinoma

Benign multilocular cyst lined by mucus-secreting epithelium

Mucinous cystadenoma

Benign GCT with elements from multiple embryonic layers; most common GCT

Mature teratoma (dermoid cyst)

Benign tumor; cells resembling bladder transitional epithelium

Brenner tumor

GCT with Schiller-Duval bodies; ↑ AFP

Yolk sac (endodermal sinus) tumor

GCT associated with struma ovarii (mature thyroid tissue)

Teratoma (monodermal)

Malignant, aggressive tumor arising from syncitiotrophoblastic cells; ↑ serum β-hCG

Choriocarcinoma

Stromal tumor associated with Meigs syndrome (ascites, hydrothorax)

Thecoma-fibroma

Benign, estrogen-secreting tumor; Call-Exner bodies

Granulosa-theca tumor

Stromal tumor secreting androgens and causing virilization	Sertoli-Leydig cell tumor
Metastatic tumor from gastric adenocarcinoma; signet ring cells	Krukenberg tumor
Most ovarian carcinomas are associated with an increase in what serologic marker?	CA-125
What two genes are associated with a predisposition to ovarian cancer?	1. *BRCA1* 2. *HNPCC*
What is the most common type of ovarian neoplasm in women older than 20 years?	Epithelial cell neoplasms (~75% of all ovarian cancers)
What is the most common type of ovarian neoplasm in women younger than 20 years?	Germ cell neoplasms

Breast Disorders

Name the breast disease associated with each of the following statements:

Benign, firm, painless, rubbery mass; most common tumor < 25-y/o	Fibroadenoma
Inflammatory lesion caused by *S. aureus*; often occurs during nursing	Acute mastitis
"Blue-domed" cysts; usually bilateral; breast tenderness during menstruation	Fibrocystic change
Benign tumor of lactiferous ducts; most common cause of serous or bloody discharge in females < 35-y/o	Intraductal papilloma
Large, malignant form of fibroadenoma	Cystosarcoma phyllodes
Invasive, malignant tumor; cells arranged in linear fashion; bloody discharge; often bilateral	Invasive lobular carcinoma
Malignant, firm mass with cells in glands; most common carcinoma of breast	Invasive ductal carcinoma
Eczematous lesion of nipple or areola containing large cells with marginal clearings	Paget disease of the breast

Name six risk factors for breast cancer:	1. Age > 45-y/o 2. Early menarche and late menopause ($\uparrow$ span of reproductive period) 3. Family history of (1° relative with history of [h/o]) premenopausal breast cancer 4. Personal h/o breast cancer 5. Inherited mutation (eg, HER-2/neu oncogene) 6. Obesity and high animal fat diet **Note:** risk is not increased by fibroadenoma or nonhyperplastic cysts.
Which disease is almost always associated with Paget disease of the breast?	Ductal carcinoma in situ
In which quadrant of the breast are most cancers located?	~50% found in upper, outer quadrant
What is the significance of estrogen/ progesterone receptors on breast cancer?	Presence of estrogen and progesterone receptors reflects good prognosis (because tumor will likely respond to hormonal therapy).
What is the single most important prognostic factor in breast cancer?	Lymph node involvement (metastatic spread)
What two tumor suppressor genes are associated with a genetic predisposition for breast cancer?	1. *BRCA1* 2. *BRCA2*
What is the general function of the *BRCA1* and *BRCA2* genes?	DNA repair
Trastuzumab (Herceptin) treatment of breast cancers is directed at the protein product of which overexpressed gene?	*HER2/neu*

Pregnancy

Name the disorder of pregnancy associated with each of the following statements:

An ovum without DNA → "honeycombed uterus" and "cluster of grapes" appearance; formed from intrauterine proliferation of trophoblasts and cystic swelling of chorionic villi; $\uparrow$ serum β-hCG	Hydatidiform mole

Tear in placental membranes → sudden peripartal respiratory distress → shock → death	Amniotic fluid embolism
Placental attachment directly to myometrium → impaired separation and massive bleeding at delivery	Placenta accreta
Placental attachment to the lower uterine segment, extending to or obstructing the inner cervical os; painless bleeding in any trimester	Placenta previa
Premature detachment of a normally situated placenta; painful bleeding often in third trimester	Abruptio placentae
Hydatidiform mole with 46,XX genotype and markedly elevated β-hCG; no embryo; paternal chromosomes	Complete mole
Hydatidiform mole with triploid genotype and ↑ β-hCG; fetal parts may be present; (2 sperm + 1 egg)	Incomplete mole
Malignant, aggressive tumor that may arise from mole, ectopic, or normal pregnancy	Gestational choriocarcinoma
Toxemia of pregnancy with triad of HTN, edema, and proteinurea	Preeclampsia
Association with preeclampsia; can lead to death by cerebral hemorrhage or ARDS	Hemolysis, Elevated LFTs, Low Platelets (HELLP syndrome)
Preeclampsia plus convulsions; DIC may be present	Eclampsia
What are some causes of polyhydramnios (> 1.5-2 L of amniotic fluid)?	Maternal diabetes, esophageal/duodenal atresia, anencephaly, Down syndrome
What are some causes of oligohydramnios (< 0.5 L of amniotic fluid) and what sequence can result?	Genitourinary obstruction (esp. posterior urethral valves in boys), bilateral renal agenesis; can result in Potter syndrome/sequence
Name the six clinically important and dangerous infections of pregnancy:	"ToRCHeS" 1. Toxoplasma 2. Rubella 3. CMV 4. **and** 5. HSV and HIV 6. Syphilis

Pituitary Disorders

Name the pituitary disorder associated with each of the following statements:

Most common pituitary adenoma	Prolactinoma (prolactin-secreting adenoma)
Deficiency of GnRH → lack of 2° sexual characteristics; associated with anosmia	Kallmann syndrome
Polyuria, polydipsia, hypernatremia from ↓ ADH; associated with a pituitary or hypothalamic injury	Central/neurogenic diabetes insipidus
Panhypopituitarism 2° to brain tumor, ischemia, or trauma	Simmonds disease. **Note:** > 75% of cells must be destroyed before clinically evident.
Hypopituitarism caused by postpartum pituitary necrosis	Sheehan syndrome
Somatotrophic adenoma causing excess GH and IGF-1	Acromegaly (adults)/gigantism (kids)
Pituitary hypersecretion of ADH→ hyponatremia, ↓ urine output, mental status changes	Syndrome of inappropriate antidiuretic hormone (SIADH)

What are the most important hormones to replace in Sheehan syndrome or pituitary apoplexy?

Cortisol and thyroid hormones

Name the endocrine/renal disorder associated with the following statements:

↓ sNa, ↑ Uosm with Uosm > Sosm	Syndrome of inappropriate ADH (SIADH)
High-normal sNa, ↑ Sosm, ↓ Uosm but no change in Uosm with H$_2$O deprivation test	Diabetes insipidus (DI)
Low-normal sNa, ↓ Uosm but ↑ Uosm toward normal w/H$_2$O deprivation test	Primary polydipsia

What are the two common presentations of a pituitary tumor?

1. Mass effect (bitemporal hemianopia, cranial nerve [CN] palsies)
2. Endocrine effects (amenorrhea, galactorrhea, hyperthyroidism, ↓ libido)

Thyroid

What are the symptoms and physical findings of hypothyroidism?	Cold intolerance, ↓ HR, hypertension, hypercholesterolemia, pericardial effusion, periorbital myxedema, hypoactive deep tendon reflexes, coarse, dry skin; hair loss, weight gain, constipation, amenorrhea, ↓ pitch of voice, depression
What are symptoms and physical findings of hyperthyroidism?	Heat intolerance, hypertension, ↑ CO, ↑ HR, palpitations, cardiomegaly (long-term), staring gaze, lid lag, ↑ sympathetic activity, fine tremor, warm, moist, and flushed skin; fine hair; Graves disease → pretibial myxedema, weight loss despite hyperphagia, ↑ motility, menstrual abnormalities, osteoporosis, anxiety

Name four laboratory findings common in hyperthyroidism:

1. ↓ TSH (in 1°)
2. ↑ free T_4
3. ↑ total T_4
4. ↑ T_3 uptake

Name four laboratory findings common in hypothyroidism:

1. ↑ TSH (very sensitive for 1°)
2. ↓ free T_4
3. ↓ total T_4
4. ↓ T_3 uptake

Name the thyroid disorder associated with each of the following statements:

Child with coarse facial features, short stature, mental retardation, and umbilical hernia	Congenital hypothyroidism (cretinism)
Goiter occurring with high frequency in iodine-deficient areas	Endemic goiter
Painless enlargement of thyroid of autoimmune etiology; Hürthle cells and germinal centers; hypothyroid	Hashimoto thyroiditis
Triad of diffuse thyroid hyperplasia, ophthalmopathy, dermopathy; hyperthyroid	Graves disease
Normal thyroid replaced by fibrous tissue; hypothyroid	Riedel thyroiditis
Postviral, painful inflammation of thyroid; associated with HLA-B35	Subacute (granulomatous, de Quervain) thyroiditis

Painless goiter that may occur in the postpartum period; lymphocytic infiltrates without germinal centers	Subacute lymphocytic (painless) thyroiditis
Thryoid-stimulating immunoglobluin (TSI) and TSH-receptor antibody (AB)	Graves disease
Thyroid peroxidase antibody	Hashimoto disease
Extreme thyroid enlargement (> 2 kg) causing mass effects; most patients euthyroid	Multinodular goiter
Most common thyroid carcinoma	Papillary carcinoma
Calcitonin-secreting tumor with amyloid deposits	Medullary carcinoma
Biopsy shows "Orphan Annie" nuclei, "fingerlike" projections, and psammoma bodies	Papillary carcinoma
Carcinoma presenting as a single nodule with uniform follicles	Follicular carcinoma
Aggressive carcinoma of older patients with pleomorphic cells; dismal prognosis	Anaplastic (undifferentiated) carcinoma
Carcinoma associated with Hashimoto thyroiditis	Lymphoma
What type of nodules is more likely to be benign: hot or cold?	Hot
Which gene is associated with medullary carcinoma of the thyroid?	*RET*
What is the function of the two genes associated with papillary carcinoma of the thyroid?	Tyrosine kinase receptors 1. *RET* 2. *NTRK1*

Name the multiple endocrine neoplasia (MEN) syndrome characterized by the following features:

Pheochromocytoma, thyroid medullary carcinoma, and parathyroid adenomas	MEN 2 (Sipple syndrome)
Tumors of the pituitary, pancreatic islet cells, and parathyroid gland	MEN 1 (Wermer syndrome)
Mutation of RET oncogene on chromosome 10q	MEN 2

Tumors in MEN 2 plus tall, thin habitus, prominent lips, and ganglioneuromas of the tongue and eyelids	MEN 3 (MEN 2b)
Mutation of *MEN 1* gene on chromosome 11q	MEN 1
Autosomal-dominant (AD) inheritance	All MEN syndromes

Parathyroid Disorders

Name the parathyroid disorder associated with each of the following statements:

Caused by chronic renal failure or ↓ vitamin D	2° hyperparathyroidism
Most commonly due to parathyroid adenomas	1° hyperparathyroidism
Etiologies include congenital gland absence, surgically induced, and autoimmune destruction	Hypoparathyroidism
Due to autonomous hormone-secreting adenoma, often occurs after correction of chronic renal failure	3° hyperparathyroidism
Autosomal-recessive (AR) end-organ resistance to PTH → short stature and short third/fourth metacarpals	Pseudohypoparathyroidism

| What four systems are primarily targeted by hyperparathyroidism? | 1. Painful bones: osteitis fibrosa cystica, osteoporosis
2. Renal stones: nephrolithiasis, nephrocalcinosis
3. Abdominal groans: constipation, peptic ulcer disease (PUD), pancreatitis
4. Psychic moans: depression, lethargy, seizures |

| Up to 20% of parathyroid adenomas are commonly associated with altered activity of which gene? | *PRAD1* |

Adrenal Disorders

Name the four etiologies for hypercorticism (Cushing syndrome):	1. Exogenous glucocorticoids (most common overall) 2. Pituitary ACTH hypersecretion (eg, adenoma) 3. Hypersecretion of cortisol (eg, adrenal hyperplasia) 4. Paraneoplastic (ectopic) ACTH secretion from a tumor
What is the most common cause of endogenous hypercortisolism?	Cushing syndrome (pituitary adenoma)
What finding specific to an ACTH-producing pituitary adenoma differentiates it from adrenal cortisol-producing and ectopic ACTH-producing tumors?	↓ Cortisol level after high-dose dexamethasone suppression test
In most cases of congenital adrenal hyperplasia, deficiency in which enzyme is associated with defective conversion of progesterone to 11-deoxycorticosterone?	21-Hydroxylase
Name nine clinical findings of Cushing syndrome:	1. Hyperglycemia (insulin resistance) 2. Virilization and menstrual irregularities in women 3. Moon facies 4. Truncal obesity 5. Buffalo hump 6. Skin changes (thinning, striae) 7. Osteoporosis 8. Immune suppression 9. Proximal muscle weakness

Name the adrenal disorder associated with each of the following statements:

Aldosterone-secreting adenoma causing HTN and hypokalemic, metabolic alkalosis	Conn syndrome (1° hyperaldosteronism)
Endotoxin-mediated massive adrenal hemorrhage	Waterhouse-Friderichsen syndrome (*N. meningitidis*)
Deficiency of aldosterone and cortisol due to adrenal atrophy or destruction	1° chronic adrenocortical insufficiency (Addison disease)

Hypothalemic pituitary axis (HPA) disturbance causing failure of ACTH secretion	2° adrenocortical insufficiency
Bilateral hyperplasia of zona glomerulosa caused by stimulation of renin-angiotensin-aldosterone (RAA) system	2° hyperaldosteronism
Results from rapid steroid withdrawal or sudden ↑ in glucocorticoid requirements	1° acute adrenocortical insufficiency (adrenal crisis)
Chromaffin cell tumor usually in adults; results in episodic hyperadrenergic symptoms	Pheochromocytoma
Malignant, "small blue cell" tumor of medulla in kids associated with N-*myc* oncogene amplification	Neuroblastoma
How are 1° and 2° adrenocortical insufficiencies differentiated?	Hyperpigmentation is absent in 2° adrenocortical insufficiency (POMC is not increased).
Measurement of what substance can differentiate between 1° and 2° hyperaldosteronism?	Renin (↑ in 2° hyperaldosteronism)
What is the drug of choice for hyperaldosteronism?	Spironolactone (aldosterone antagonist)
What is the "rule of 10's" for pheochromocytomas?	10% malignant 10% bilateral 10% extra-adrenal 10% pediatric 10% familial 10% calcified
Besides MEN, name three familial syndromes associated with pheochromocytomas:	1. Sturge-Weber syndrome 2. von Recklinghausen syndrome 3. von Hippel-Lindau syndrome
What substances are secreted from pheochromocytomas and how are they detected?	Epinephrine and norepinephrine; detected by ↑ urinary secretion of catecholamines and their metabolites (metanephrine, VMA, and so forth)

Adrenogenital Syndromes

Name the enzyme deficiency
responsible for each of the following
androgenital syndromes:

↓ Sex hormones, ↓ cortisol,
↑ mineralocorticoids; HTN,
hypokalemia, phenotypic
female without maturation

17α-Hydroxylase deficiency

↓ Cortisol, aldosterone, and
corticosterone; ↑ sex hormones;
virilization, HTN

11β-Hydroxylase deficiency

↓ Cortisol, aldosterone, and
corticosterone; ↑ sex hormones;
virilization, hypotension,
hyperkalemia, "salt wasting"

21-Hydroxylase deficiency

What is the phenotypic result
of androgen insensitivity syndrome
(testicular feminization)?

"Hairless woman"; XY with undescended
testes but female/ambiguous genitalia

List the three syndromes associated
with 21-hydroxylase deficiency:

1. Salt-wasting adrenogenitalism
2. Simple virilization adrenogenitalism
   (ambiguity and adrenal hyperplasia)
3. Asymptomatic

Diabetes

Describe the acute presentation of
type 1 diabetes mellitus (DM).

Polydipsia, polyuria, polyphagia,
weight loss, and diabetic ketoacidosis
(DKA) if extreme

What causes hyperglycemia in
type 1 DM?

Lack of insulin from decreased
β-cell mass

What is the proposed mechanism
of islet cell destruction in type 1 DM?

Environmental triggering of
autoimmunity to islet β-cells

What is the theorized cause of
type 2 DM?

Obesity increases insulin resistance and
causes derangement of β-cell insulin
secretion.

What are three ways to diagnose DM?

1. Fasting serum glucose > 126
   (100-126 = impaired fasting glucose)
2. Oral glucose tolerance test > 200
   (148-200 = impaired glucose
   tolerance)
3. Symptoms + random glucose > 200

What is HbA$_{1c}$ and what is it used for?

Percent of glycosylated hemoglobin in blood; correlates with glycemic control over the last 90 to 120 days

Type 1 or type 2 DM?

Relatively common in the US population	Type 2
Younger average age of onset	Type 1
Strong, polygenic predisposition	Type 2
Associated with obesity	Type 2
Insulin treatment required from the time of diagnosis	Type 1
Associated with HLA-DR3 and -DR4	Type 1
May present with hyperosmolar coma	Type 2
May present initially as DKA	Type 1
Amyloid deposition in the islets	Type 2

What two cleavage products of proinsulin are stored in the granules of β-islet cells?

1. Insulin
2. C-peptide

Which membrane protein mediates glucose uptake by β-islet cells?

GLUT-2

Increased cytoplasmic concentration of which ion stimulates the secretion of insulin?

Calcium

By what mechanism is the cytoplasmic concentration of calcium increased in β-cells following uptake of glucose?

Decreased activation of adenosine triphosphate (ATP)-sensitive potassium channels leads to membrane depolarization, resulting in an influx of extracellular calcium via a voltage-dependent calcium channel.

Glucose uptake in which organ is independent of insulin?

The brain

What signal transduction pathway mediates the mitogenic effects of insulin binding?

MAP-kinase pathway

Activation of the PI-3K signal transduction pathway by insulin results in the translocation of what molecule to the surface of myocytes in order to transport glucose into myocytes?

GLUT-4

List four potential effects of advanced glycation end products (AGEs) in type 1 diabetes:	1. Cross-linking of collagen 2. Accumulation of extracellular matrix proteins resistant to proteolytic degradation 3. Generation of reactive oxygen species 4. NF-κB activation
What is the most common cause of death in diabetics?	Myocardial infarction (MI) due to accelerated atherosclerosis
What is the most common morphologic change in the microvasculature of a diabetic?	Diffuse thickening of the basement membrane

Describe the long-term effect(s) of DM on each of the following organ systems:

Cardiovascular (large vessels)	Atherosclerosis → cerebrovascular accident (CVA), MI, peripheral vascular disease (PVD)
Renal/urinary	**Glomerular:** glomerulosclerosis, proteinuria **Vascular:** arteriosclerosis → HTN, chronic renal failure **Infectious:** UTIs, pyelonephritis, necrotizing papillitis
Nervous	Motor and sensory peripheral neuropathy, autonomic degeneration
Eye	Retinopathy, cataract formation
Skin	Xanthomas, cutaneous infections, poor wound healing, fungal infections
Name four causes of 2° DM:	1. Pancreatic disease (eg, hemochromatosis, pancreatitis, pancreatic carcinoma) 2. Pregnancy (gestational diabetes) 3. Cushing syndrome 4. Other endocrine disorders (eg, acromegaly, glucagonoma, hyperthyroidism)

Pancreatic Endocrine Tumors

Name the islet cell tumor associated with each of the following statements:

Most common islet cell tumor	Insulinoma (β-cell tumor)
2° DM, necrolytic migratory erythema	Glucagonoma (α-cell tumor)

Associated with Zollinger-Ellison syndrome	Gastrinoma
Associated with watery diarrhea, hypokalemia, and achlorhydria (WDHA) syndrome	VIPoma
2° DM, cholelithiasis, steatorrhea	Somatostatinoma (δ-cell tumor)
Clinically characterized by Whipple triad	Insulinoma (β-cell tumor)
Name the clinical findings of Whipple triad:	Hypoglycemia, concurrent central nervous system (CNS) dysfunction, and reversal of symptoms with glucose
What is Zollinger-Ellison syndrome?	Hypersecretion of gastric HCl, recurrent PUD, and hypergastinemia

PHARMACOLOGY

Pituitary

For each of the following drugs, provide:
1. **The mechanism of action (MOA)**
2. **Indication(s) (IND)**
3. **Significant side effects and unique toxicity (TOX) (if any)**

Octreotide	**MOA:** somatostatin analog
	IND: acromegaly, secretory diarrhea from VIPoma, carcinoid symptoms, high-output fistulas
Leuprolide	**MOA:** GnRH analog. **Note:** given pulsatile = agonist; given continuous = antagonist
	IND: *continuous* → prostate cancer, endometriosis, uterine fibroids. *Pulsatile* → infertility
	TOX: antiandrogenic effects, nausea, vomiting
Oxytocin	**MOA:** ↑ uterine contraction
	IND: induce/reinforce labor; control uterine hemorrhage
	TOX: uterine rupture, hypertensive crisis

Desmopressin

MOA: vasopressin analog

IND: central diabetes insipidus, nocturnal enuresis

TOX: HTN, overhydration, coronary constriction

Thyroid and Parathyroid

For each of the following drugs, provide:
1. The mechanism of action (MOA)
2. Indication(s) (IND)
3. Significant side effects and unique toxicity (TOX) (if any)

Levothyroxine (T_4)

MOA: synthetic $T_4 \rightarrow$ converted to T_3

IND: hypothyroidism (maintenance replacement)

TOX: nervousness, palpitations, $\uparrow$ HR, heat intolerance

Propylthiouracil/methimazole

MOA: blocks thyroid peroxidase, propylthiouracil also $\downarrow$ peripheral conversion of $T_4 \rightarrow T_3$

IND: hyperthyroidism (propylthiouracil okay in pregnancy)

TOX: rash, agranulocytosis (rare), +ANCA vasculitis, hepatotoxicity, lupuslike syndrome

Risedronate

MOA: bisphophonate (inhibits osteoclastic function)

IND: osteoporosis, Paget disease, metastatic bone cancer, hyperparathyroidism

TOX: GI upset, esophagits

Calcitonin

MOA: $\downarrow$ bone resorption, $\downarrow$ serum Ca^{2+} and phosphate

IND: acute hypercalcemia, Paget disease, osteoporosis

Which other drug is used to treat the symptoms of hyperthyroidism?

Propanolol (β-blocker)

Diabetes

Sulfonylureas (eg, tolbutamide, glyburide, chlorpropamide)

MOA: pancreas, closes K^+ channels in β-cell membrane → depolarization → ↑ Ca^{2+} influx → insulin release

IND: type 2 diabetes (not used in type 1 because it requires some residual β-cell activity)

TOX: hypoglycemia, weight gain

Metformin (Glucophage)

MOA: liver, ↓ gluconeogenesis; ↑ glycolysis; ↓ postprandial glucose

IND: newly diagnosed diabetic (no islet cell function required)

TOX: potentially life-threatening lactic acidosis, ↓ vitamin B_{12} absorption, contraindicated in renal insufficiency

Glitazones (eg, rosiglitazone, pioglitazone)

MOA: ↑ target cell response to insulin

IND: type 2 diabetes (monotherapy or combination)

TOX: hepatotoxicity (troglitazone), upper respiratory infection (URI), weight gain, edema, congestive heart failure, and anemia (rosiglitazone)

α-Glucosidase inhibitor (eg, acarbose)

MOA: inhibits α-glucosidase at brush border →↑ glucose absorption

IND: type 2 diabetes

TOX: GI upset (flatulence, diarrhea)

Insulin

MOA: tyrosine kinase activity →↑ glycogen and protein synthesis, triglyceride (TG) storage, and K^+ uptake

IND: type 1 and refractory type 2 diabetes; life-threatening hyperkalemia

TOX: hypoglycemia and rare hypersensitivity reaction

For each of the following types of insulin, state the peak and duration of action:

    Insulin lispro

Peak = 30 to 60 minutes; duration = 3 to 4 hours

    NPH insulin

Peak = 8 to 12 hours; duration = 18 to 24 hours

Lente insulin	Peak = 8 to 12 hours; duration = 18 to 24 hours
Ultralente insulin	Peak = 8 to 16 hours; duration = 18 to 28 hours
Insulin glargine	Peak = none (peakless); duration 20 to 24+ hours

Adrenal Gland

| Describe the mechanism of action of corticosteroids: | Corticosteroids bind to cytoplasmic receptors, pass into the nucleus complexed with their receptors, and act as transcription factors for specific target genes. |
| How do glucocorticoids affect arachidonic acid metabolism? | Glucocorticoids inhibit phospholipase A2, blocking the release of arachidonic acid and ↓ production of prostaglandins and leukotrienes. |

Select the most appropriate corticosteroid for each of the following clinical situations:

Diagnosis of Cushing syndrome	Dexamethasone
Autoimmune disorder	Prednisone
Addison disease	Hydrocortisone (+/− fludrocortisone)
Relief of inflammation	Prednisone, cortisone
Asthma/allergies	Beclomethasone or triamcinolone aerosol
Used to ↑ fetal lung maturity	Betamethasone
Cancer chemotherapy	Prednisone

List the effect of glucocorticoids on each of the following systems:

Metabolic	↑ Gluconeogenesis; net ↑ in fat deposition in prototypical areas
Muscle	↑ Muscle protein catabolism; myopathy → weakness
Bone	↑ Bone catabolism
Immune	Inhibits cell-mediated immunity; ↑ PMNs; ↓ lymphocytes, basophils, eosinophils, and monocytes; ↓ leukocyte migration

Psych	Behavioral changes, psychoses
GI	↓ Resistance to ulcers
Vascular	↓ Capillary permeability →↓ edema at sites of inflammation

What is the consequence of abrupt discontinuation of corticosteroid use?

Acute adrenal insufficiency syndrome (potentially lethal)

Name eight commonly observed effects of long-term corticosteroid use:

1. Osteoporosis
2. HTN
3. Insulin resistance
4. Edema
5. Psychoses
6. Peptic ulcers
7. ↑ Susceptibility to infections
8. Cataracts

What classic toxicity is associated with excess corticosteroid use?

Iatrogenic Cushing syndrome

For each of the following drugs, provide:
1. **The mechanism of action (MOA)**
2. **Indication(s) (IND)**
3. **Significant side effects and unique toxicity (TOX) (if any)**

Spironolactone

MOA: spironolactone binds estrogen receptors

IND: hirsutism (eg, in PCOS), prostate/breast cancer

TOX: gynecomastia, thrombocytopenia, hepatotoxicity

Clomiphene

MOA: blocks negative feedback →↑ GnRH →↑ LH and FSH → ovulation

IND: infertility

TOX: ovarian enlargement, multiple births, hot flashes

Tamoxifen

MOA: competes for estrogen receptors → blocks binding to ER ⊕ cells

IND: breast cancer

TOX: ↑ risk of endometrial carcinoma, hot flashes

Finasteride

MOA: 5α-reductase inhibitor →↓ DHT

IND: benign prostatic hyperplasia (BPH), hair loss

TOX: impotence, gynecomastia

Flutamide	**MOA:** competitive androgen receptor blocker
	IND: prostatic carcinoma
Mifepristone (RU486)	**MOA:** competitive progesterone receptor blocker
	IND: abortion
	TOX: GI upset, metrorrhagia
Dinoprostone	**MOA:** PGE_2 analog causes cervical dilation and uterine contraction
	IND: induction of labor; abortion
Ritodrine, terbutaline	**MOA:** β_2-agonists relax the uterus
	IND: preterm labor
	TOX: maternal and fetal tachycardia, fluid retention, and hyperglycemia
Sildenafil, vardenafil	**MOA:** inhibits phosphodiesterase type 5 →↑ cGMP → smooth muscle relaxation of corpus cavernosum
	IND: erectile dysfunction
	TOX: hypotension if also taking a nitrate, priapism, headache, color vision changes
Name five benefits of oral contraceptives (OCPs):	1. ↓ Risk of ovarian and endometrial cancer 2. ↓ Genitourinary infections 3. Regulates menstrual cycle 4. Low failure rate (if taken appropriately) 5. ↓ Risk of ectopic pregnancy
Name five disadvantages of OCPs:	1. Requires daily pill ingestion 2. Not protective against STDs 3. ↑ Triglycerides 4. ↑ Risk of hepatic adenoma 5. Induces hypercoagulable state
Name four contraindications to OCPs:	1. Pregnancy 2. H/o thromboembolism or stroke 3. H/o breast cancer or endometrial cancer 4. Smoking (in women > 35-y/o)

CHAPTER 9

Renal and Genitourinary

EMBRYOLOGY

Name the structure(s) derived from each of the following:

Nephrogenic cord (three structures)
1. Pronephros
2. Mesonephros
3. Metanephros

Ureteric bud
C CUP (*"see you pee"*): Collecting tubules, Calyces, Ureter, Pelvis

Genital Ridge
Gonads

Reproductive structures from the mesonephric (Wolffian) duct
"SEED" (in males *only*): Seminal vesicles, Epididymis, Ejaculatory duct, Ductus deferens

Reproductive structures from the paramesonephric (Müllerian) duct
In women *only*: Fallopian tubes, uterus, superior portion of vagina

Metanephros
Definitive adult kidney

Name the embryologic tissue layer that following components of the genitourinary system develop from:

Kidneys (ie, nephrons)
Mesoderm (intermediate mesoderm)

Collecting tubules, calyces, pelvis, ureters
Mesoderm (intermediate mesoderm)

Bladder, urethra
Endoderm (cloaca)

Name the parts of the external genitalia in males and females derived from the following embryologic structures:

Genital tubercle

Males: glans penis; females: glans clitoris

Urogenital sinus

Males: corpus spongiosum, bulbourethral (Cowper) glands, prostate gland; females: vestibular bulbs, Bartholin and Skene glands

Urogenital folds

Males: ventral shaft of penis; females: labia minora

Labioscrotal swelling

Males: scrotum; females: labia majora

Describe the following congenital disorders:

Exstrophy of the bladder

Congenital defect in the anterior wall of the bladder and adjacent abdominal wall causing the bladder to be exposed at birth; associated with epispadias

Horseshoe kidney

Fusion of the lower (or upper) poles of kidneys → kidney fails to ascend → often malrotated and remains in pelvis

Hypospadias

Penile abnormality resulting in urethra opening on the ventral (inferior) side of penis; most common congenital penile abnormality

Epispadias

Penile abnormality resulting in urethral opening on the dorsal (superior) side of penis; associated with bladder exstrophy

Renal agenesis

Results from failure of the ureteric bud to form; associated with Potter syndrome

Potter syndrome

Renal agenesis → oligohydramnios → limb deformities and pulmonary hypoplasia

What structure limits the ascent of a fused horseshoe kidney?

Inferior mesenteric artery

What substance secreted by the testes

Suppresses development of paramesonephric ducts in males?

Müllerian-inhibiting substance

Promotes development of the mesonephric ducts?

Fetal androgens

Describe the gonads and external genitalia of the following:

Female (XX) infant with congenital adrenal hyperplasia (CAH)	Female gonads with masculinized genitalia
Male (XY) infant with androgen-insensitivity syndrome	Male gonads with female external genitalia, but no uterus or fallopian tubes

ANATOMY

Name the structures contained in the retroperitoneal space:	Ureters, kidneys, adrenals, pancreas, duodenum (2nd, 3rd, and 4th parts), ascending/descending colon, rectum, aorta, IVC
What is the approximate vertebral level of the kidneys?	T12 to L3 (The right kidney is slightly lower because of liver.)
Name the renal blood vessel that runs posterior to the superior mesenteric artery (SMA) and anterior to the aorta:	Left renal vein
What vessel does the left gonadal vein drain into?	Left renal vein
What important structures do the ureters pass *under* on their way to the bladder?	Females: uterine artery; males: ductus deferens; *water* (ureters) *under the bridge* (uterine artery, ductus deferens)
Which terminal vessels carry blood toward the glomerulus?	Afferent arterioles
What specialized cells are found between the afferent and efferent glomerular arterioles and have receptors for angiotensin II (AT II) and atrial natriuretic peptide (ANP)?	Lacis cells (extraglomerular mesangial cells)
What makes up the juxtaglomerular apparatus (JGA)?	JG cells, lacis cells, and the macula densa
What hormone do the JG cells secrete?	Renin
What anatomic feature makes stress incontinence more common in women?	External urethral sphincter does not completely surround female urethra.
Name the sensory and motor components of the micturition reflex:	Pelvic splanchnic nerves (parasympathetic S2-S4)

PHYSIOLOGY

What percentage of body weight is total body water (TBW)?

~60%

What proportion of TBW is accounted for by intracellular fluid (ICF) and extracellular fluid (ECF)?

Two-thirds ICF, one-third ECF (60 = 40 + 20. Rule: 40% body weight is ICF, 20% is ECF.)

Name the major cations and anions found in ICF:

Cations = K^+, Mg^{2+}; anions = proteins, organophosphates (eg, ADP, ATP)

Name the major cations and anions found in ECF:

Cations = Na^+; anions = Cl^-, HCO_3^-

What are the relative proportions of plasma and interstitial fluid in ECF?

One-fourth plasma volume, three-fourths interstitial volume

What is considered normal ECF osmolality?

~290 mOsm

Clearance of what chemical can be used to measure glomerular filtration rate (GFR)?

Inulin (Inulin is freely filtered, but neither secreted nor reabsorbed.)

What is a useful clinical measure to estimate GFR?

Creatinine clearance

What is considered normal GFR?

~120 mL/min

Effective renal plasma flow (ERPF) can be measured by calculating the clearance of what substance?

Para-aminohippuric acid (PAH). PAH is filtered and secreted.

Complete the following calculations:

$U_x V/P_x$ (urine concentration × urine volume/plasma concentration) =

Renal clearance (C_x)

ERPF/(1 − hematocrit) =

Renal blood flow (RBF)

GFR/RPF (renal plasma flow) =

Filtration fraction (FF)

GFR × (plasma$_x$) =

Filtered load

$V_{urine\ flow} − (U_{osm} V/P_{osm}) =$

Free water clearance

Define GFR using the Starling formula.

$K_f[(P_{GC} − P_{BS}) − (\pi_{GC} − \pi_{BS})]$, where $K_f =$ filtration coefficient, GC = glomerular capillary, BS = Bowman space

List the three components of the glomerular filtration barrier:	1. Fused basement membrane (negative charge barrier) 2. Fenestrated capillary endothelium (size barrier) 3. Epithelial or podocyte foot process layer
If C_x > GFR then there is net ...	tubular secretion of substance X
If C_x < GFR then there is net ...	tubular absorption of substance X
If C_x = GFR then there is ...	no net tubular absorption or secretion of substance X
What proportion of total cardiac output does RBF account for?	~25%
How is RBF maintained at a constant level?	Autoregulation (via myogenic response to stretch and the activity of the JGA)
How do the following substances affect the renal arterioles, RPF, GFR, and FF?	
Prostaglandins	Prostaglandins dilate afferent arterioles: ↑ RPF, ↑ GFR, thus FF stays constant
AT II	AT II constricts efferent arterioles: ↓ RPF, ↑ GFR, thus FF increases
What effect do the following have on RPF, GFR, and FF?	
Afferent arteriole constriction	Decreased RPF and GFR, no change in FF
Efferent arteriole constriction	Decreased RPF, increased GFR, increased FF
Increased plasma protein concentration	No change in RPF, decreased GFR and FF
Decreased plasma protein concentration	No change in RPF, increased GFR and FF
What is the maximum plasma glucose concentration at which glucose will no longer be reabsorbed?	~200 to 250 mg/dL (Concentrations of > 250 mg/dL glucose will be lost in the urine.)
What is the transport maximum (T_m) for glucose?	At 350 mg/min, carriers are saturated (T_m = renal threshold/GFR).
What factors cause K^+ to shift out of cells?	↓ Insulin, β-blockers, acidosis, digitalis, extreme exercise, cell lysis, hyperosmolarity

What factors cause K$^+$ to shift into cells?	Insulin, β-agonists, alkalosis
List four causes of decreased distal K$^+$ secretion:	1. Low-K$^+$ diet 2. Hypoaldosteronism 3. Acidosis 4. K$^+$-sparing diuretics
List six causes of increased distal K$^+$ secretion:	1. High-K$^+$ diet 2. Hyperaldosteronism 3. Alkalosis 4. Thiazide diuretics 5. Loop diuretics 6. Luminal anions

Describe a clinical scenario which might lead to each of the following physiologic changes:

Isosmotic volume contraction	Diarrhea
Isosmotic volume expansion	Isotonic fluid infusion (eg, normal saline IV)
Hyperosmotic volume contraction (two scenarios)	1. Profuse sweating 2. Diabetes insipidus
Hyperosmotic volume expansion	High NaCl intake, infusion of hypertonic saline
Hypo-osmotic volume contraction	Adrenal insufficiency (hypoaldosteronism)
Hypo-osmotic volume expansion	Syndrome of inappropriate antidiuretic hormone (SIADH)

FUNCTIONAL REGIONS OF THE NEPHRON

Name the part of the nephron where each of the following processes occur:

Site of reabsorption of all glucose and amino acids, and the majority of bicarbonate, sodium, and water	Proximal convoluted tubule (PCT)
Site of active reabsorption K$^+$, Na$^+$, Cl$^-$	Thick ascending loop of Henle
Site of 50% of urea reabsorption	PCT (passively)
Site of active reabsorption of Na$^+$, Cl$^-$	Early distal convoluted tubule (DCT)
Site of action of thiazide diuretics	DCT
Site of action of K$^+$-sparing diuretics	Collecting tubules

Sections that are impermeable to water	Thick ascending loop of Henle, collecting ducts (in absence of ADH)
Site where ammonia is excreted to act as a buffer for secreted H^+ ions	PCT
Portion of the nephron which is impermeable to Na^+ and passively reabsorbs water	Thin descending loop of Henle
Aldosterone-sensitive site where Na^+ is exchanged for K^+ or H^+	Collecting tubules
Site of active Ca^{2+} reabsorption that is controlled by PTH	Early DCT
Site of action of loop diuretics	Thick ascending loop of Henle
Section where reabsorption of water is regulated by vasopressin (ADH)	Collecting tubules
Site of action of carbonic anhydrase inhibitors	PCT
Section which contains principal cells and intercalated cells	Collecting tubules
Site of 85% of all phosphate reabsorption (via cotransport)	PCT

ENDOCRINE FUNCTIONS OF THE KIDNEYS

List the four main endocrine functions of the kidneys:	1. PTH-mediated conversion of 25-OH vitamin D to 1, 25-OH vitamin D by 1α-hydroxylase 2. Secretion of renin by JG cells in response to arterial pressure changes and in response to Na^+ and Cl^- delivery to the macula densa 3. Secretion of prostaglandins (to increase GFR by dilating afferent arteriole) 4. Secretion of erythropoeitin in response to hypoxia by peritubular endothelial cells
Name the effect of each of the following on the kidneys:	
ANP	↓ Na^+ reabsorption, ↑ GFR
Aldosterone	↑ Na^+ reabsorption, ↑ K^+ secretion, ↑ H^+ secretion in collecting tubule

Vasopressin (ADH)	$\uparrow Na^+ /K^+/2Cl^-$ transporters in thick ascending limb, $\uparrow$ water permeability in principal cells (via aquaporins), $\uparrow$ urea absorption in collecting duct
Where is angiotensin-converting enzyme (ACE) primarily found?	Lung capillaries
Briefly describe the renin-angiotensin-aldosterone cascade:	$\downarrow$ BP ($\downarrow$ stretch of cells in afferent arterioles) $\rightarrow$ secretion of renin $\rightarrow$ conversion of angiotensinogen to angiotensin I (AT I) $\rightarrow$ AT I converted to AT II by ACE
What is the function of AT II?	Increases intravascular volume and $\uparrow$ vascular tone $\rightarrow \uparrow$ BP
Name six specific actions of AT II:	1. Causes potent vasoconstriction 2. Releases vasopressin and adrenocorticotropic hormone (ACTH) from the pituitary 3. Promotes release of aldosterone from adrenal cortex 4. Stimulates hypothalamus to increase thirst 5. Stimulates catecholamine release from the adrenal medulla 6. Increases Na^+ and HCO_3^- reabsorption in proximal tubule
What cells in the kidneys produce and secrete erythropoietin?	Peritubular capillary cells
What stimulates erythropoietin production and release?	Hypoxia

PATHOLOGY

Polycystic Kidney Disease

Name the disease characterized by multiple 3 to 4 cm renal cysts, bilateral enlargement of the kidneys, and chronic renal failure in adults:	Autosomal dominant (adult) polycystic kidney disease (ADPKD)
What are the signs and symptoms of ADPKD?	Flank pain, hypertension, hematuria, and UTI
Which gene is most commonly associated with ADPKD?	PKD1 (85% of cases)

Name three extra renal manifestations of ADPKD:

1. Liver cysts (40%)
2. Berry aneurysms (10%-30%)
3. Mitral valve prolapse (25%)

What is the prognosis of patients with autosomal recessive polycystic kidney disease (ARPKD)?

Poor; majority die in infancy or early childhood

What type of renal lesions are characteristic of ARPKD?

Multiple cylindrical cysts found perpendicular to cortex in an enlarged kidney

Which of the cystic renal diseases is associated with an increased risk of renal cell carcinoma?

Dialysis-associated cystic disease

Nephrotic and Nephritic Syndromes

What are the classic features of the following:

    Nephrotic syndrome

Massive proteinuria (>3.5 g/d), hypoalbuminemia, hyperlipidemia, edema

    Nephritic syndrome

Hypertension, azotemia, RBC casts, oliguria, hematuria

Glomerulonephropathies

What term describes the type of immune deposits found outside of the glomerular BM (GBM) but within the podocytes?

Subepithelial

What term describes the type of immune deposits found outside the endothelium but inside the GBM?

Subendothelial

Name the immunofluorescence pattern of deposition of immunoglobulins and/or complement associated with the following diseases:

    Membranous glomerulonephritis (GN)

Granular or "starry-sky"

    Goodpasture syndrome

Linear

    IgA nephropathy (Berger disease)

Mesangial

    Poststreptococcal

Granular or "starry-sky"

Name the electron microscopic (EM) appearance of the immunoglobulin and/or complement deposits in the following diseases:

Membranous GN

"Spike and dome" subepithelial deposits

Membranoproliferative GN (MPGN)

Subendothelial humps, "tram track"

Poststreptococcal GN

Subepithelial humps

Name the glomerulopathy most closely associated with each of the following statements:

X-linked syndrome of glomerulonephritis, lens dislocation, nerve deafness, and posterior cataracts

Alport syndrome

Nodular glomerulosclerosis, glomerular capillary basement membrane thickening

Diabetic glomerulosclerosis (Kimmelstiel-Wilson disease)

Commonly associated with HIV infection, heroin abuse, sickle cell disease, and obesity

Focal-segmental glomerulonephritis (FSGN)

Diffuse loss of foot processes of the visceral epithelial cells on EM, but normal appearance on light microscopy

Minimal change disease (lipoid nephrosis)

Apple green birefringence on Congo red stain

Amyloidosis

C-ANCA

Wegener granulomatosis

Most common cause of nephrotic syndrome in kids

Minimal change disease (lipoid nephrosis)

Electron dense deposits in the GBM proper and autoantibody to C3 nephritic factor

MPGN type II (aka dense deposit disease)

Crescents seen in glomeruli on light microscopy

Rapidly progressive glomerulonephritis (RPGN)

Most common cause of end-stage renal disease

Diabetic glomerulosclerosis

Basement membrane thickening and splitting (*train tracks*)

MPGN type I

Syndrome of hematuria and hemoptysis caused by anti-GBM antibodies	Goodpasture syndrome
Mesangial widening, recurrent hematuria, and proteinuria	IgA nephropathy
Associated with hepatitis C	MPGN
Responds well to steroids	Minimal change disease (aka steroid responsive nephropathy)
X-linked recessive defect in collagen type IV	Alport syndrome
Asymptomatic familial hematuria	Thin membrane disease (GBM is only 50%-60% of normal thickness.)
"Wire loop lesions"	Systemic lupus erythematosus (SLE)—lupus nephropathy (diffuse proliferative pattern)
Henoch-Schönlein purpura	IgA nephropathy
Irregularly thick GBM with splitting of lamina densa seen on EM	Alport syndrome
Upper respiratory vasculitis and granulomas	Wegener granulomatosis

Renal Tubular Acidosis

Name the type of renal tubular acidosis (RTA) associated with the following statements:

Decreased bicarbonate reabsorption	Type II (proximal)
Dysfunction of principal cells	Type IV
Decreased acidification and acid excretion	Type I (distal)
Hyperkalemia	Type IV
Nongap metabolic acidosis	Types I, II, IV
Fanconi syndrome	Type II (proximal)
Aldosterone deficiency/resistance	Type IV
Most common RTA	Type IV

Acid-Base Disturbances

Name the simple acid/base disturbance
and the associated compensatory
response:

pH > 7.4, P_{CO_2} > 40 mm Hg

Metabolic alkalosis → hypoventilation

pH < 7.4, P_{CO_2} > 40 mm Hg

Respiratory acidosis → renal HCO_3^-
reabsorption

pH > 7.4, P_{CO_2} < 40 mm Hg

Respiratory alkalosis → renal HCO_3^-
secretion

pH < 7.4, P_{CO_2} < 40 mm Hg

Metabolic acidosis → hyperventilation

What is the formula for calculating
anion gap?

$Na^+ - (Cl^- + HCO_3^-)$

What is a normal anion gap range?

8 to 12 mEq/L

List three common causes of nongap
metabolic acidosis:

1. Diarrhea
2. Renal tubular acidosis
3. Hyperchloremia

Name the most common cause of
respiratory acidosis:

Hypoventilation (which can be
caused by acute/chronic lung
disease, sedatives, weakening of
respiratory muscles)

List three common causes of respiratory
alkalosis:

1. Hyperventilation
2. Early aspirin ingestion
3. Gram-negative sepsis

List five common causes of metabolic
alkalosis:

1. Excessive vomiting
2. Diuretic abuse
3. Antacid use
4. Hyperaldosteronism
5. Cushing syndrome

List nine possible causes of anion
gap metabolic acidosis:

"MUD PILERS"

1. Methanol
2. Uremia
3. Diabetic ketoacidosis
4. Paraldehyde
5. Isoniazid (INH) or Iron tablet
   overdose
6. Lactic acidosis
7. Ethylene glycol or Ethanol
8. Rhabdomyolysis (massive)
9. Salicylate toxicity

Acute Renal Failure

List the three main types of acute renal failure (ARF):	1. Prerenal 2. Intrinsic 3. Postrenal
List four common prerenal causes of ARF:	1. Hypovolemia 2. Decreased RBF (eg, decreased cardiac output, renal artery stenosis) 3. High peripheral vascular resistance 4. Drugs (eg, diuretics, NSAIDs)
List five common causes of intrinsic ARF:	1. Acute tubular necrosis (ischemic, nephrotoxic, sepsis) 2. Acute glomerulonephritis 3. Autoimmune vasculitis (eg, lupus, scleroderma) 4. Interstitial nephritis 5. Hemolytic uremic syndrome (children)
What is the general mechanism for the development of postrenal ARF?	Any outflow obstruction (benign prostatic hyperplasia [BPH], bladder-neck, stones, prior gynecologic surgery, bilateral ureteric). **Note:** postrenal ARF accounts for <5% of all causes of ARF.

Name the type of ARF associated with each of the following:

Oliguria and $Fe_{Na} < 1\%$	Prerenal
Oliguria and $Fe_{Na} > 1\%$	Intrinsic
Hyaline urine casts	Prerenal
Muddy brown/granular casts	Intrinsic (muddy brown casts are particularly associated with ATN)
Blood urea nitrogen (BUN): creatinine ratio > 20	Prerenal
Urine osmolality > 500 mOsm	Prerenal

List the effects of uremia on each of the following organs or systems:

Nervous system	Asterixis, confusion, seizures, coma
Cardiovascular system	Fibrinous pericarditis
Hematologic system	Coagulopathy, immunosuppression
Gastrointestinal system	Nausea, vomiting, gastritis
Skin	Pruritis
Endocrine system	Glucose intolerance

List six nonuremic complications of renal failure:	1. Metabolic acidosis 2. Hyperkalemia → arrhythmias 3. Na^+ and H_2O excess → pulmonary edema and congestive heart failure (CHF) 4. Hypocalcemia → osteodystrophy (from failure to secrete active vitamin D) 5. Anemia (↓ EPO secretion) 6. Hypertension (from renin hypersecretion)
Which type of ATN often causes GBM rupture?	Ischemic
What substances cause direct injury to the proximal tubules?	Nephrotoxins: drugs (aminoglycosides), toxins, and massive amounts of myoglobin (typically in the setting of a crush injury or strenuous exercise)

Renal Infections

What infection commonly presents with flank pain, costovertebral angle tenderness, fever, dysuria, pyuria, bacteriuria?	Acute pyelonephritis
What are the two major causes of pyelonephritis?	1. Ascending infection 2. Hematogenous seeding
What are the most common organisms responsible for acute pyelonephritis?	*Escherichia coli* (most common), *Proteus, Klebsiella, Enterobacter, Pseudomonas.* (Think enteric gram-negative rods.)
What is the greatest risk factor for pyelonephritis?	Vesicoureteric reflux (or incompetence)
List five possible sequelae of acute pyelonephritis:	1. Abscess 2. Necrotizing papillitis 3. Renal scars 4. Perinephric abscess 5. Pyonephrosis
What condition is characterized by broad renal scarring, deformed calyces, progressive loss of renal parenchyma, and thyroidization of kidneys?	Chronic pyelonephritis
What finding on microscopic examination of urine is pathognomonic for pyelonephritis?	WBC casts

Tubulointerstitial Diseases

Name the tubulointerstitial disease associated with each of the following clinical scenarios:

Abuse of phenacetin-containing compounds

Renal papillary necrosis

Penicillin and NSAID use; associated with eosinophilia

Interstitial nephritis

AR syndrome characterized by dysfunction of proximal tubules, leading to impaired reabsorption of amino acids, glucose, phosphate, and bicarbonate

Fanconi syndrome

AR disease characterized by impaired tryptophan reabsorption; clinically resembles pellagra

Hartnup disease

AR syndrome characterized by impaired active chloride reabsorption in the loop of Henle; clinically mimics the actions of loop diuretics

Bartter syndrome

Name the five diseases associated with renal papillary necrosis:

1. Diabetes mellitus
2. Acute pyelonephritis
3. Analgesic nephropathy
4. Sickle cell disease
5. Urinary tract obstruction

Renal Vascular Disease

Name the renal vascular pathology associated with each of the following statements:

Macroscopically, kidneys have a fine granular surface; hyaline arteriolosclerosis, interstitial fibrosis, glomerular sclerosis

Benign nephrosclerosis

Hyperplastic arteriolitis (onion-skinning); presents with diastolic BP > 130, encephalopathy, proteinuria, hematuria, and papilledema

Malignant nephrosclerosis

Pediatric syndrome characterized by ARF, microangiopathic hemolytic anemia, thrombocytopenia, and hypertension

Classic hemolytic-uremic syndrome (HUS)

Syndrome characterized by ARF, microangiopathic hemolytic anemia, hypertension, fever, and mental status changes; associated with ADAMTS-13 defect	Thrombotic thrombocytopenic purpura (TTP)
What is the most common cause of HUS?	*Escherichia coli* O157:H7 (75% of cases)
What three groups of patients are at increased risk of developing renal failure from benign nephrosclerosis?	1. African Americans 2. Diabetics 3. Patients with hypertension
What type of infarction typically occurs in the kidneys?	"White," due to end-organ type arterial supply of kidneys
What conditions are associated with diffuse cortical necrosis?	Obstetric catastrophes (eg, severe placental abruption) and septic shock
Name two major causes of renal artery stenosis (RAS):	1. Atherosclerosis (70%) 2. Fibromuscular dysplasia (30%)
What group of people are most likely to have secondary hypertension due to fibromuscular dysplasia-induced RAS?	Women in their 20's and 30's

Urolithiasis

Name the type of renal calculi associated with each of the following statements:

Radiopaque (two types)	1. Calcium stones 2. Struvite stones
Staghorn calculi	Struvite (aka ammonium magnesium phosphate)
Infection with urease-positive bacteria	Struvite (think *Proteus*)
Most common type of calculus	Calcium
Gout (or any other hyperuricemic condition)	Uric acid stones
Elevated PTH	Calcium
Secondary to inherited defect of amino acid transporter	Cystine (due to cystinuria)
What are the signs and symptoms associated with urinary stone disease?	Renal colic (flank pain radiating to groin), hematuria, and pyelonephritis

Renal and Urinary Tract Tumors

What must be ruled out in an older adult with hematuria?

Urinary tract malignancies (renal and bladder)

Name the renal or urinary neoplasm associated with each of the following statements:

Large, palpable flank mass in a toddler

Wilms tumor (aka nephroblastoma) or neuroblastoma

Most common tumor of the renal pelvis

Transitional cell carcinoma

Benign tumor of kidney often associated with tuberous sclerosis

Angiomyolipoma

Most common renal malignancy

Renal cell carcinoma

Clear cells

Renal cell carcinoma

Associated with phenacetin abuse, cigarette smoking, cyclophosphamide, and aniline dyes

Transitional cell carcinoma

Large, benign tumor of kidney, composed of eosinophilic cells; arises from the intercalated cells of collecting duct

Oncocytoma

Secondary polycythemia

Renal cell carcinoma

Associated with *Schistosoma haematobium*

Squamous cell carcinoma of the bladder

Invades renal vein and sometimes IVC

Renal cell carcinoma

Painless hematuria in an older patient who smokes

Transitional cell carcinoma of the bladder

Classically manifests clinically with hematuria, flank pain, and a flank mass

Renal cell carcinoma

Which gene is most commonly altered in clear cell carcinomas?

VHL (von Hippel-Lindau) gene (mutated or hypermethylated)

Which gene is most commonly altered in papillary renal cell carcinomas?

MET

Which hormone is secreted by 5% to 10% of all renal cell carcinomas?

Erythropoeitin

Renal cell carcinomas (RCC) are associated with ectopic production of which other hormones?	ACTH, renin, parathyroid hormone receptor protein (PTHrp), prolactin
Why is RCC often refractory to chemotherapy?	Expression of P-glycoprotein, a marker of multidrug resistance

Name the syndrome characterized by Wilms tumor plus each of the following findings:

Gonadal dysgenesis, nephropathy associated with *WT1* gene mutations	Denys-Drash syndrome
***WT1* gene mutation, aniridia, GU malformations, and mental/ motor retardation**	**WAGR** complex
Organomegaly, hemihypertrophy, macroglossia, gigantism, neonatal hypoglycemia associated with the *WT2* gene	Beckwith-Wiedemann syndrome

Name the most common genetic defect associated with each of the following:

Transitional cell carcinoma	Chromosome 9p and 9q alterations
Renal cell carcinoma	Alterations of chromosome 3 affecting the *VHL* gene
Wilms tumor	Deletion of *WT1* gene (tumor suppressor gene on 11p13)
Beckwith-Wiedemann syndrome	*WT2* gene deletion (11p15.5)
What is the inheritance pattern of Beckwith-Wiedemann syndrome?	Genomic (paternal) imprinting

Urinary System

Name the urinary disease associated with each of the following statements:

Michaelis-Gutmann bodies	Malakoplakia
Fibrous masses over the sacrum and lower aorta that encroach on the ureters causing obstruction and hydronephrosis	Sclerosing retroperitonitis
Disease characterized by chronic bacterial cystitis with yellow and gray plaques in the mucosa of the bladder	Malakoplakia

How does chronic urinary outlet obstruction affect the bladder wall?

Chronic obstruction causes bladder wall hypertrophy

What are the common symptoms of lower urinary tract infection (cystitis)?

Dysuria, frequency, urgency

What is the most common source of bacteria that causes cystitis?

Colon (*E. coli* = 80%)

Why are women at 10 times the risk of men for developing a urinary tract infection (UTI)?

The female urethra is shorter and more likely to be colonized with fecal flora.

List the most common UTI organisms:

"SEEKS PP"

Serratia marcescens

Escherichia coli

Enterobacter cloacae

Klebsiella pneumoniae

Staphylococcus saprophyticus

Proteus mirabilis

Pseudomonas aeruginosa

Which UTI-causing bacterium is frequently nosocomial, drug-resistant, and may produce a red pigment?

Serratia marcescens

Isomorphic red cells in the urine suggest bleeding from what portion of the urinary tract?

Lower urinary tract (ie, nonglomerlular bleeding)

What type of trauma commonly causes extravasation of urine into the superficial perineal space?

Straddle injury (rupture of urethra below urogenital diaphragm)

Name the four types of urinary incontinence:

1. Stress
2. Urge
3. Overflow
4. Total

Name the type of voiding dysfunction or incontinence associated with the following characteristics:

A small urinary bladder and detrusor overactivity resulting in bladder wall thickening

Hypertonic neurogenic bladder

A large urinary bladder and detrusor areflexia that may result in overflow incontinence

Atonic neurogenic bladder

Small amounts of urine leakage associated with coughing, laughing, or straining

Stress incontinence

Leakage of urine associated with sudden, strong need to urinate

Urge incontinence

PHARMACOLOGY—RENAL

For each of the following drugs, provide the following:
1. The mechanism and location of action (MLOA)
2. Indication(s) (IND)
3. Significant side effects and unique toxicity (TOX) (if any)

Furosemide, ethacrynic acid

MLOA: inhibitor of $Na^+/K^+/2Cl^-$ cotransporter in thick ascending loop of Henle

IND: diuresis, hypertension, CHF, and other edematous states (ascites, nephrotic syndrome, etc.)

TOX: "CHIA DOG"

Calciuria

Hypokalemic metabolic alkalosis

Interstitial nephritis

Allergy to sulfa

Dehydration

Ototoxicity

Gout

Spironolactone

MLOA: competitive aldosterone receptor antagonist; acts in collecting duct (CD)

IND: diuresis, CHF

TOX: hyperkalemic metabolic acidosis, gynecomastia, antiandrogen effects

Triamterene and amiloride

MLOA: block Na^+/K^+ channels in collecting duct

IND: used in combination with other diuretics (especially loop and thiazide diuretics) for their K^+-sparing properties

TOX: leg cramps (triamterene)

Acetazolamide	**MLOA:** carbonic anhydrase inhibitor (CAI) $\rightarrow\downarrow$ HCO_3^- reabsorption in PCT $\rightarrow\uparrow$ urine osmolarity **IND:** diuresis, glaucoma **TOX:** metabolic acidosis, ammonia toxicity, neuropathy. **Note:** sulfa allergy
Mannitol	**MLOA:** $\uparrow$ tubular fluid osmolarity $\rightarrow\uparrow$ urine flow; acts in PCT, thin descending limb, and CD **IND:** diuresis, elevated intracranial pressure (ICP) **TOX:** pulmonary edema, dehydration
Thiazides—chlorothiazide, hydrochlorothiazide	**MLOA:** inhibitor of NaCl reabsorption in early DCT $\rightarrow\uparrow$ urine osmolarity **LOA:** DCT **IND:** hypertension, CHF **TOX:** may cause hyperglycemia, hyperlipidemia, hypercalcemia, and allergic response in patients sensitive to sulfa drugs
ACE inhibitors—captopril, lisinopril, enalapril	**MLOA:** inhibitor of ACE $\rightarrow\downarrow$ levels of AT II ($\rightarrow\uparrow$); prevents inactivation of bradykinin (potent vasodilator) **IND:** hypertension, renal protective effects in diabetics, CHF **TOX: "CAPTOPRIL"** Cough Angioedema Proteinuria Taste changes HypOtension Pregnancy issues (fetal renal toxicity) Rash Increased renin and K^+ Lowers AT II **Contraindicated in bilateral RAS**
Losartan	**MLOA:** AT II receptor antagonist **IND:** hypertension **TOX:** dizziness, headache; teratogenic
Demeclocycline	**MLOA:** ADH antagonist in CD **IND:** SIADH

Name the diuretic of choice in the following situations:

Diuresis in sulfa-allergic patient	Ethacrynic acid
Hypercalcemia	Loop diuretics (eg, furosemide)
Hyperaldosteronism	Spironolactone
Nephrogenic DI	Thiazide diuretics (eg, chlorothiazide)
Severe edematous states	Loop diuretics (eg, furosemide)
Elevated ICP	Mannitol
Altitude sickness	Acetazolamide
Calcium stones	Thiazide diuretics (eg, chlorothiazide)
Used in shock to maintain RBF	Mannitol

Which diuretics decrease blood pH? CAIs and K^+-sparing diuretics

Which diuretics increase blood pH? Loop and thiazide diuretics

Which diuretics increase urinary Ca^{2+}? Loop diuretics and spironolactone

Which diuretics decrease urinary Ca^{2+}? Thiazide diuretics and amiloride

Which diuretics increase urinary NaCl? All classes

CHAPTER 10

Hematology and Oncology

EMBRYOLOGY

From what embryonic layer are angioblasts derived?

Mesoderm

Name the site(s) of red blood cell (RBC) production during each of the following developmental phases:

First trimester

Yolk sac

Second trimester

Liver and spleen

Third trimester

Central and peripheral skeleton

Postpartum

Axial skeleton

PATHOLOGY

Coagulopathy

What is the most common inherited hypercoagulable state?

Factor V Leiden

The factor V Leiden mutation inhibits factor V cleavage by which protein?

Protein C

What is the effect of estrogen, endogenous or exogenous, on thrombosis?

Estrogen induces a hypercoagulable state.

What clotting factors require vitamin K for their synthesis?

Factors II, VII, IX, X, and proteins C and S

What common laboratory test is used to assess the intrinsic coagulation system?

Partial thromboplastin time (PTT)

What common laboratory test is used to assess the extrinsic coagulation pathway?

Prothrombin time (PT)

What commonly used anticoagulant interferes with the extrinsic pathway?

Warfarin. **Remember: "WEPT"**— Warfarin affects the Extrinsic pathway and is monitored by **PT**.

The use of the chelator, ethylene diamine tetra acetate (EDTA), as an anticoagulant, in tubes is designed to inactivate what factor in the blood?

Calcium

What inhibitor of the coagulation cascade inactivates factors Va and VIIIa?

Protein C

What are the two major functions of von Willebrand factor?

1. Transport of factor VIII
2. Linkage of platelets and collagen

Dysfunction of what clotting component results in mucous membrane hemorrhage, petechiae, purpura, and prolonged bleeding time?

Platelet abnormalities

Dysfunction of what clotting component results in hemarthroses, purpura, and prolonged PT and/or PTT?

Coagulation factor abnormalities

Name the coagulopathy associated with the following clinical and pathologic features:

Most common hereditary bleeding disorder

von Willebrand disease

Most common type of hemophilia

Hemophilia A (factor VIII deficiency)

Most common cause of acquired platelet dysfunction

Aspirin use

Autosomal dominant (AD) disorder causing increased bleeding time

von Willebrand disease

Autosomal recessive (AR) defect in platelet adhesion caused by lack of GpIIb/IX

Bernard-Soulier disease

AR defect in platelet aggregation caused by deficiency of GpIIb/ GpIIIa, a membrane receptor responsible for binding fibrinogen	Glanzmann thrombasthenia
Common presentation includes hemarthroses and easy bruising, ↑ PTT, normal PT	Hemophilia (A and B)
Prolonged bleeding time with normal platelet count, normal PT, and ↑ PTT	von Willebrand disease
Prolonged PT, PTT, ↑ bleeding time, thrombocytopenia, presence of fibrin split products	Disseminated intravascular coagulation (DIC)
Normal PT, PTT, normal platelet count, ↑ bleeding time	Aspirin use
Syndrome characterized by antiplatelet antibodies (commonly anti-Ib-IX or IIb-IIIa), often post-viral infections	Idiopathic thrombocytopenia (ITP)
Syndrome characterized by thrombocytopenia, microangiopathic hemolytic anemia, fever, and neurologic symptoms	Thrombotic thrombocytopenic purpura (TTP)
Widespread hyaline microthrombi in arterioles and capillaries causing schistocytes and helmet cells	Microangiopathic hemolytic anemia
Splenomegaly, epistaxis, petechiae, generalized tender lymphadenopathy, serum antibodies (+)	SLE-autoimmune thrombocytopenia

Anemias

List five of the most common causes of microcytic anemia:	1. Iron deficiency 2. Lead poisoning 3. Chronic disease (sometimes normocytic) 4. Sideroblastic 5. Thalassemia
List four of the most common causes of normocytic anemia:	1. Sickle cell anemia 2. Aplastic anemia 3. Acute blood loss 4. Hemolytic anemia

List five of the most common causes of macrocytic anemia:	1. Liver disease 2. Vitamin B_{12} deficiency 2. Folate deficiency 4. Alcoholism 5. Hypothyroidism
What is the primary site of iron absorption? Vitamin B_{12}? Folate?	Duodenum; terminal ileum (need intrinsic factor); jejunum (respectively)
What is the major cause of iron deficiency anemia in adults?	Menorrhagia or gastrointestinal (GI) bleeding (ie, colon cancer, ulcers)
What are two common clinical complaints in an anemic patient?	1. Dyspnea on exertion 2. Fatigue
Which amino acid substitution in the β-globin gene is most commonly seen in sickle cell anemia?	Glu6 → Val
What is the major type of hemoglobin in homozygous sickle cell anemia?	HbS
In sickle cell disease, what is the mechanism of ischemic necrosis of the bones, lungs, liver, brain, spleen, or penis?	↓ O_2 tension → abnormal RBCs sickle → microvascular occlusions
What is the major regulatory enzyme in heme biosynthesis?	Aminolevulinate (ALA) synthase
What two common enzyme deficiencies can cause hemolytic anemia?	1. Glucose-6-phosphate dehydrogenase (G6PD) 2. Pyruvate kinase
What hemolytic anemia is associated with exposure to oxidant stress?	G6PD deficiency
What two common RBC membrane defects can cause hemolytic anemia?	1. Hereditary spherocytosis 2. Paroxysmal nocturnal hematuria (PNH)
What common cause of atypical pneumonia is associated with cold autoimmune hemolytic anemia?	*Mycoplasma pneumoniae*
What type of anemia is caused by lack of intrinsic factor (IF) secretion by gastric parietal cells?	Pernicious anemia (vitamin B_{12} deficiency)

What two autoimmune diseases of the GI tract can cause megaloblastic anemia?

1. Pernicious anemia (due to lack of IF production)
2. Crohn disease of the distal ileum (due to lack of IF-B_{12} complex reabsorption)

What parasites are capable of causing megaloblastic anemia?

Diphyllobothrium latum (by depleting B_{12}) and *Giardia lamblia* (by depleting folate)

How does gastric resection cause megaloblastic anemia?

Parietal cells, which are responsible for IF production may be removed when the gastric fundus is resected.

What type of malignancy is associated with pernicious anemia?

Gastric carcinoma

Name three medications capable of causing autoimmune hemolytic anemia:

1. Penicillin
2. Cephalosporins
3. Quinidine

What types of malignancies are associated with autoimmune hemolytic anemia?

Leukemias and lymphomas

What laboratory tests are seen in hemolytic anemia?

↑ Unconjugated bilirubin, ↑ urine urobilinogen, ↓ hemoglobin, hemoglobinuria, ↓ haptoglobin, hemosiderosis

Name two commonly used medications that can cause aplastic anemia:

1. Nonsteroidal anti-inflammatory drugs (NSAIDs)
2. Chloramphenicol

What happens to the total iron binding capacity (TIBC), serum iron concentration, and percent saturation of transferrin in each of the following diseases?

Iron deficiency anemia

↑ TIBC, ↓ serum iron, ↓ % saturation

Anemia of chronic disease

↓ TIBC, ↓ serum iron, normal saturation

Iron overload

Normal TIBC, ↑ serum iron, maximal saturation

Name the type(s) of anemia associated with the following clinical and pathologic features:

Most common type of anemia

Iron deficiency anemia

Abnormal Schilling test

Pernicious anemia

ABO incompatibility, lymphoid neoplasm, Raynaud phenomena, anti-i antibodies	Cold autoimmune hemolytic anemia
Atrophic glossitis	Pernicious anemia
Autosplenectomy	Sickle cell anemia
Basophlilic stipling of erythrocytes, blue/gray discoloration at gumline, wrist/foot drop	Anemia from lead poisoning
Celiac sprue	Folate deficiency anemia (megaloblastic)
Chronic atrophic gastritis	Pernicious anemia
Colon cancer	Iron deficiency anemia (early) and anemia of chronic disease (late)
Crescent-shaped erythrocytes and Howell-Jolly bodies	Sickle cell anemia
Deficiency of α- or β-*globin* gene synthesis	Thalassemia
Deficiency of decay accelerating factor	Paroxysmal nocturnal hemoglobinuria
Demyelination of the dorsal and lateral tracts of the spinal cord	Pernicious anemia
End-stage liver disease	Macrocytic anemia
Helmet cells, burr cells, triangular cells	Microangiopathic anemia (2° to DIC, thrombotic thrombocytopenic purpura-hemolytic-uremic syndrome [TTP-HUS], or mechanical heart valves)
Hypersegmented polymorphonuclears (PMNs)	Vitamin B_{12} or folate deficiency anemia
Increased serum lactate dehydrogenase (LDH)	Hemolytic anemia
Microcytosis, atrophic glossitis, esophageal webs (Plummer-Vinson syndrome)	Iron deficiency anemia
Pancytopenia and fatty infiltration of bone marrow	Aplastic anemia
Systemic lupus erythematosus (SLE), chronic lymphocytic leukemia (CLL), lymphomas, drugs; + direct Coombs test (due to IgG autoantibodies)	Warm autoimmune hemolytic anemia
AD deficiency of spectrin, positive osmotic fragility test	Hereditary spherocytosis

Reduced erythropoietin	Anemia of chronic disease
Ringed sideroblasts	Sideroblastic anemia
Susceptibility to infection by encapsulated organisms	Sickle cell anemia (from splenic autoinfarction)
Transient normocytic anemia	Anemia of acute blood loss

What is the genetic defect in thalassemias?

Splicing defect, causing decreased α or β sub-chain production

Name the type of thalassemia responsible for each of the following findings:

β-Thalassemia associated with growth retardation, frontal bossing, and hepatosplenomegaly (HSM) (from extramedullary hematopoesis), jaundice, and iron overload (2° to transfusions), and ↑ Hgb F

β-Thalassemia major (β–/β–); **Note:** β-thalassemia minor (β+/β–), typically asymptomatic

α-Thalassemia associated with mild microcytic anemia, usually asymptomatic

α-Thalassemia minor (two alleles affected); **Note:** when only one allele involved (carrier state) → no anemia

α-Thalassemia associated with pallor, splenomegaly, chronic hemolytic anemia, and intraerythrocytic inclusions

Hgb H disease (three alleles affected)

α-Thalassemia associated with stillborn fetus

Hydrops fetalis (all four alleles affected)

White Blood Cell (WBC) Neoplasms

What are the two major categories of lymphoma?

1. Hodgkin disease (HD)
2. Non-Hodgkin lymphoma (NHL)

Name the general type of lymphoma (HD or NHL) associated with the following clinical and pathologic features:

Interleukin (IL)-5 secreting Reed Sternberg (RS) cells	HD
Commonly arises from B cells	NHL
Constitutional symptoms including fever, night sweats, weight loss	Both
Mediastinal lymphadenopathy, contiguous spread	HD

Many cases associated with Epstein-Barr virus (EBV)	HD
Peripheral lymphadenopathy, noncontiguous spread	NHL
Bimodal age distribution, but most common in young men	HD
Peak incidence from 20 to 40 years of age	NHL
Associated with immunosuppression including AIDS	NHL
Painful lymphadenopathy with alcohol consumption	HD

Name the type of HD associated with each of the following clinical and pathologic findings:

Most common type	Nodular sclerosis
Abundance of RS cells	Mixed cellularity
Lacunar cells and collagen banding	Nodular sclerosis
Commonly seen in older patients with HD	Mixed cellularity
Widely disseminated disease with poor prognosis	Lymphocyte depletion
More common in females	Nodular sclerosis
Abundance of lymphocytes	Lymphocyte predominance
Commonly seen in men < 35 years presenting with cervical or axillary lymphadenopathy	Lymphocyte predominance
High proportion of RS cells relative to lymphocytes	Lymphocyte depletion

Name the type of NHL associated with each of the following clinical and pathologic findings:

Overexpression of cyclin D1	Mantle cell lymphoma
Starry-sky appearance on histopathology	Burkitt lymphoma
Clinically similar to CLL; characterized by nodules of small lymphocytes	Small cell lymphocytic lymphoma
Older adults with *BCL2* gene mutations	Follicular lymphoma

Often appears at extranodal sites and can cause small bowel obstruction	Diffuse large cell lymphoma
Child presenting with enlarging mandibular mass	Burkitt lymphoma
Common in children who present with a mediastinal mass and a syndrome similar to that of acute lymphocytic leukemia (ALL)	Lymphoblastic lymphoma
TdT+ lymphocytes	Precursor B- or T-cell acute lymphoblastic leukemia/lymphoma
Endemic in Africa and associated with EBV	Burkitt lymphoma

Name the specific leukemia associated with the following age brackets:

0 to 14 years old	ALL
15 to 39 years old	AML
40 to 59 years old	AML and CML
> 60 years old	CLL

Name the specific leukemia associated with each of the following findings:

Very high white cell counts, often > 200,000	Chronic myelogenous leukemia (CML)
Isolated lymphocytosis	CLL
TdT+ lymphoblasts	ALL
Large, immature myeloblasts predominate	Acute myelogenous leukemia (AML)
Neoplastic pre-T or pre-B lymphocytes, CD10 ⊕	ALL
CD19/CD20 and CD5 ⊕ malignant cells	CLL
Bone marrow is replaced with myeloblasts	AML
Philadelphia chromosome t(9:22)	CML
Auer rods	AML (M3 > M2 > M1)
Low leukocytic alkaline phosphatase	CML (also seen in paroxysmal nocturnal hematuria)
Associated with fatigue, thrombocytopenia, signs of anemia, frequent infections, leukemia cutis, and DIC	AML (M3)

Bone pain, fever, generalized lymphadenopathy, HSM, and signs of central nervous system (CNS) spread	ALL
Excellent prognosis if treated early	ALL
May progress to AML	CML
Most responsive to therapy	ALL
Associated with prior exposure to radiation	CML
Peripheral leukocytes containing tartarate-resistant acid phosphatase (TRAP) and cytoplasmic projections	Hairy cell leukemia (**Remember:** *"TRAP the Hairy beast")*

Myeloproliferative Disorders

Name the four chronic myeloproliferative disorders:	1. CML 2. Polycythemia vera 3. Essential thrombocytosis 4. Myelofibrosis with myeloid metaplasia

Name the myeloproliferative disorder associated with each of the following clinical and pathologic findings:

↑ RBC mass and low/normal erythropoietin	Polycythemia vera
Tear drop deformity of erythrocytes, bone marrow hypercellularity	Myelofibrosis with myeloid metaplasia
Plethoric complexion, pruritus after showering, blurred vision, splenomegaly, and epistaxis	Polycythemia vera
Erythromelalgia (throbbing or burning of hands and feet)	Essential thrombocytosis
Basophilia	Polycythemia vera
Widespread extramedullary hematopoesis with megakaryocytic proliferation in the bone marrow	Myelofibrosis with myeloid metaplasia
Hyperviscosity syndrome	Polycythemia vera and essential thrombocytosis
Peripheral thrombocytosis, bone marrow megakaryocytosis, and splenomegaly	Essential thrombocytosis

Name the plasma cell disorder associated with the following clinical and pathologic findings:

Bone pain, osteopenia, pathologic fractures, and "punched-out" lytic lesions on x-ray	Multiple myeloma
Russel bodies and "plymphocytes" (plasmacytoid lymphocytes)	Waldenstrom macroglobulinemia
Bence-Jones proteinuria	Multiple myeloma and Waldenstrom macroglobulinemia
Small M-spike on plasma electrophoresis in an otherwise healthy patient	Monoclonal gammopathy of undetermined significance (MGUS)
Hypercalcemia; renal insufficiency	Multiple myeloma
Hyperviscosity syndrome	Waldenstrom macroglobulinemia
Large M-spike on plasma electrophoresis	Multiple myeloma and Waldenstrom macroglobulinemia
Primary amyloidosis	Multiple myeloma

Peripheral Blood Smear

Name the condition associated with each of the following peripheral blood smear findings:

Defective PMN degranulation → accumulation of giant granules in PMNs and other leukocytes	Chediak-Higashi anomaly
Atypical lymphocytes	Infectious mononucleosis
Large numbers of Auer rods (Faggot cells)	AML (M3 subtype)
Basophilic stippling	Lead poisoning
Burr cells (echinocytes)	Burns, uremia
Dumbbell-shaped bilobed nuclei	Pelger-Huet anomaly
Giant platelets	Bernard-Soulier disease, May-Hegglin anomaly
Heinz bodies, bite cells	G6PD deficiency
Helmet cells, schistocytes	Microangiopathic hemolytic anemia (DIC, TTP, HUS)
Howell-Jolly bodies	Asplenia
Hypersegmented PMN nuclei	Megaloblastic anemia
Intracytoplasmic rings	Malaria, babesiosis

Lymphocytic cerebriform nuclei	Sézary syndrome
Nucleated erythrocytes	Hemolytic anemia
Rouleau formation	Multiple myeloma and Waldenstrom macroglobulinemia
Small platelets	Wiskott-Aldrich syndrome
Smudge cells	CLL
Spherocytes	Hereditary spherocytosis
Spur cells (acanthocytes)	Abetalipoproteinemia, liver disease
Target cells (codocytes)	Thalassemias, iron deficiency anemia, liver disease, sickle cell anemia
Teardrop cells (dacryocytes)	Myelofibrosis
Toxic granulations in leukocytes (Dohle bodies)	Sepsis

Chromosomal Translocations

Name the neoplasm associated with the following chromosomal translocations and genes/gene products:

t(11:14) protooncogene under Ig promoter	Mantle cell lymphoma
t(11:22) EWS (EWS-FLI1 fusion protein)	Ewing sarcoma
t(14:18) *BCL2*	Follicular lymphoma
t(15:17) (PML/RAR-β [retinoic acid receptor alpha])	AML (M3 subtype, treated with retinoic acid)
t(3:6) VHL	von Hippel-Lindau syndrome (t[3:8] and t[3:11] are two common variants seen in VHL)
t(8:14) c-myc and IgH	Burkitt lymphoma (t[8:22] and t[2:8] are two common variants seen in Burkitt lymphoma)
t(9:22) bcr-abl fusion protein	CML (treated with imatinib)

Tumor Markers

Name the neoplasm associated with the following tumor markers:

α_1-AT	Liver cancer, yolk-sac tumors
α-Fetoprotein (AFP)	Germ cell tumors, hepatocellular carcinoma

Alkaline phosphatase	Metastatic bone involvement, Paget disease
β-HCG	Hydatiform moles, Choriocarcinoma, Gestational trophoblastic tumors
CA-125	Ovarian cancers
Carcinoembryonic antigen (CEA)	Colon, pancreatic, and other cancers of the GI tract
Prostate-specific antigen (PSA)	Prostate cancer
S-100	Melanoma, neural tumors

Cancer Genetics

For each of the following tumor suppressor genes, state the function and the malignancy/malignancies they are associated with:

APC	**Function:** regulation of β-catenin in the Wnt/β-catenin signaling pathway—promotes cell adhesion and regulates cell proliferation **Associated malignancies:** familial adenomatosis polyposis (FAP) and many GI cancers
BRCA1 and *BRCA2*	**Function:** DNA repair and transcriptional regulation **Associated malignancies:** breast and ovarian cancers
NF1 and *NF2*	**Function:** regulates signal transduction through the ras pathway **Associated malignancies:** neurofibromas, schwannomas; (NF-2 also associated with meningioma)
p16	**Function:** regulates cell cycle by inhibiting cyclin-dependent kinases **Associated malignancies:** pancreatic and esophageal carcinomas and malignant melanoma
p53	**Function:** regulates cell death and proliferation in response to DNA damage **Associated malignancies:** most human cancers

Rb

Function: regulates transition from G1 to S in the cell cycle by sequestering E2Fs, a family of transcription factors

Associated malignancies: retinoblastoma, osteosarcoma

WT1

Function: inhibits transcription of genes promoting cell proliferation

Associated malignancies: Wilms tumor

For each of the following oncogenes, state the function and the malignancy/ malignancies they are associated with:

abl

Function: promotes cell proliferation through tyrosine kinase activity

Associated malignancies: CML, ALL

BCL2

Function: overexpression prolongs cell survival by inhibiting apoptosis

Associated malignancies: follicular and undifferentiated lymphomas

cyclin D

Function: promotes cell proliferation by stimulating the phosphorylation of pRb

Associated malignancies: lymphoma, breast, liver, and esophageal cancers

CDK4

Function: promotes cell proliferation by phosphorylating pRb

Associated malignancies: sarcoma, glioblastoma multiforme, malignant melanoma

HER2/neu

Function: amplification promotes cell proliferation by enhancing growth factor signal transduction

Associated malignancies: breast, ovarian, lung, stomach cancers

myc

Function: promotes cell proliferation by transcriptional activation of specific genes

Associated malignancies: Burkitt lymphoma, small cell carcinoma of the lung, neuroblastoma

ras

Function: signal transduction through the MAP kinase pathway

Associated malignancies: colon cancer and many other human cancers

ret	**Function:** receptor tyrosine kinase that promotes cell proliferation in response to growth factors
	Associated malignancies: multiple endocrine neoplasia 2A and 2B; familial medullary thyroid carcinoma
sis	**Function:** β-chain of PDGF which promotes cell proliferation
	Associated malignancies: astrocytomas, osteosarcomas

Miscellaneous Oncology

Name the type of neoplasm associated with the following diseases:

Actinic keratosis	Squamous cell carcinomas of skin
AIDS	Aggressive malignant lymphomas, Kaposi sarcoma, brain lymphomas
Barrett esophagitis	Esophageal adenocarcinoma
Chronic atrophic gastritis	Gastric adenocarcinoma
Cirrhosis	Hepatocellular carcinoma
Down syndrome	ALL
Dysplastic nevus	Malignant melanoma
Immunodeficiency states	NHL
Myasthenia gravis	Thymoma
Paget disease of bone	Secondary osteosarcoma and fibrosarcoma
Plummer-Vinson syndrome	Squamous cell carcinomas of esophagus
Tuberous sclerosis	Astrocytoma and cardiac rhabdomyosarcoma
Ulcerative colitis	Colonic adenocarcinoma
Xeroderma pigmentosa	Squamous and basal cell carcinomas of skin

List the four major differences between benign and malignant neoplasms:

1. Differentiation and anaplasia
2. Rate of growth
3. Local invasion
4. Metastases (most important difference)

What are the three ways a tumor can spread?	1. Invasion of lymphatic system (eg, carcinoma of the breast) 2. Hematogenous (typical of sarcomas) 3. Seeding of body cavity (eg, ovarian cancer)
What four classes of genes are the primary targets for genetic mutation leading to cancer?	1. Protooncogenes (promote cellular growth) 2. Tumor suppressor genes (inhibit cellular growth) 3. Genes that regulate and mediate apoptosis 4. Genes that regulate and mediate DNA repair
What three genetic mechanisms can lead to the activation of protooncogenes?	1. Point mutations 2. Chromosomal rearrangements 3. Amplification
What three chromosomal abnormalities are characteristic of tumor cells?	1. Amplification 2. Deletion 3. Translocation
What three factors influence tumor growth?	1. Doubling time of tumor cells 2. Cell proliferation 3. Cell death (apoptosis)
Name the six small, round, blue cell tumors of childhood:	1. Ewing sarcoma 2. Lymphoma 3. Neuroblastoma 4. Medulloblastoma 5. Rhabdomyosarcoma 6. Primitive neuroectodermal tumors

Chemical Carcinogens

What are the two steps in the process of chemical carcinogenesis?	1. Initiation: cells undergo irreversible genetic mutation. 2. Promotion: chemicals promote growth of initiated cells.
Name the neoplasm associated with each of the following chemical, viral, and microbial carcinogens and types of radiant energy:	
Aflatoxin	Hepatocellular carcinoma
Aniline dyes	Bladder cancer
Aromatic hydrocarbons	Lung cancer (aromatic hydrocarbons found in cigarettes)

Asbestos	Malignant mesothelioma
EBV	Burkitt lymphoma, nasopharyngeal cancer, B-cell lymphoma in AIDS patients, some types of HD
Estrogen	Breast carcinoma and endometrial carcinoma
Helicobacter pylori	Gastric adenocarcinoma and marginal zone lymphoma (MALToma)
Hepatitis B virus	Hepatocellular carcinoma
Human papilloma virus	Cervical squamous cell carcinoma and genital warts
Human T-cell lymphocytic virus-1 (HTLV-1)	T-cell leukemia/lymphoma
Ionizing radiation	Myeloid leukemias and thyroid cancers
Nitrosamines	Gastric cancer
Polyvinylchloride (PVC) assembly	Hepatic hemangiosarcoma
Ultraviolet radiation	Skin cancers
Schistosoma haematobium	Squamous cell carcinoma of the urinary bladder

Paraneoplastic Syndromes

Name the process of profound weight loss and weakness due to muscle and fat loss in a patient with an advanced neoplasm:	Cancer cachexia
Name the tumor associated with the following paraneoplastic syndromes:	
Acanthosis nigracans	Many types of visceral malignancies
Carcinoid syndrome	Carcinoid and neuroendocrine carcinomas of the bronchi or GI tract
Clubbing of fingers	Pulmonary or thoracic malignancies
Cushing syndrome	Adrenocorticotropic hormone (ACTH)-secreting pituitary adenoma or a cortisol-secreting adrenal adenoma
DIC	AML (M3)
Hypercalcemia	Parathyroid hormone (PTH)-secreting squamous cell carcinoma of the lung
Lambert-Eaton myasthenic syndrome	Small cell carcinoma of the lung

Thrombophlebitis

Pancreatic or lung adenocarcinoma

Syndrome of inappropriate antidiuretic hormone (SIADH)

Antidiuretic hormone (ADH)-secreting small cell carcinoma of the lung

PHARMACOLOGY

Medication for Anemia

Name the drug of choice for each of the following groups of anemic patients:

Adolescent girls with heavy periods and pregnant women

Iron

Patients on methotrexate who develop megaloblastic anemia

Folate

Elderly patients with atrophic gastritis who develop megaloblastic anemia

Cyanocobalamin (vitamin B_{12})

Patients with anemia secondary to end-stage renal disease

Erythropoietin

Patients with extremely low WBC count and prone to infection

G-CSF, GM-CSF

Chemotherapeutic Agents

For each of the following drugs, provide:
1. **The mechanism of action (MOA)**
2. **Indication(s) (IND)**
3. **Significant side effects and unique toxicity (TOX) (if any)**

Methotrexate

MOA: folate analog that inhibits dihydrofolate reductase and, consequently, S phase of the cell cycle

IND: leukemia, lymphoma, carcinoma, sarcoma

TOX: myelosuppression (reversible with leucovorin)

5-Fluorouracil

MOA: inhibits pyrimidine synthesis which inhibits S phase progression

IND: colon cancer and other solid tumors

TOX: myelosuppression and phototoxicity

Cytarabine

MOA: inhibits pyrimidine synthesis which inhibits S phase progression

IND: acute leukemias

TOX: neurotoxicity

6-Mercaptopurine or 6-thioguanine

MOA: inhibits purine synthesis which inhibits S phase progression

IND: leukemia, lymphoma

TOX: myelosuppression, hepatotoxicity

Busulfan

MOA: DNA alkylating agent

IND: palliative role in CML treatment

TOX: pulmonary fibrosis, hyperpigmentation

Cyclophosphamide

MOA: DNA alkylating agent

IND: NHL, breast and ovarian carcinomas

TOX: hemorrhagic cystitis (prevented with mesna), myelosuppression

Nitrosureas (carmustine, lomustine, streptozocin)

MOA: DNA alkylating agent capable of crossing the blood-brain barrier

IND: brain tumors

TOX: CNS toxicity including dizziness and ataxia

Cisplatin

MOA: DNA alkylating agent

IND: testicular cancer, female reproductive tract cancers, bladder and testicular cancers

TOX: nephrotoxicity and acoustic nerve damage

Doxorubicin/adriamycin

MOA: intercalates into DNA and inhibits DNA replication

IND: Hodgkin disease, myeloma, sarcoma, solid tumors

TOX: cardiotoxicity, alopecia, myelosuppression

Bleomycin

MOA: intercalates into DNA and causes DNA strand breaks

IND: testicular cancer, lymphomas

TOX: pulmonary fibrosis, myelosuppression

Etoposide

MOA: inhibits topoisomerase, causing double-stranded breaks in DNA

IND: small cell carcinoma of lung, prostate cancer, testicular cancer

TOX: Bone marrow suppression, hypotension

Prednisone

MOA: may trigger apoptosis

IND: CLL, HD, lymphomas

TOX: cushingoid reaction, immunosuppression, cataracts, acne, osteoporosis, hypertension (HTN), peptic ulcers, hyperglycemia

Tamoxifen/raloxifene

MOA: estrogen receptor agonist/ antagonist

IND: breast cancer

TOX: increased risk of endometrial cancer

Vinblastine/vincristine

MOA: binds tubulin to inhibit formation of the mitotic spindle

IND: HD, lymphoma, Wilms tumor, choriocarcinoma

TOX: vincristine: peripheral neuropathy and paralytic ileus; vinblastine: myelosuppression

Paclitaxel

MOA: binds tubulin and prevents disassembly of the mitotic spindle

IND: ovarian and breast cancers

TOX: myelosuppression, hypersensitivity

Anticoagulants

What test is used to monitor anticoagulation in a patient treated with heparin?

PTT

What test is used to monitor anticoagulation in a patient treated with warfarin?

PT

Warfarin

MOA: causes synthesis of dysfunctional vitamin K-dependent clotting factors (II, VII, IX, X)

IND: chronic treatment and prophylaxis of DVT

TOX: hemorrhage, teratogenic, osteoporosis

Heparin

MOA: increases PTT by activating antithrombin III

IND: acute treatment of DVT, pulmonary embolus, angina, myocardial infarction (MI), ischemic stroke

TOX: hemorrhage, Heparin-Induced Thrombocytopenia Syndrome (**HITS**)

Low-molecular-weight heparin (LMWH) (eg, enoxaparin)

MOA: similar to heparin

IND: anticoagulation outside of the hospital, commonly for DVT

Thrombolytics (streptokinase, urokinase, tissue plasminogen activator, anistreplase)

MOA: facilitate the conversion of plasminogen to plasmin, which cleaves thrombin and fibrin clots

IND: acute therapy for MI and ischemic stroke

TOX: hemorrhage

Clopidogrel and ticlopidine

MOA: antiplatelet agent that blocks adenosine diphosphate (ADP) receptors to inhibit platelet aggregation

IND: acute coronary syndrome, interventional cardiology procedures, transient ischemic attacks, and stroke

TOX: hemorrhage, leukopenia, diarrhea

Eptifibatide and tirofiban

MOA: prevent platelet aggregation by blocking glycoprotein IIb/IIIa receptors

IND: acute coronary syndromes

TOX: hemorrhage

CHAPTER 11

Skin and Connective Tissues

EMBRYOLOGY/ANATOMY/HISTOLOGY

Name the embryonic structures that
give rise to each of the following:

    Epidermis

    Ectoderm

    Melanocytes

    Neural crest cells

Name the layers of the epidermis:

"Californians Like Girls in String
Bikinis" (from surface → base)

Stratum Corneum

Stratum Lucidum (lacking in thin skin
of face and genitalia)

Stratum Granulosum

Stratum Spinosum

Stratum Basalis

What epidermal dendritic cells are
responsible for antigen presentation?

Langerhans cells

Name the type of collagen described
by the following statements:

    Found in Bone, tendons, skin, fascia,
cornea, and dentin; replaces reticulin
later in wound repair

    Type I (**Remember:** bONE)

    Found in Cartilage, nucleus pulposus,
and ocular vitreous body

    Type II (**Remember:** carTWOlage)

    Found in skin, blood vessels, uterus,
fetal tissues, and involved in early
wound repair (granulation tissue)

    Type III (Reticulin)

    Component of Basement membrane
or basal lamina

    Type IV (**Remember:** type IV, under the
floor/basement membrane)

Found at epiphyseal plates	Type X
Accounts for ~90% of collagen in the body	Type I

Mnemonic for collagen types I to IV	"Be Cool, Read Books"

Name the epithelial cell specialization described by the following statements:

Allows adjacent cells to communicate via connexons	Gap junction. **Note:** missing in cancer cells
Connects cells to underlying extracellular matrix	Hemidesmosomes
Extends around entire perimeter; contains E-cadherin and actin filaments	Zona adherens
Prevents diffusion across intracellular space; extends around entire perimeter	Zona occludens (tight junction)
Small, discrete sites of attachment; contains desmoplakin and keratin	Macula adherens (desmosome)

Helical array of polymerized dimmers of α and β tubulin	Microtubules

How are the internal structures of cilia organized?	9 + 2 arrangement of microtubules (9 doublets around 2 central microtubules)

Which enzyme causes bending of cilia and how does it work?	Dynein is an adenosine triphosphatase (ATPase) that links the 9 doublets and causes bending by differential sliding.

Name the cytoskeletal elements that perform the following functions:

Microvilli, muscular contraction, cytokinesis, adhering junction	Actin and myosin
Cilia, flagella, mitotic spindle, neurons, centrioles	Microtubules
Vimentin, desmin, cytokeratin, glial fibrillary acid protein, neurofilaments	Intermediate filaments

Where are apocrine sweat glands found?	Axilla, mons pubis, and anal regions

PATHOLOGY

Give the dermatologic term for each
of the following descriptions:

Flat, nonpalpable, circumscribed lesion < 1 cm in diameter; different color than surrounding skin	Macule
A macule > 1 cm in diameter	Patch
Palpable, solid, elevated skin lesion ≤5 mm in diameter	Papule
A papule > 5 mm in diameter	Plaque
Fluid-containing blister < 0.5 cm in diameter	Vesicle
Fluid-containing blister > 0.5 cm in diameter	Bulla
Pus-filled, raised area	Pustule
Solid, round lesion; diameter = thickness, > 5 mm in diameter	Nodule

Name the dermatologic disorder
characterized by the following
descriptions:

Autosomal recessive (AR) defect in melanin synthesis → predisposition to multiple skin disorders	Albinism (oculocutaneous)
Acquired loss of epidermal melanocytes → depigmented white patches	Vitiligo
Masklike facial hyperpigmentation associated with pregnancy	Melasma
Tan-brown, evenly pigmented, localized overgrowth of melanin-forming cells of the skin present at birth with benign behavior and variable histology	Nevocellular nevus (mole)
Often multiple, atypical, irregularly pigmented lesions and on non-sun-exposed skin, that have the potential to transform into malignant melanoma	Dysplastic nevus
Eruption of comedones and pustules; ↑ during puberty and adolescence; associated with proliferation of *Propionibacterium*	Acne vulgaris

Umbilicated, pearly, dome-shaped papules typically occurring in the genitals; caused by poxvirus infection	Molluscum contagiosum
Benign papilloma caused by HPV infection, most commonly found on dorsum of hand; koilocytes are characteristic	Verruca vulgaris (common wart)
Common benign neoplasm of older adults; sharply demarcated, tan-brown plaques with a "pasted on" appearance	Seborrheic keratosis (senile keratosis)
Benign, flesh-colored, dome-shaped, > 1 cm nodule with central keratin-filled plug-craterlike that resembles squamous cell carcinoma; may resolve without treatment	Keratoacanthoma
Yellowish papules or nodules that tend to occur on the eyelids; associated with hypercholesterolemia	Xanthoma (on the eyelids = xanthelasma)
Accumulation of excessive dermal collagen that can occur following skin trauma; results in large, raised tumorlike scar	Keloid
Proliferation of Langerhans cells; electron microscopy (EM) shows Birbeck granules	Histiocytosis X
A T-cell lymphoproliferative disease arising in the skin; initially simulates eczema or other inflammatory dermatoses	Mycosis fungoides (cutaneous T-cell lymphoma)
Rough, scaling epidermal lesion, usually < 1 cm, due to chronic sunlight exposure; may be a precursor for squamous cell carcinoma	Actinic keratosis
Thickened, hyperpigmented skin in the flexural areas; may be suggestive of visceral malignancy	Acanthosis nigricans
Capillary hemangioma appearing as a purple-red area on the face or neck	Port-wine stain

Name the inflammatory dermal lesion
associated with each of the following
findings:

Pruritic, inflammatory disorders due to infection, atopy, chemicals, UV light, or repeated trauma	Dermatitis
Characteristic "target" macule or papule; associated with infections, drugs, cancers, and autoimmune disease	Erythema multiforme
Silvery scaling plaques over the knees, elbows, and scalp	Psoriasis
"Saw toothing" of rete ridges	Lichen planus
Munro microabscesses in the stratum corneum	Psoriasis
Pruitic eruption commonly on flexor surfaces. Associated with asthma and allergic rhinitis	Atopic dermatitis (eczema)
Wickham stria	Lichen planus
Purple, pruritic, polygonal, papules	Lichen planus
Characteristic rete elongation and parakeratosis	Psoriasis
Fever combined with erosions and hemorrhagic crusting of mucosal surfaces	Stevens-Johnson syndrome
Type IV hypersensitivity reaction following exposure to allergens such as poison ivy or poison oak	Allergic contact dermatitis
Sometimes associated with severe destructive rheumatoid arthritis-like lesions of the fingers	Psoriasis (psoriatic arthritis)

Name the blistering dermal disease
associated with each of the following
descriptions:

Subepidermal bullae causing detachment of the entire thickness of the epidermis	Bullous pemphigoid
Pruritic subepidermal blisters occurring in groups; eosinophils and IgA deposits at tips of dermal papillae; seen in patients with celiac disease	Dermatitis herpetiformis

Intraepidermal/suprabasal blisters that often rupture; may be fatal	Pemphigus vulgaris
Immunofluorescence demonstrates linear deposition of complement and antibodies to hemidesmosome proteins BPAG1 and BPAG2	Bullous pemphigoid
IgA and IgG antibodies to gluten	Dermatitis herpetiformis
Antibodies (Abs) to the desmosomal protein desmoglein 3 in the macula adherens	Pemphigus vulgaris

Name the neurocutaneous syndrome characterized by each of the following features:

Port-wine stains of the face, ipsilateral glaucoma, retinal lesions, and hemangiomas of the meninges	Sturge-Weber syndrome
Hypopigmented macules (ash-leaf spots), adenoma sebaceum, seizures, and mental retardation	Tuberous sclerosis
Multiple organ hemangioblastomas, cysts, and paragangliomas throughout the body	von Hippel-Lindau disease
Café au lait spots, acoustic neuromas, and meningiomas	Neurofibromatosis

Which syndrome is characterized by mycosis fungoides, erythema, and scaling?	Sézary syndrome, cutaneous T-cell lymphoma

Connective Tissue Disorders

Name the connective tissue disorder characterized by each of the following descriptions:

Immune complex deposition in almost any organ, characteristic butterfly malar rash, wire loop lesions in kidney, Libman-Sacks endocarditis, ANA, anti-dsDNA, anti-Smith antibodies	Systemic lupus erythematous
Calcinosis, Raynaud phenomenon, esophageal dysfunction, sclerodactyly, telangiectasias; anticentromere antibodies	CREST syndrome

Autosomal dominant (AD) mutation in the *fibrillin-1* gene (*FBN1*) on chromosome 15q	Marfan syndrome
Most common form is an AD defect in collagen type I synthesis; may be confused with child abuse	Osteogenesis imperfecta
Proximal muscle weakness, elevated serum creatine kinase, less often associated with malignancy	Polymyositis
Abnormal collagen synthesis causing bleeding tendency, hypermobile joints, and hyperextensible skin	Ehlers-Danlos syndrome
Blue sclera and brittle bones	Osteogenesis imperfecta
Proximal muscle weakness, heliotrope rash, more often associated with malignancy	Dermatomyositis
Antinuclear ribonucleoprotein (anti-nRNP) antibodies	Mixed connective tissue disease
Widespread visceral involvement; anti-Scl-70 antibodies	Diffuse scleroderma
Triad of xeropthalmia (dry eyes), xerostomia (dry mouth), arthritis; anti-Ro, anti-La antibodies	Sjögren syndrome

Skin Cancer

Name the skin malignancy associated with each of the following statements:

The most common skin malignancy	Basal cell carcinoma
Associated with excessive sunlight exposure; may arise from dysplastic nevus cells	Malignant melanoma
Actinic keratosis is a precursor lesion	Squamous cell carcinoma
Locally aggressive, ulcerating, and hemorrhagic; almost never metastases	Basal cell carcinoma
Occurs in sun-exposed areas and tends to involve the *lower* part of the face	Squamous cell carcinoma
Occurs in sun-exposed areas and tends to involve the *upper* part of the face	Basal cell carcinoma

Histopathology characterized by "keratin pearls"	Squamous cell carcinoma
Histopathology shows darkly staining cells with palisading nuclei	Basal cell carcinoma
Radial phase precedes vertical growth phase	Malignant melanoma
Associated with arsenic and radiation exposure	Squamous cell carcinoma
What are the characteristics worrisome for malignant melanoma?	ABCDE's Asymmetry Border (irregular) Color Diameter Evolving
What is the most important prognostic factor in malignant melanoma?	Depth of invasion
What clinical variant of malignant melanoma has the poorest prognosis?	Nodular melanoma
What clinical variant of malignant melanoma often appears on the hands and feet of dark-skinned people?	Acral-lentiginous melanoma

Miscellaneous Skin Disorders

Name the dermatologic finding(s) associated with each of the following diseases:

Gastric adenocarcinoma	Acanthosis nigricans
Addison disease	Hyperpigmentation and striae
Rheumatic fever	Erythema marginatum
Kawasaki syndrome	Erythematous palms and soles; dry, red lips; desquamation of fingertips
Insulin resistance, diabetes mellitus type 2	Acanthosis nigricans
Sézary syndrome	Mycosis fungoides (lymphoma of the skin-simulating eczema)
Severe chronic renal failure	Uremic frost
Bacterial endocarditis	Osler nodes (tender, raised lesions on pads of fingers or toes) and Janeway lesions (small, erythematous lesions on palms or soles)

Xeroderma pigmentosum	Dry skin and melanoma
Henoch-Schönlein purpura	Purpuric lesions on extensor surfaces of arms, legs, buttock
Hypothyroidism	Cool, dry skin with coarse brittle hair
Graves disease	Warm, moist skin with fine hair; pretibial myxedema
Graft-versus-host disease	Maculopapular rash
von Recklinghausen disease (NF-1)	Multiple café au lait spots
Familial hypercholesterolemia	Xanthomas
Systemic lupus erythematosus	Malar rash and photosensitivity
Pellagra	Dermatitis

Name the dermatologic finding(s) associated with each of the following infectious diseases:

Anthrax	Vesicular papules covered by black eschar
Parvovirus B19	Erythema infectiosum (*slapped cheek* appearance)
Lyme disease	Erythema chronicum migrans
Primary syphilis	Painless chancre
Secondary syphilis	Rash over palms and soles, condyloma latum
Rocky Mountain spotted fever	Rash over palms and soles (migrates centrally)
Congenital cytomegalovirus	Pinpoint petechial "blueberry muffin" rash
HPV (in genital region)	Condylomata acuminata
Herpes simplex virus (type 1)	Painful vesicles (at border of lips)
Leprosy	Hypopigmented, anesthetic skin patches

CHAPTER 12

Musculoskeletal

ANATOMY

Name the peripheral nerve or region
of the brachial plexus injured in each
of the following scenarios:

Erb-Duchenne or Waiter's tip palsy	Upper trunk of the brachial plexus (C5, C6)
Klumpke injury due to sudden upward jerk of the arm; associated with Horner syndrome	Lower trunk of the brachial plexus (C8, T1)
Claw hand (impaired wrist flexion and adduction)	Ulnar nerve
Wrist drop	Radial nerve
Vague pain in wrist with tingling, burning sensation in hand (carpal tunnel syndrome)	Median nerve
Deltoid paralysis	Axillary nerve
Winged scapula after mastectomy (paralyzed serratus anterior)	Long thoracic nerve
Foot drop	Common peroneal nerve
Loss of ability to plantarflex	Tibial nerve
Anterior shoulder dislocation	Axillary nerve
Positive distal tingling on percussion of anterior wrist (Tinel) and tingling on forced flexion (Phalen) tests	Median nerve (at wrist)
Anterior hip dislocation resulting in loss of adduction of the thigh	Obturator nerve
Loss of ability to rise from a seated position or climb stairs due to loss of gluteus maximus function	Inferior gluteal nerve

Positive Trendenlenburg sign (when contralateral leg is raised, contralateral hip falls secondary to ipsilateral gluteus medius weakness)	Superior gluteal nerve
Posterior hip dislocation	Sciatic nerve

Name the fracture associated with the following statements:

Laceration of the deep brachial artery and/or radial nerve	Midshaft fracture of the humerus
Greatest risk of upper extremity compartment syndrome in children (Volkman contracture)	Supracondylar fracture of the humerus
Young person with fall on outstretched hand, tenderness in the anatomic snuffbox	Scaphoid fracture
Caused by closed fist striking a hard object	Boxer's fracture or fracture of the fifth metacarpal
Elderly woman falling on an outstretched hand with the wrist extended	Colles fracture (fracture of the distal radius with dorsal displacement of hand)
Associated with foot drop due to injury of common peroneal nerve	Fracture of fibular neck
Lower extremity fracture caused by landing on foot from a large vertical drop	Calcaneal fracture (must check lumbar spine x-rays for associated fracture)
List the muscles that make up the hypothenar eminence:	**O**pponens digiti minimi, **A**bductor digiti minimi, **F**lexor digiti minimi (**OAF**)
List the muscles that make up the thenar eminence:	**O**pponens pollicis, **A**bductor pollicis brevis, **F**lexor pollicis brevis
What are the functions of the thenar and hypothenar muscles?	**O**ppose, **A**bduct, and **F**lex
What muscles ADduct at the metacarpophalangeal (MCP) joints?	Palmar interosseous muscles (**PAD**)
What muscles ABduct at the MCP joints?	Dorsal interosseous muscles (**DAB**)
What ligaments make up the borders of the anatomic snuffbox?	Extensor pollicis longus, extensor pollicis brevis, abductor pollicis longus

What artery passes through the anatomic snuffbox?	Radial artery
How can one test for radial or ulnar artery patency?	Allen test (used before arterial blood sampling from the radial artery)
What structures are damaged by lateral impact to the knee/twisting injury?	The terrible triad: anterior cruciate ligament (ACL), medial collateral ligament (MCL), and medial mensicus
What does a positive anterior drawer/ Lachman sign suggest?	Torn ACL
What does abnormal passive abduction (valgus instability) of the leg suggest?	Torn MCL
What is the most common site for a clavicular fracture?	Middle one-third
What is the term for increased pressure within a fascial compartment that causes damage to muscles and neurovascular structures?	Compartment syndrome

What are the six P's of compartment syndrome?

1. Pain out of proportion/pain with passive stretch
2. Parasthesias
3. Paralysis
4. Pallor
5. Pulselessness
6. Poikilothermia (cold)

What ligaments can be stretched or torn by inversion of the ankle?	Anterior talofibular ligament (most common, "Always Tears First"), calcaneofibular (second most common), posterior talofibular ligament (least common)
What common carpal bone fracture can lead to avascular necrosis?	Scaphoid fracture
What are the muscles of the rotator cuff?	Supraspinatus, Infraspinatus, Teres minor, Subscapularis (SITS) muscles
What term is used to describe the syndrome of pain on extension of the wrist and fingers?	Lateral epicondylitis (tennis elbow)

Name the syndrome characterized by sensory loss of the medial forearm and hand, disappearance of radial pulse on turning head away from affected side, with atrophy of thenar, hypothenar, and interosseous muscles:

Thoracic outlet syndrome (often due to cervical accessory rib)

Fracture that presents with leg in abduction, external rotation, and appearing shorter than the contralateral leg

Femoral neck fracture

Injury that presents with an internally rotated and adducted leg appearing shorter than the contralateral leg?

Posterior dislocation of the hip

PHYSIOLOGY

State the key cellular events in excitation-contraction coupling in skeletal muscle:

1. Action potentials cause depolarization of T tubules.
2. Ca^{2+} release from sarcoplasmic reticulum.
3. Ca^{2+} binds troponin C, causes conformational change.
4. Tropomyosin moves to expose actin-binding site.
5. Actin and myosin interact to generate contractile force.
6. Ca^{2+} reuptake by sarcoplasmic reticulum.

How does Ca^{2+} activate contraction in smooth muscle cells?

By binding to calmodulin, activating myosin light-chain kinase (MLCK)

Name the type(s) of muscle fiber associated with each of the following cellular or histologic features:

Peripherally located nucleus

Skeletal muscle fibers

Centrally located nucleus

Smooth and cardiac muscle fibers

Distinct banding pattern

Cardiac and skeletal muscle fibers; bands are appearance of sarcomeres

Capacity to regenerate

Smooth muscle fibers

Z-lines

Cardiac and skeletal muscle fibers; Z-lines are borders that separate sarcomeres

Gap junctions	Smooth muscle fibers
Intercalated disks	Cardiac muscle fibers
Synapse with peripheral nerves	Skeletal muscle fibers
Inositol triphosphate (IP$_3$)-mediated calcium release	Smooth muscle fibers
Ca^{2+}-mediated calcium release	Cardiac muscle fibers
Voltage-mediated, T-tubule-mediated calcium release	Skeletal muscle fibers
Troponin is the major calcium-binding protein	Cardiac and skeletal muscle fibers

Name the type of skeletal muscle fiber associated with each of the following features:

Slow twitch	Type 1—*one slow*
Fast twitch	Type 2
Abundant lipid stores	Type 1—*fat*
Red color	Type 1—*red*
White color	Type 2
Primarily uses anaerobic metabolism, few mitochondria	Type 2
Primarily uses aerobic metabolism, many mitochondria	Type 1—*ox*
Abundant glycogen stores	Type 2
Generation of a sustained force	Type 1
Generation of a sudden movement	Type 2
Mneumonic for type 1 fibers	**Remember:** "One Slow, Fat, Red Ox"

MUSCULOSKELETAL AND CONNECTIVE TISSUE PATHOLOGY

Nonneoplastic Bone Disorders

Name the bone disease associated with the following clinical and pathologic features:

AD disorder characterized by short limbs due to narrow epiphyseal plates, normal torso, enlarged head, frontal bossing, and bow legs	Achondroplasia, most common cause of dwarfism

A group of disorders characterized by abnormalities of type 1 collagen	Osteogenesis imperfecta
Inadequate proline and lysine hydroxylation of procollagen	Scurvy
Vitamin D deficiency → failure of bone mineralization	Rickets (children) or osteomalacia (adults)
Vitamin C deficiency → bone lesions, bleeding from gums. and petechial hemorrhages	Scurvy
Associated with blue sclera and multiple fractures	Osteogenesis imperfecta
↑ Parathyroid hormone (PTH) → "Brown tumor" of bone (fibrosis, giant cells, osteoclasts hemorrhagic debris, and cyst formation)	Osteitis fibrosa cystica (von Recklinghausen disease of bone)
Slow paramyxovirus infection of osteoblasts and osteoclasts that results in multiple fractures and ↑ serum alkaline phosphatase	Paget disease of bone (osteitis deformans)
Marrow fibrosis, moth-eaten bones on x-ray (XR), and metastatic calcifications	Osteitis fibrosa cystica (von Recklinghausen disease of bone), caused by hyperparathyroidism
Multiple lytic lesions of spine and skull	Multiple myeloma
Progressive decrease in bone mass most pronounced in menopausal women	Osteoporosis
Hereditary disorder of increased bone density caused by defective osteoclast function and bone overgrowth	Osteopetrosis
Lateral curvature of spine, usually with rotational component; most common in adolescent females	Scoliosis
Subperiosteal hemorrhage, failure of ephiphyseal cartilage replacement by osteoid, osteoporosis	Scurvy (vitamin C deficiency)
Delayed fontanelle closure, "Rachitic rosary" (thickening of costochondral junction), and Harrison groove	Rickets (vitamin D deficiency)
Marked cortical thinning and attenuation of bone trabeculae	Osteogenesis imperfecta

Poor calcification of bone leading to skeletal abnormalities, including bowing of legs, craniotabes, and pigeon breast deformity in children	Rickets
Mosaic pattern of lamellar bone, increased serum alkaline phosphatase	Paget disease of bone (osteitis deformans)
Bone infection → sequestrum and involucrum around the inflammatory focus	Pyogenic osteomyelitis
Infarction of osteocytes leading to joint pain and osteoarthritis	Avascular necrosis
Avascular necrosis of the head of the femur; typically presents with painless limp in obese adolescent	Legg-Calve-Perthés disease
Partial avulsion of tibial tuberosity; typically presents as knee pain in an active adolescent	Osgood-Schlatter disease
Bacterial infection of bone, causing an acute febrile illness and localized pain and inflammation at the site of infection	Pyogenic osteomyelitis
Granulomatous disease caused by spread of tuberculosis to spine	Pott disease
Vertebral compression fractures causing pain, kyphosis, and loss of height in the elderly	Osteoporosis

What is the most likely etiology of Paget diease?

Slow reaction to paramyxovirus infection of osteoblasts

What are the three phases of Paget disease of bone?

1. Osteolytic phase: bone reabsorption by large osteoclasts
2. Mixed phase: osteoblastic and osteoclastic activity results in mosaic pattern of bone
3. Burnt-out phase: osteoblastic activity predominates

Name six complications of Paget disease of bone:

1. High-output cardiac failure due to intraosseous atrioventricular (AV) shunting
2. Hearing loss
3. Leonitiasis ossea
4. Osteosarcoma
5. Osteoarthritis
6. Bone pain from fractures

Osteomyelitis

Name the most common organism(s)
responsible for pyogenic osteomyelitis
in each of the following patients:

    Otherwise healthy adult   *Staphylococcus aureus*

    Intravenous drug user   *Pseudomonas* spp.

    Sickle cell anemia patient   *Salmonella*

    Newborn   *Streptococci* spp. or *Escherichia coli*

    Child   *Staphylococcus aureus*

    Most common mechanism   *Traumatic*
    of seeding for adults

    Most common mechanism   *Hematogenous*
    of seeding for children

Neoplasia of Bone

Name the bone tumor associated
with the following clinical
and pathologic findings:

    Most common bone tumor   Metastatic tumors to bone

    Most common primary bone tumor   Multiple myeloma

    Most common benign tumor of bone   Osteochondroma or exostosis

    Most common primary malignant   Osteosarcoma
    tumor of bone

    Benign sessile tumor attached   Osteoma
    to the bone surface, usually
    affecting skull and facial bones

    Benign tumor (< 2 cm) that is   Osteoid osteoma
    painful at night (due to excess PGE_2),
    relieved with aspirin and common
    in males < 25 years old (y/o)

    Malignant tumor typically occurring   Osteosarcoma
    in the metaphyseal region prior
    to epiphyseal closure in patients
    < 25 y/o

    Mushroom-shaped, laterally   Osteochondroma or exostosis
    protruding tumor that may result
    from lateral displacement of the
    growth plate

    Benign tumor composed primarily   Chondroma
    of mature hyaline cartilage

Benign tumor composed of fibrous trabeculae of woven bone resembling Chinese characters	Fibrous dysplasia
Nodule of hyaline cartilage encased in reactive bone	Enchondroma
Malignant, painful, *small round blue cell tumor of childhood* occurring typically in the appendicular skeleton (may also affect ribs)	Ewing sarcoma/primitive neuroectodermal tumor (PNET)
Malignant tumor composed of multinucleated giant cells within a fibrous stroma, occurring in the epiphyses of long bones	Giant cell tumor of bone
Lacelike pattern of bone produced by tumor cells	Osteosarcoma
Homer-Wright pseudorosettes, onion skin appearance on x-ray	Ewing sarcoma/PNET
Malignant tumor of cartilage found in the central skeleton	Chondrosarcoma
Double bubble or soap bubble appearance on XR	Giant cell tumor of bone
Benign but painful bone tumor that appears as a radiolucent nidus surrounded by dense bone	Osteoid osteoma or osteoblastoma
Codman triangle on x-ray forms as tumor, causing periosteal elevation	Osteosarcoma
Onion skin appearance on x-ray	Ewing sarcoma
What is the most common genetic defect associated with Ewing sarcoma/PNET?	t(11;22)(q24;q12) translocation (85%) associated with an *EWS-FLI1* fusion gene product
Mutation of what gene increases the risk of osteosarcoma by 1000 × x?	*Rb* gene
What malignancies are most likely to metastasize to bone?	Breast, lung, thyroid, kidney, and prostate (BLT with a Kosher pickle)
What pediatric disease is characterized by the triad of skull lesions, diabetes insipidus, and exophthalmos?	Hand-Schüller-Christian disease or histiocytosis X
What pediatric disease is characterized by polyostotic fibrous dysplasia, café au lait spots, precocious puberty, and other endocrine disorders?	McCune-Albright syndrome

Arthritis

Name the arthritic joint disease associated with the following clinical and pathologic findings:

Most common type of arthritis	Osteoarthritis
Most common type of infective arthritis and most common cause of arthritis in sexually active adults	Gonococcal arthritis
Anti-IgG Fc antibodies	Rheumatoid arthritis (RA); anti-IgG Fc antibodies are called rheumatoid factor
Subcutaneous rheumatoid nodules	RA
Heberden (DIP) and Bouchard (PIP) nodes	Osteoarthritis
PIP and MCP involvement	RA (**Note:** RA almost never affects DIP)
Most commonly affects great toe (podagra)	Gout
Presents as pain in weight-bearing joints after use, improves with rest	Osteoarthritis
Infrequent complication of psoriasis asymmetrically affecting DIP and PIP joints in the lower extremities	Psoriatic arthritis
Swan-neck and boutonniere deformity	RA
Chronic low back pain, rigidity, fixation of spine causing a condition referred to as bamboo spine	Ankylosing spondylitis
Infection causing migratory polyarthritis and erythema chronicum migrans; may lead to pericarditis and aseptic meningitis	Lyme disease
Arthritic joint disease associated with inflammatory bowel disease	Ankylosing spondylitis
Presents as morning stiffness improving with use, symmetric joint involvement, systemic symptoms	RA
Arthritis in the absence of systemic symptoms	Osteoarthritis
Extraskeletal manifestations of this arthritic disease include pulmonary fibrosis, aortic insufficiency, and cauda equina syndrome	Ankylosing spondylitis

Triad of conjunctivitis or anterior uveitis, urethritis, and arthritis	Reactive arthritis, previously know as Reiter syndrome (**Remember:** *can't see, can't pee, can't climb a tree*)
Tophi (nodules of fibrous tissue) and crystals may be found on Achilles tendon or at external ear	Gout
Osteophyte formation at edge of articular surface and at sites of ligamentous attachment	Osteoarthritis
Filling of the joint space by granulation tissue (ie, a pannus)	RA
Frayed fragments of cartilage and osteophytes released into synovium forming "joint mice"	Osteoarthritis
Associated with hyperuricemia, thiazide diuretic use, and urate kidney stones	Gout
Eburnation of bone due to cartilage erosion	Osteoarthritis
Marginal erosion of subchondral bone	RA
Cystic changes in bones underlying affected joints	Osteoarthritis
Precipitation of urate crystals in joints resulting in an inflammatory response	Gout
Precipitation of calcium pyrophosphate dihydrate crystals in joints → inflammatory response	Pseudogout (aka calcium pyrophosphate deposition disease [CPPD])
Infective arthritis common in individuals with complement deficiencies; associated with ↑ susceptibility to meningitis	Gonococcal arthritis
Associated with deficiency of hypoxanthine guanine phosphoribosyl transferease (HGPRT)	Lesch-Nyhan syndrome (X-linked disease which may include gout as one of its manifestations)
Positively birefringent, rhomboid-shaped crystals	Pseudogout = Positively birefringent
Negatively birefringent, needle-shaped crystals in synovial fluid	Gout
Infective monoarticular arthritis typically causing knee pain and a pustular rash	Gonococcal arthritis

Infective polyarticular arthritis caused by *Borrelia burgdorferi*	Lyme disease
Monoarticular arthritis with gram-positive organisms on synovial fluid analysis	Nongonococcal septic arthritis
Stress, alcohol binge, or a large meal may precipitate an attack of this type of arthritis	Gout
Treatment for acute gout attack	Indomethacin (NSAID), Colchicine (use limited by GI side effects)
Treatment for chronic gout	Allopurinol (inhibits xanthine oxidase), probenecid (inhibits reabsorption of uric acid)
Anticytokine therapy for RA is directed at which two cytokines?	1. Interleukin (IL)-1 2. Tumor necrosis factor (TNF)
What is the factor produced by activated T cells and fibroblasts that promotes bone destruction by osteoclasts?	Receptor Activator of Nuclear Factor κ B Ligand (RANKL), also known as TNF-related activation-induced cytokine (TRANCE)
What group of diseases is associated with high incidence (90%) in HLA-B27-positive patients?	Seronegative spondyloarthropathies (ankylosing spondylitis, reactive arthritis, arthritis associated with inflammatory bowel disease [IBD])
Name four extra-articular manifestations of RA:	1. Pleural and pericardial effusions 2. Acute vasculitis 3. Inflammatory lesions of lungs, pleura, myocardium, pericardium, peripheral nerves, and eyes 4. Amyloidosis (in severe, long-term disease)
What chemotactic factors are generated by urate crystal activation of complement?	C3a and C5a
How is tissue injury mediated in gout?	Release of lysosomal enzymes from neutrophils
Why are leukemia, multiple myeloma, and other neoplastic processes associated with gout?	High cell turnover releases uric acid and predisposes to an attack of gout.
What is the renal complication of long-standing gout?	Urate nephropathy

Which syndrome is characterized by cutaneous pigmentation, leg ulcerations, splenomegaly, neutropenia, and RA?

Felty syndrome

What two bacteria most commonly cause nongonococcal septic arthritis?

Staphylococcus aureus and *Streptococcus* spp.

CHAPTER 13

Behavioral Sciences

LIFE CYCLE

Development

At what age is an average child expected to do each of the following:

Hold his/her head up	3 months
Sit up without support	6 months
Crawl	9 months
Walk	12 months
Ride a tricycle	36 months (tricycle at 3 years)
Display stranger anxiety	7 months
Use a pincer grasp	9 months (**Remember:** an upside-down pincer grasp forms the number "9")
Say their first word	12 months (1 word at 1 year)
Use two-word combinations	24 months (2 words at 2 years)
Use three-word sentences	36 months (3 words at 3 years)
Understand object permanence	12 to 24 months
Toilet training	30 to 36 months
"No" phase, repeated temper tantrums	24 months (address tantrums by ignoring behavior)
Show abstract reasoning (formal operations)	Adolescence/puberty

At what age are the following reflexes considered normal:

Babinski	0 to 12 months
Palmar	0 to 2 months
Rooting	0 to 3 months

Name the components of the Apgar score:

APGAR (0, 1, or 2 in each category)

Appearance/color (blue/pale, trunk pink, all pink)

Pulse (0, <100, >100)

Grimace (0, grimace, grimace + cough)

Activity/muscle tone (limp, some, active)

Respiratory effort (0, irregular, regular)

Determine the Apgar score for these patients:

  Newborn with a pink trunk, heart rate (HR) = 50, a grimace and cough when stimulated, strong muscle tone, and an irregular respiratory effort

7

  A blue newborn, HR = 30, a grimace when stimulated, appears limp, and has no respiratory effort

2

What is the definition of low birth weight?

Less than 2500 g

Name four sequelae of low birth weight:

1. Infections
2. Respiratory distress syndrome
3. Persistent fetal circulation
4. Necrotizing enterocolitis

What term describes the act of a child reverting to a more primitive mode of behavior due to stress?

Regression

Name four long-term effects of depriving affection from infants:

The 4 W's:

1. Weak
2. Wordless
3. Wary
4. Wanting

What term describes depression in an infant due to sustained separation from the caregiver?

Anaclitic depression (results in impaired social, emotional, and physical development)

Name three findings that are suggestive of each type of abuse listed below:

  Physical child abuse

1. Fractures at different stages of healing
2. Cigarette burns
3. Retinal hemorrhage/detachment (32% of kids < 5 years old [y/o] are physically abused)

Sexual child abuse	1. Genital/anal trauma 2. STDs 3. UTIs (25% of kids < 8 y/o are sexually abused)
Elder abuse	1. Evidence of depleted finances 2. Poor hygiene 3. Spiral fractures

Aging

Name the changes found in the elderly in each of the following categories:

Psychiatric	Depression and anxiety more common; ↑ suicide rate
Sexual	Men: slower erection/ejaculation, ↑ refractory period; women: vaginal shortening, thinning, and dryness **Note:** sexual interest does *not* decrease.
Sleep patterns	↓ Rapid eye movement (REM), slow-wave sleep; ↑ sleep latency, awakenings
Cognitive	↓ Learning speed; intelligence stays the same

Name three conditions that would qualify normal bereavement as pathologic grief:	1. Prolonged grief (> 1 year) 2. Excessively intense grief (sleep disturbances, significant weight loss, suicidal ideations) 3. Grief that is delayed, inhibited, or denied
Name the Kübler-Ross stages of dying:	Denial, anger, bargaining, depression, acceptance. **Note:** one or more stages can occur at once and not necessarily in this order.

PHYSIOLOGY

Sleep

Name the sleep stage associated with each of the following descriptions:

Light sleep, peacefulness, ↓ HR and BP	Stage 1
Deepest non-REM sleep; sleepwalking, bedwetting	Stages 3 and 4
Deeper sleep; EEG shows sleep spindles and K-complexes; occupies ~half of total sleep time in young adults	Stage 2

Beta waves (↑ frequency, ↓ amplitude) only	Awake (eyes open) and alert
Beta, alpha, and theta waves → "sawtoothing"	REM
Alpha waves	Awake (eyes closed)
Dreaming, loss of motor tone, ↑ brain O_2 use, erections; occurs every 90 minutes	REM
Delta (slow) waves (↓ frequency, ↑ amplitude)	Stages 3 and 4

Name the sleep disorder described in each of the following statements:

Abnormal behavior associated with sleep or sleep-wake transitions (eg, sleep terrors, enuresis, somnabulism)	Parasomnia
Disturbance in amount, quality, or timing of sleep (eg, insomnia, narcolepsy)	Dyssomnia
Nighttime respiratory effort against an impeded airway, resulting in 10-second lapses in breathing and chronic fatigue	Obstructive sleep apnea

What is a useful drug for night terrors and sleepwalking?

Benzodiazepines (shortens stage 4 sleep)

Which drug treats enuresis in children by decreasing stage 4 sleep?

Imipramine

What is the main neurotransmitter involved in REM sleep?

Acetylcholine (ACh)

Name four physiologic changes that occur in REM sleep:

1. Increased and variable pulse
2. Increased and variable BP
3. Penile/clitoral tumescence
4. Rapid eye movements

Name four clinical findings of narcolepsy:

1. Sleep paralysis (brief paralysis upon awakening)
2. Hypna**go**gic (**go**ing to sleep) and hypnopompic (waking) hallucinations
3. ↓ REM latency (sleep episodes all start in REM)
4. Cataplexy (sudden loss of muscle tone, especially with extreme emotion)

How is narcolepsy treated?

Stimulants (eg, amphetamines), scheduled naps

What three sleep pattern changes are typical of depressed patients?

1. Reduced slow-wave sleep
2. ↓ REM latency
3. "Terminal insomnia" (early-morning awakenings)

Sexuality

Name the four stages of the sexual response cycle:

1. Excitement
2. Plateau
3. Orgasm
4. Resolution

Name three possible etiologies of sexual dysfunction:

1. Drugs (eg, selective serotonin reuptake inhibitors [SSRIs], ethanol [ETOH], antihypertensives)
2. Disease (eg, depression, diabetes, myocardial infarction [MI])
3. Psychologic (eg, aversion, hypoactive desire, premature ejaculation)

What disorder of sexual function is characterized by painful spasm of the outer one-third of the vagina during intercourse or pelvic examination?

Vaginismus

What is a paraphilia?

Unusual sexual activities or sexual desire for unusual objects (eg, pedophilia, voyeurism, and so forth)

Behavioral Neurochemistry

For each of the following diseases, describe the associated neurotransmitter activity:

Schizophrenia

↑ Dopamine (DA) and 5-hydroxytryptamine (5-HT)

Depression

↓ Norepinephrine (NE) and 5-HT

Anxiety

↑ NE, ↓ γ-aminobutyric acid (GABA), and 5-HT

Alzheimer dementia

↓ ACh in Alzheimer dementia

Parkinson disease

↓ DA

Huntington disease

↓ GABA and ACh

SUBSTANCE ABUSE

What is the lifetime prevalence of substance abuse/dependence?	13%
How is "dependence" defined?	Withdrawal occurs if substance is stopped and patient has tolerance to substance.
Excluding tobacco and caffeine, what is the most commonly abused substance?	Alcohol
What is a short, useful alcoholism screening tool?	"CAGE" questions Have you felt the need to Cut down? Have you ever felt Annoyed by criticism of your drinking? Have you ever felt Guilty about drinking? Have you ever had an Eye opener?
What is the major complication of alcohol withdrawal and when is it most likely to occur?	Delirium tremens (DTs); peak occurrence is 2 to 7 days. **Note:** DTs are a medical emergency.
What is the mortality rate of DTs?	15% to 20%
Name three gastrointestinal (GI) complications of alcoholism:	1. GI bleeding (from ulcers, gastritis, esophageal varices, or Mallory-Weiss tears) 2. Pancreatitis 3. Liver disease
Which syndrome of anterograde amnesia, confabulations, ataxia, and nystagmus results from thiamine deficiency in chronic alcoholics?	Wernicke-Korsakoff syndrome—**Remember: W**obbly-**K**onfabulations (associated with bilateral mammillary body necrosis)

What am I high on?

Central nervous system (CNS) and respiratory depression, euphoria, pinpoint pupils, nausea, and ↓ GI motility	Opioids; inspect for track marks along veins
Psychomotor agitation, dilated pupils, euphoria, ↑ HR and BP, prolonged wakefulness and attention, delusions, ↑ pain threshold	Amphetamines
All of the above, plus tactile hallucinations, angina, and sudden cardiac death	Cocaine

Belligerence, psychomotor agitation, nystagmus, ataxia, homicidality, psychosis, delirium, ↑ HR, and fever — Phencyclidine hydrochloride (PCP)

Delusions, visual hallucinations, postuse "flashbacks" — Lysergic acid diethylamide (LSD)

Euphoria, ↑ appetite, dry mouth, paranoid delusions, erythematous conjunctiva — Marijuana

Disinhibition, emotional lability, slurred speech, ataxia, blackouts, coma — Alcohol

What is the drug of choice for opioid overdose? — Naloxone and naltrexone (competitively inhibit opioid receptors)

Which drug is used for heroin detoxification? — Methadone (long-acting oral opioid)

PSYCHOLOGY

What are the three parts of Freud's structural theory of the mind?
1. Id
2. Superego
3. Ego

Which of these parts is described by the following statements:

Represents conscience and moral values — Superego

Controlled by primitive wishes and pleasures; represents instinctive sexual and aggressive drives — Id

Bridges unconscious mind and external world — Ego

What Freudian term encompasses repressed sexual feelings of a child for the opposite-sex parent, plus a rivalry with the same-sex parent? — Oedipus complex

What type of insight therapy, developed by Freud, may be useful for chronic personality problems? — Psychoanalysis

What describes a scenario in which a patient's unconscious feelings from past relationships are experienced in the present relationship with the physician? — Transference reaction

What reaction occurs when the physician unconsciously reexperiences feelings about his/her parents (or other important persons) with the patient?

Countertransference reaction

Name the four mature ego defense mechanisms:

1. Suppression
2. Altruism
3. Sublimation
4. Humor

Note: defense mechanisms are automatic and unconscious.

Name the type of learning that is described by each of the following statements:

Reflexive response is elicited by a learned stimulus

Classical conditioning

Tendency of an organism to follow the first thing they see after birth

Imprinting

Behavior is eliminated when not reinforced

Extinction

Behavior is determined by its consequences

Operant conditioning

Unwanted behavior is paired with painful stimulus

Aversive conditioning

Type of classical conditioning where the subject learns that it cannot escape a painful stimulus

Learned helplessness

In what type of reinforcement schedule is a reward presented after a random, unpredictable number of responses?

Variable ratio (slowest extinction when not rewarded); example = slot machine

In what type of reinforcement schedule is a reward presented after every response?

Continuous (rapid extinction when not rewarded); example = vending machine

Criteria for mental retardation begin below what IQ level?

Less than 70 (2 SD below the mean of 100)

PSYCHIATRY

Name the type of amnesia described below:

Inability to remember things that occurred before insult to CNS

Retrograde amnesia

Inability to remember things that occurred after a CNS injury → no new memory formation	Anterograde amnesia
Complication of electroconvulsive therapy (ECT)	Retrograde amnesia
Thiamine deficiency causing bilateral mammillary body necrosis; seen in alcoholics	Korsakoff (anterograde) amnesia

Delirium or dementia?

Waxing and waning level of consciousness	Delirium
Rapid onset; transient	Delirium
Characterized by memory loss	Dementia (think deMEMtia)
Associated with disturbances in sleep-wake cycle	Delirium
Often irreversible	Dementia
Associated with changes in sensorium (hallucinations and illusions)	Delirium

Name four major causes of delirium:	"HIDE": 1. Hypoxia 2. Infection (often UTIs) 3. Drugs 4. Electrolyte abnormalities
What is the most common etiology for dementia?	Dementia of Alzheimer type (DAT) = 70% to 80% of cases
Name some other etiologies for dementia:	"DEMENTIASS" Degenerative diseases (Parkinson, Huntington) Endocrine (thyroid, pituitary, parathyroid) Metabolic (electrolytes, glucose, hepatorenal dysfunction, ETOH) Exogenous (CO poisoning, drugs, heavy metals) Neoplasia Trauma Infection (encephalitis, meningitis, cerebral abscess, syphilis, prion diseases, HIV, Lyme disease) Affective disorders (depression may mimic dementia)

Stroke (multi-infarct dementia, ischemia, vasculitis). **Note:** vascular causes ~10% of dementias

Structure (normal-pressure hydrocephalus [NPH]).

Note: NPH is one of the few reversible causes of dementia.

Mood Disorders

Name the nine key features of major depressive disorder (MDD):

"SIG E CAPSS"

1. Sleep changes (insomnia/hypersomnia)
2. Inability to experience pleasure, Interest decreases
3. Guilt or feelings of worthlessness
4. Energy ↓ (fatigue)
5. Concentration ↓, indecisiveness increases
6. Appetite disturbance with weight change (> 5% body weight in 1 month)
7. Psychomotor changes (agitation or retardation)
8. Suicidal ideations
9. Sadness (depressed mood for most of day)

What features are required to make the diagnosis of MDD?

Two episodes (involving five of the above nine including # 1 or 2) of impaired functioning for **2 weeks,** separated by **2 months**

What is the suicide rate in MDD?

Approximately 15% to 30%

Name the risk factors for suicide:

"SAD PERSONS"

Sex—male (women > attempts; men > actual suicides)

Age (↓ 15-24 and the elderly)

Depression

Previous attempts = #1 risk factor

Ethanol

Rational thought

Sickness

Organized plan

No spouse

Social support lacking

What is the first-line pharmacotherapy for MDD?	SSRIs
Name two other alternate pharmacotherapies:	1. Tricyclic antidepressants (TCAs) 2. Monoamine oxidase inhibitors (MAOIs)
What is a safe, effective treatment for refractory MDD?	ECT
What is the distinctively abnormal, elevated, expansive mood that lasts > 1 week *or* is severely impairing (eg, requiring hospitalization)?	Manic episode
What are the seven key features of mania?	"DIG FAST" (at least three of the following for diagnosis): 1. Distractibility 2. Insomnia 3. Grandiosity 4. Flight of ideas or racing thoughts 5. Psychomotor Agitation 6. Speech that is pressured (hyperverbal) 7. Thoughtlessness (↑ pleasurable activities with ↑ consequences)

Name the following mood disorders:

Chronic disorder > 2 years (alternating hypomania and mild depression); no period of euthymia > 2 months and *no* significant impairment	Cyclothymia
Less severe features for several days that are *not* impairing; no psychotic features	Hypomania
History of major depressive episodes and at least one hypomanic episode	Bipolar II disorder
Manic episodes that often alternate with depressive episodes	Bipolar I disorder

Somatoform Disorders

Name the somatoform disorder associated with each of the following descriptions:

Preoccupation with an imagined physical defect, causing significantly impaired social and occupational functioning	Body dysmorphic disorder

Multiple, unrelated physical complaints leading to excessive medical attention seeking and severely impaired functioning	Somatization disorder (requires four pain, two GI, one sexual/GU, and one pseudoneurologic complaints). **Note:** cannot be intentional or fake
Prolonged preoccupation with concerns of having a serious illness (despite negative medical work-ups) and exaggerated attention to bodily or mental sensations	Hypochondriasis
Conscious simulation of physical or psychologic illness solely to receive attention from medical personnel	Factitious disorder (Munchausen syndrome). **Note:** technically *not* a somatoform disorder because it is intentional
Intentionally simulating illness for personal gain (usually financial)	Malingering. **Note:** also *not* a somatoform disorder; suspect in cases involving litigation
Sudden onset of motor/sensory neurologic disorder following traumatic emotional event	Conversion disorder

Name the type of gain associated with each of the following descriptions:

Interpersonal or social advantages gained indirectly from illness	Secondary gain
Benefits of illness on the patient's internal psychic economy	Primary gain
Advantage gained by the caretaker	Tertiary gain

Name the type of anxiety disorder associated with each of the following:

Maladaptive reaction to environmental or psychologic stress that interferes with functioning and does not remit after the stress ends	Adjustment disorder
Marked, persistent fear of an object/situation that is excessive and unreasonable → stimulus is avoided; patient has insight (treat by exposure therapy)	Specific phobia
Occurs after a person is subjected to a traumatic event; lasts >1 month; may be debilitating	Posttraumatic stress disorder (PTSD)
Symptoms of PTSD that occur within 4 weeks of the stressor and last < 4 weeks	Acute stress disorder

Moments of intense fear characterized by palpitations, choking sensation, GI upset, perspiration, chest pain, and chills	Panic disorder
Excessive worrying for the majority of days over the past 6 months that causes significant impairment	Generalized anxiety disorder
Recurrent, intrusive, senseless thoughts and impulses; plus the repetitive behaviors driven by the will to decrease the anxiety caused by them	Obsessive-compulsive disorder (OCD)

Name the dissociative disorder characterized by the following statements:

Two or more separate personalities in one individual; ↑ in women and sexually abused	Dissociative identity disorder (formerly multiple personality disorder)
A complete, often transient, inability to remember important personal information	Dissociative amnesia
Amnesia plus sudden wandering from home and taking on a different identity	Dissociative fugue

Psychoses

Give the appropriate term for each of the following psychotic symptoms:

False belief or wrong judgment held with conviction despite incontrovertible evidence to the contrary	Delusion
False perception of an actual external stimulus	Illusion
Thought disorder whereby ideas are not logically connected to those that occur before or after	Loose association
Misinterpreting others' actions or environmental cues as being directed toward one's self when, in fact, they are not	Ideas of reference
Subjective perception of an object or event when no such external stimulus exists	Hallucination

Name the psychotic disorder characterized by each of the following findings:

Two or more psychotic symptoms and disturbed behavior for > 6 months; results in impaired functioning

Schizophrenia

Psychotic symptoms lasting 1 to 6 months

Schizophreniform disorder

Psychotic symptoms lasting > 1 day, but < 1 month (often with obvious precipitating psychosocial stressor)

Brief psychotic disorder

Fixed, nonbizarre delusional system; without other thought disorders or impaired functioning

Delusional disorder

Symptoms of major mood disorder as well as of schizophrenia (with psychotic features occurring before mood disturbance); chronic social and occupational impairment

Schizoaffective disorder

Clouded consciousness, predominantly visual hallucinations, often occurring in inpatient setting

Psychotic disorder due to a general medical condition

Adopting the delusional system of a psychotic person

Shared psychotic disorder (Folie-à-deux)

Name the five subtypes of schizophrenia:

1. Disorganized
2. Catatonic
3. Paranoid
4. Undifferentiated
5. Residual

Give two examples of positive symptoms of schizophrenia:

1. Hallucinations
2. Delusions

Positive symptoms respond best to what type of drugs?

Typical antipsychotics

Give four examples of negative symptoms that are characteristic of schizophrenia:

The 4 A's:

1. Affect flat
2. Alogia
3. Anhedonia
4. Avolition

Negative symptoms respond best to what type of drugs?

Atypical antipsychotics. **Note:** worse prognosis if negative symptoms predominate

Childhood Disorders

Name the disorder of childhood described by each of the following statements:

Repetitive behaviors (in patient < 18 y/o) that violate social norms; may exhibit physical aggression, cruelty to animals, vandalism, and robbery, along with truancy, cheating, and lying	Atypical antipsychotics. **Note:** worse actions)
Recurrent pattern of negativistic, hostile, and disobedient behavior toward authority figures; loss of temper and defiance (but not theft or lying)	Oppositional defiant disorder (predominantly **words**)
Developmentally inappropriate degrees of inattention, impulsiveness, and hyperactivity at home, in school, and in social situations	Attention deficit hyperactivity disorder (ADHD)
Pervasive developmental disorder (PDD) with stereotyped movements and nonprogressive impairments in social interactions, communication, and behavior	Autism
Progressive syndrome of autism, dementia, ataxia, and purposeless hand movements; regression of development; mainly in girls	Rett syndrome
PDD with severe impairment in social skills and repetitive behaviors, leading to impaired social and occupational functioning but without significant delays in language development	Asperger disorder

Personality Disorders

List the three cluster A personality disorders:	"Weird" 1. Paranoid 2. Schizoid 3. Schizotypal
List the four cluster B personality disorders:	"Wild" 1. Histrionic 2. Borderline 3. Antisocial 4. Narcissistic

List the three cluster C personality disorders:

"Worried"
1. Avoidant
2. Obsessive-compulsive
3. Dependent

Name the personality disorder characterized by each of the following statements:

Socially inhibited, sensitive to rejection, feels inferior

Avoidant (C)

Peculiar appearance, interpersonal awkwardness, "magical" or odd thought patterns, no psychosis

Schizotypal (A)

Impulsive, unstable mood, chaotic relationships, feels empty and alone, self-mutilation, females >> males

Borderline (B)

Sense of entitlement, grandiosity, lacks empathy for others, insists on special treatment when ill

Narcissistic (B)

Suspicious and distrustful, uses projection as primary defense mechanism

Paranoid (A)

Lacks self-confidence, submissive, and clingy

Dependent (C)

Unable to maintain intimate relationships, extroverted, melodramatic, sexually provocative

Histrionic (B)

Disregards and violates rights of others, criminality, males > females; if < 18 y/o = conduct disorder

Antisocial (B)

Lifelong pattern of voluntary social withdrawal, no psychosis, shows minimal emotions

Schizoid (A)

PHARMACOLOGY—PSYCHOPHARMACOLOGY

For each of the following drugs, provide:

1. The mechanism of action (MOA)
2. Indication(s) (IND)
3. Significant side effects and unique toxicity (TOX) (if any)

Antidepressants

TCAs (imipramine, clomipramine, amitriptyline, desipramine, nortriptyline, doxepin, amoxapine)	**MOA:** prevents reuptake of NE and 5-HT **IND:** depression, enuresis (imipramine), depression in elderly (nortriptyline), OCD (clomipramine), depression with psychotic features (amoxapine), neurologic pain **TOX:** sedation (desipramine is least sedating), anticholinergic effects, lethal in overdose → respiratory depression, hyperpyrexia, and **Tri-C's:** **C**ardiac arrhythmia, **C**onvulsions, **C**oma
SSRIs (fluoxetine, paroxetine, sertraline, citalopram, fluvoxamine, escitalopram)	**MOA:** selectively blocks reuptake of 5-HT (usually requires 2-3 weeks to take effect) **IND:** depression, premenstrual syndrome (fluoxetine), OCD (fluvoxamine) **TOX:** agitation, insomnia, sexual dysfunction, "serotonin syndrome" with MAOIs (muscle rigidity, hyperthermia, cardiovascular collapse)
Bupropion	**MOA:** heterocyclic agent, mechanism not well known **IND:** depression, smoking cessation **TOX:** agitation, seizures, insomnia (↓ sexual side effects)
Trazodone	**MOA:** mainly inhibits serotonin reuptake **IND:** depression **TOX:** postural hypotension, sedation, priapism
Venlafaxine	**MOA:** inhibits 5-HT and NE reuptake **IND:** depression, generalized anxiety disorder **TOX:** stimulant effects, minimal effects on P-450
Mirtazapine	**MOA:** 5-HT_2 receptor antagonist and α_2-antagonist →↑ NE and 5-HT release **IND:** depression **TOX:** sedation, ↑ appetite, ↑ cholesterol

MAOIs (TIP: T ranylcypromine, I socarboxazid, phenelzine)	**MOA:** nonselective MAOIs
	IND: atypical depressions, anxiety disorders, pain disorders, eating disorder
	TOX: hypertensive crisis with tyramine or meperidine ingestion, "serotonin syndrome" with SSRIs
Lithium	**MOA:** prevents generation of inositol triphosphate (IP_3) and diacylglycerol (DAG) 2° messenger systems
	IND: bipolar disorder (prevents and treats acute mania)
	TOX: hypothyroidism, nephrogenic DI, teratogenesis (Ebstein anomaly)
Carbamazepine	**MOA:** blocks sodium channels and inhibits action potentials
	IND: bipolar disorder, mixed episodes, and rapid cycling form
	TOX: hematologic SEs, elevated LFTs, teratogenesis (neural tube defects)
Valproic acid	**MOA:** increases CNS levels of GABA
	IND: bipolar disorder, mixed manic episodes, and rapid cycling form
	TOX: hepatotoxicity, thrombocytopenia, teratogenesis (neural tube defects)

Antipsychotics

What is the name for the stereotyped oral-facial movements that occur as a result of long-term antipsychotic use?	Tardive dyskinesia
Describe the chronology of extrapyramidal side effects from neuroleptic medications:	**Rule of 4's: 4** hours—acute dystonia, **4** days—akinesia, **4** weeks—akathesia, **4** months—tardive dyskinesia (usually irreversible)
What is the characteristic triad of neuroleptic malignant syndrome (NMS)?	Muscle rigidity, autonomic instability, and hyperpyrexia
What is the treatment for NMS?	Dantrolene and DA agonists

For each of the following drugs, provide:

1. The mechanism of action (MOA)
2. Indication(s) (IND)
3. Significant side effects and unique toxicity (TOX) (if any)

Typical antipsychotics—high potency (haloperidol, perphenazine, trifluoperazine)	**MOA:** block D_2 DA receptors (less blockade of α_2, muscarinic, and histaminic receptors) **IND:** schizophrenia, psychosis (especially positive symptoms) **TOX:** ↑ neurologic (eg, extrapyramidal) SEs, NMS, tardive dyskinesia, Parkinsonism, hyperprolactinemia
Typical antipsychotics—low potency (chlorpromazine, thioridazine)	**MOA:** block D_2 DA receptors (more blockade of α_2, muscarinic, and histaminic receptors) **IND:** schizophrenia, psychosis **TOX:** ↓ neurologic SEs, ↑ anticholinergic and endocrine SEs; cardiac conduction defects and retinal pigmentation (thioridazine), corneal and lenticular deposits (chlorpromazine)
Atypical antipsychotics (clozapine, risperidone, olanzapine, quetiapine)	**MOA:** block $5\text{-}HT_2$; block D_4 and $D_1 > D_2$ receptors **IND:** schizophrenia, psychosis (especially negative symptoms); OCD/anxiety disorder (olanzapine) **TOX:** ↓ anticholinergic and extrapyramidal symptoms (EPS); metabolic syndrome (hyperlipidemia, glucose intolerance), agranulocytosis (clozapine)

MEDICAL ETHICS

What are four key components to informed consent?	The patient must: 1. Understand the health implications of their diagnosis 2. Be informed of risks, benefits, and alternatives to treatment 3. Be aware of outcome if they do not give their consent 4. Have the right to withdraw consent at any time

Name four exceptions to informed consent:	1. Patient not legally competent to make decisions 2. In an emergency (implied consent) 3. Patient waives the right to informed consent 4. Therapeutic privilege—withholding info that would severely harm the patient or undermine decision-making capacity if revealed
What are five situations in which parent/ legal guardian consent is not required to treat a minor?	1. Emergencies 2. STDs 3. Prescription of contraceptives 4. Treatment of ETOH/drug treatment 5. Care during pregnancy
What four criteria qualify a minor as emancipated?	1. Self-supporting 2. In the military 3. Being married 4. Having children that they support
What type of directive is based on the incapacitated patient's prior statements and decisions?	Oral advance directive (substituted judgment standard)
What type of written advance directive gives instructions for the patient's future health care should he/she become incompetent to make decisions?	Living will
What type of document allows the patient to designate a surrogate to make medical decisions in case the patient loses decision-making capacity?	Durable power of attorney
Name the ethical responsibility of the physician described by each of the following statements:	
Requires physicians to "do no harm"	Nonmaleficence
Requires physicians to act in the best interests of the patient	Beneficence (may conflict with patient autonomy)
Demands respect for patient privacy and autonomy	Confidentiality
Name five exceptions to confidentiality:	1. Suspected child and/or elder abuse 2. Suicidal/homicidal patient 3. Impaired automobile driver 4. Specific infectious diseases—physician duty to report to public officials or individuals at risk

5. Tarasoff decision–law requiring physician to directly inform/protect potential victim from harm

What elements are required in order to prove a malpractice claim?

The **"4 D's"**: must prove that the physician showed **D**eriliction (deviation from standard of care) of a **D**uty that caused **D**amages **D**irectly to the patient

What is the legal standard of death?

Failure to meet cardiorespiratory criteria and irreversible cessation of all brain functions (including brainstem)

BIOSTATISTICS

For each description, name the proper term and the equation used to calculate the value described below:

Probability that a person without the disease will be correctly identified

Specificity

$TN/(TN + FP)$

Probability that a person who tests positive actually has the disease

Positive predictive value

$TP/(TP + FP)$

Probability that a person who has a disease will be correctly identified

Sensitivity

$TP/(TP + FN)$

Total number of cases in a population at any given time

Prevalence

$TP + FN/\text{(entire population)}$

Number of new cases that arise in a population over a given time interval

Incidence

Prevalence $\times$ duration of disease (approximately)

Used in case-control studies to approximate the relative risk if the disease prevalence is too high

Odds ratio

$TP \times TN/FP \times FN$

Used in cohort studies to compare incidence rate in exposed group to that in unexposed group

Relative risk

$(TP/[TP + FP])/(FN/[FN + TN])$

Probability that patient with a negative test actually has no disease

Negative predictive value

$TN/(FN + TN)$

How are incidence and prevalence related?

Incidence $\times$ disease duration = prevalence

Prevalence > incidence for chronic diseases; prevalence = incidence for acute diseases

What quality is desirable for a screening tool?

High sensitivity (**SNOUT**—**S**e**N**sitivity rules **OUT**)

What quality is desirable for a confirmatory test?

High specificity (**SPIN**—**S**pecificity rules **IN**)

Name four ways to reduce bias:

1. Use of placebo
2. Blinded studies (single, double)
3. Crossover studies (each subject is own control)
4. Randomization

Name the type of statistical distribution described below:

Asymmetry with tail to the right

Positive skew

Two peaks

Bimodal

Scores cluster in the high end

Negative skew

Bell-shaped

Normal (Gaussian)

What percent of the area under a normal curve falls within 1, 2, and 3 standard deviations (SD) of the mean?

68% (1 SD), 95% (2 SD), 99.7% (3 SD)

How is standard error of the mean (SEM) calculated?

$\sqrt{(SD)}$/square root of sample size

Name the term for each of the following descriptions:

Refers to the reproducibility of a test

Reliability

Refers to the appropriateness of a test (whether the test measures what it is supposed to)

Validity

Absence of random variation in a test; consistency and reproducibility of a test

Precision

Closeness of a measurement to the truth

Accuracy

Test that compares the difference between two means

t-test

Test that analyzes the variance of three or more variables

Analysis of variance (ANOVA)

Test that compares percentages or proportions

χ^2 (chi-squared test)

Absolute value that indicates the strength of a relationship

r (always between −1 and 1)

Observational study where the sample is chosen based on presence/absence of risk factors	Cohort study (eg, prospective, historical)
Experimental study comparing benefits of *two* or more alternative treatments	Clinical trial
Observational study where the sample is chosen based on disease presence/absence	Case-control study (usually retrospective)
Assembling data from multiple studies to achieve great statistical power	Meta-analysis
Hypothesis postulating that there is no difference between groups	Null hypothesis (H_0)
Error of mistakenly rejecting H_0 (stating that there is a difference when there really is not)	Type I error (α)
Error of failing to reject H_0 (stating there is no difference when there really is)	Type II error (β)
Probability of rejecting H_0 when it is in fact false	Power ($1-\beta$)
Probability of making an α error	*P* value

PUBLIC HEALTH/EPIDEMIOLOGY

Name four reportable STDs:	1. Gonorrhea 2. Syphilis 3. Hepatitis B 4. Acquired immunodeficiency syndrome (AIDS) (nonreportable = HIV, chlamydia, genital herpes)
What is the leading cause of mortality in each of the following age groups:	
< 1 y/o	Congenital anomalies
1 to 14 y/o	Unintentional injuries
15 to 24 y/o	Unintentional injuries (mostly car accidents)
25 to 64 y/o	Cancer (#1 lung, #2 breast/prostate, #3 colon)
65 years and older	Heart disease

What is 1° disease prevention?

Aims to prevent disease occurrence (eg, vaccination, education)

What is 2° disease prevention?

Early detection of disease; screening programs

What is 3° disease prevention?

Reduces disability resulting from disease (eg, physical therapy for stroke)

What is the current definition of "obese"?

BMI> 30, BMI> 25 is overweight

Approximately what percentage of the US population is obese?

~30%, > 50% overweight

What is the divorce rate in the United States?

~50%

Name three risk factors for divorce:

1. Teenage marriage
2. Mixed religions
3. Low SES. **Note:** peaks during second and third years

What is the criterion to qualify for hospice care?

Medically anticipated death within 6 months

What federal program addresses health care needs of the elderly?

MedicarE **(Elderly)**

What federal and state program addresses health care needs of the underprivileged?

MedicaiD **(Destitute)**

What 1996 law helps to protect rights to health coverage during events such as changing or losing jobs, pregnancy, moving, or divorce?

Health insurance portability and accountability act (HIPAA)

CHAPTER 14

Make the Diagnosis

NUTRITION

1-year-old (y/o) impoverished child presents with lethargy and poor wound healing; physical examination (PE): low-grade fever, pallor, oral mucosal petechiae, and bleeding gums.	Scurvy
50-y/o with history of (h/o) long-term treatment of psoriasis with methotrexate presents with nausea and fatigue; PE: within normal limits (WNL); workup (W/U): MCV > 100, hypersegmented neutrophils, and normal vitamin B_{12} levels.	Folic acid deficiency
42-y/o alcoholic presents with ataxia and shortness of breath (SOB); PE: nystagmus, cardiomegaly with flow murmur, ↓ DTRs, ↓ peripheral sensation, and hepatomegaly.	Beriberi
48-y/o Scandinavian woman presents with weakness, ataxia, and SOB; PE: ↓ balance and vibratory sensation in lower extremities; W/U: MCV > 100, hypersegmented PMNs, and positive Schilling test.	Pernicious anemia

MICROBIOLOGY AND INFECTIOUS DISEASES

4-y/o with a superficial skin infection consisting of erythematous pustules with honey-colored scabs.	Impetigo, most commonly due to *Staphylococcus aureus*

6-y/o child with poor hygiene presents with complaints of severe perianal itching that is worse at night; W/U: a "scotch tape test" reveals eggs visualized under the microscope.	Pinworm infection
36-y/o man presents with flu-like symptoms since moving to a farm in Ohio 2 months ago; PE: fever and generalized lymphadenopathy; chest x-ray (CXR): bilateral hilar adenopathy.	Histoplasmosis
Patient with recent h/o antibiotic use presents with fever, bloody diarrhea, and abdominal pain; PE: tender abdominal examination, guiaic + stool; complete blood count (CBC): leukocytosis; colonoscopy: tan nodules seen attached to erythematous bowel wall with superficial erosions.	Pseudomembranous colitis (*Clostridium difficile* colitis)
18-y/o student returns to clinic with a rash after being treated with ampicillin for fever and sore throat; PE: tonsilar exudates and enlarged posterior cervical lymph nodes; W/U: ↑ lymphocytes and ⊕ heterophile antibody test.	Infectious mononucleosis due to Epstein Barr virus (EBV)
28-y/o with h/o treatment for 2° syphilis 5 hours ago with intramuscular (IM) penicillin presents with fever, chills, muscle pain (myalgias), and headache.	Jarisch-Herxheimer reaction
33-y/o northern European with h/o eating raw fish presents with shortness of breath and weakness; W/U: megaloblastic anemia, operculated eggs on stool examination.	*Diphyllobothrium latum* infection (with vitamin B_{12} deficiency)
17-y/o swimmer presents with pain and discharge from the left ear; PE: movement of tragus is extremely painful; Gram stain shows gram-negative rods.	Otitis externa (most likely due to *Pseudomonas aeruginosa*)
10-y/o with sickle cell disease and recent h/o prodromal illness presents with sudden-onset pallor, fatigue, and tachycardia; CBC: pancytopenia with reticulocytes < 1%.	Parvovirus B19 aplastic crisis

44-y/o parrot owner presents with fever, chills, headache, and cough; PE: Horder spots on abdomen and splenomegaly; CXR: bilateral, interstitial infiltrates.

Psittacosis

33-y/o epileptic with recent loss of consciousness presents with fever and cough with purulent, putrid sputum; W/U: Gram stain reveals mixed oral flora; CXR: consolidation of right lower lobe.

Aspiration pneumonia

50-y/o man presents with a fever of unknown origin. One month ago he had a dental procedure. He has a history of rheumatic heart disease; PE: significant for a heart murmur, splinter hemorrhages, Janeway lesions, Roth spots, and Osler nodes.

Subacute bacterial endocarditis due to *Streptococcus viridans*

9-y/o with recent viral prodomal illness presents to ER vomiting and lethargic after being given aspirin for fever; W/U: impaired liver function; computed tomography (CT): cerebral edema.

Reye syndrome

15-y/o new pet owner presents with painful axillary lumps and fever; PE: cervical lymphadenopathy.

Catscratch disease

2-month-old with maternal h/o rash and flu in first trimester presents with a rash and failure to attain milestones; PE: microcephaly, cataracts, jaundice, continuous machinery-like murmur at left upper sternal border, and hepatosplenomegaly (HSM).

Congenital rubella

8-y/o from Connecticut presents with fever, rash, headache, and joint pain after playing in the woods; PE: distinctive macule with surrounding 6 cm target-shaped lesion.

Lyme disease

35-y/o man with h/o urinary catheterization presents with fever, chills, dysuria, and perineal pain; PE: swollen, tender, hot prostate; urinalysis (UA): WBCs and culture ⊕ for *Escherichia coli*.

Acute bacterial prostatitis

38-y/o man with h/o asthma presents with recurrent fever, wheezing, and cough productive of brown mucous plugs; CBC: eosinophilia, high IgE titers; CXR: mucoid impaction of dilated central bronchi.	Allergic bronchopulmonary aspergillosis
6-y/o unvaccinated child presents with rhinorrhea, cough, conjunctivitis; PE: oral lesions are noted which are bluish with an erythematous border.	Measles
37-y/o man with a recent h/o upper respiratory infection (URI) presents with fever and severe chest pain; PE: friction rub and Kussmauls sign; W/U: ↑ ESR, normal cardiac enzymes, and diffuse ST elevations on ECG.	Acute pericarditis
4-y/o presents with barking cough, fever, and rhinorrhea; PE: respiratory distress and tachypnea; x-ray of soft tissues of neck reveals "steeple sign."	Croup
18-y/o sexually active woman with h/o treatment for purulent vaginitis presents with a fever and tenderness, warmth, and swelling of her right knee.	Gonococcal arthritis
Newborn presents with rash and maternal h/o intrauterine growth retardation (IUGR) and flu during first trimester; PE: petechial rash, chorioretinitis, microcephaly, ↓ hearing, and HSM; W/U: ↓ platelets and periventricular calcifications on head CT.	Congenital cytomegalovirus (CMV)
25-y/o West Virginian man presents with fever, headache, myalgia, and a petechial rash that began peripherally but now involves his whole body, even his palms and soles; W/U: shows +OX19 and OX2 Weil-Felix reaction.	Rocky Mountain spotted fever
10-y/o presents with fevers and a pruritic rash spreading from the trunk to the arms; PE: vesicles of varying stages.	Varicella
29-y/o athlete presents with a red, pruritic skin eruption with an advancing peripheral, creeping border on the forearm; W/U shows septate hyphae in KOH scraping.	Tinea corporis (ringworm)

8-y/o presents with fever, photophobia, stiff neck, and headache; PE: ⊕ Kernig and Brudzinski signs; lumbar puncture shows normal glucose and ↓ WBCs.

Viral meningitis

21-y/o presents with nausea, vomiting, bloating, and foul-smelling stools on returning from a camping trip; W/U: binucleate, flagellated trophozoites in stool.

Giardiasis

14-y/o adolescent boy with h/o recent travel to Mexico now presents with jaundice and dark yellow urine; PE: icterus and firm hepatomegaly; W/U: ↑ bilirubin (BR), ↑ LFTs with alanine transaminase (ALT) > aspartate transaminase (AST).

Hepatitis A infection

26-y/o sexually active, native Caribbean presents with painless, beefy-red ulcers of the genitalia and inguinal swelling; W/U: Donovan bodies on Giemsa-stained smear.

Granuloma inguinale

Patient presents with sudden onset of severe watery diarrhea, vomiting, and abdominal discomfort 4 hours after eating potato salad at a picnic; the symptoms resolve spontaneously within 24 hours.

Staphylococcus aureus-induced diarrhea

6-y/o with recent h/o sore throat presents with multiple joint pain and swelling, fever, and SOB; PE: erythema marginatum, subcutaneous nodules, and apical systolic murmur; W/U: ↑ ESR and CRP.

Acute rheumatic fever

25-y/o woman presents with malodorous vaginal discharge; W/U: visualization of the discharge under the microscope demonstrates multiple vaginal epithelial cells covered in bacteria.

Bacterial vaginosis due to *Gardenella vaginalis*

73-y/o presents with a painful, unilateral, vesicular rash in the distribution of the CN V_1; cornea shows diminished sensation and stains with fluorescein.

Herpes zoster ophthalmicus

29-y/o missionary with h/o travel to rural India presents with high fever and right upper quadrant (RUQ) pain; PE: severe hepatomegaly and dullness over right lower lung; abdominal CT: large, cavitating lesion in liver.

Amebic liver abscess

25-y/o sexually active man presents with dysuria, irritation, and cloudy discharge; W/U: a Gram stain of the discharge reveals neutrophils, but no organisms are visualized.

Nongonococcal urethritis, most likely due to *Chlamydia trachomatis*

31-y/o obese woman presents with pruritis in her skin fold beneath her pannus; PE: whitish curd-like concretions beneath the abdominal panniculus; W/U shows budding yeast on 10% KOH preparation.

Cutaneous candidiasis

NEUROSCIENCE

55-y/o man presents with lower extremity weakness and muscle atrophy; PE: positive Babinski reflex, upper extremity hyperreflexia, and spasticity.

Amyotrophic lateral sclerosis (ALS)

65-y/o presents with a gradual decline in memory and inability to complete activities of daily living; W/U: CT shows marked enlargement of ventricles and diffuse cortical atrophy.

Alzheimer disease

65-y/o woman with h/o spinal metastases from breast cancer presents with pain radiating down the back of her leg, saddle anesthesia, urinary retention; PE: absent ankle jerk reflexes; W/U: CT shows large bony fragment in lumbar spinal canal.

Cauda equina syndrome

65-y/o man with h/o carotid atherosclerosis presents with aphasia and right-sided weakness; PE: dense right-hemiparesis, positive Babinski on right; W/U: CT shows left middle cerebral artery (MCA) territory infarction and edema.

Left MCA cerebrovascular accident

20-y/o presents with nausea, vomiting, and headache 2 hours after being hit in the temple with a baseball; patient lost consciousness initially but recovered quickly; W/U: CT shows lens-shaped, right-sided hyperdense mass adjacent to temporal bone.

Epidural hematoma

40-y/o with h/o *Campylobacter* enteritis 1 week ago presents with ascending symmetric muscle weakness; CSF shows ↑ protein, normal cellularity (albuminocytologic dissociation).

Guillain-Barré syndrome

37-y/o man with family history (FH) of a father who died at 45 with worsening tremor and dementia presents with poor memory, depression, choreiform movements, and hypotonia; W/U: MRI demonstrates marked atrophy of the caudate nucleus.

Huntington disease

25-y/o with h/o bilateral temporal lobe contusions 1 week ago presents with a sudden increase in appetite, sexual desire, and hyperorality.

Klüver-Bucy syndrome

30-y/o woman with insidious onset of diplopia, scanning speech, paresthesias, and numbness of right upper extremity and urinary incontinence; W/U: MRI shows discrete areas of periventricular demyelination and CSF analysis is positive for oligoclonal bands.

Multiple sclerosis

65-y/o woman with h/o neurofibromatosis type 2 presents with headache, right-sided leg jerking, and worsening mental status; PE: papilledema and right-sided pronator drift; W/U: CT scan shows dural-based, enhancing, left-sided softball-sized tumor.

Meningioma

55-y/o with a h/o squamous cell carcinoma of the lung presents with nausea, vomiting, headache, and diplopia; PE: papilledema, left oculomotor palsy, right pronator drift; MRI: multiple round, hyperintense cortical and cerebellar lesions.

Metastases to brain

30-y/o woman presents with unilateral throbbing headache, nausea, photophobia, scotoma; similar symptoms occur monthly at the same time of her menstrual cycle.	Migraine
65-y/o with urinary incontinence, loss of short-term memory, and dementia; PE: wide based, magnetic gate; W/U: CT scan shows massively dilated ventricular system.	Normal pressure hydrocephalus
60-y/o presents with gradual onset of pill-rolling tremor; PE: masked facies, stooped posture, festinating gait, cogwheel muscle rigidity.	Parkinson disease
30-y/o presents with loss of libido, galactorrhea, and irregular menses; PE: bitemporal hemianopia; W/U: negative beta human chorionic gonadotropin (β-hCG).	Prolactinoma (prolactin-secreting pituitary adenoma)
45-y/o presents with the gradual onset of sharp pain radiating from his buttocks down his leg that began 2 weeks ago when he began to lift a heavy box; PE: positive straight leg raise test.	Sciatica from acute herniation of a lumbar disc
50-y/o with h/o polycystic kidney disease presents with "worst headache of life," photophobia, nausea; PE: right eye deviated down and out; W/U: CSF is xanthrochromic.	Subarachnoid hemorrhage from ruptured berry aneurysm
32-y/o man with h/o Arnold-Chiari malformation presents with bilateral upper extremity muscle weakness; PE: loss of pain and temperature sensation, ↓ DTR in upper extremities and scoliosis; MRI shows central cavitation of the thoracic spinal cord.	Syringomyelia
75-y/o alcoholic man on warfarin for h/o atrial fibrillation presents with declining mental status, headache, and papilledema; CT shows crescenteric, hypodense, 2 cm fluid collection along convexity.	Chronic subdural hematoma

36-y/o woman with family h/o renal cell carcinoma presents with gait disturbance and blurred vision; PE: retinal hemangiomas, nystagmus, cerebellar ataxia, dysdiadokinesia; MRI shows two cerebellar cystic lesions.	von Hippel-Lindau disease
A 50-y/o with h/o alcoholism presents with psychosis, opthalmoplegia, and ataxia; MRI: mamillary body atrophy and diffuse cortical atrophy.	Wernicke encephalopathy

CARDIOVASCULAR

56-y/o woman presents with dyspnea on exertion (DOE); PE: loud S_1, delayed P_2, and a diastolic rumble; W/U: transesophageal echocardiogram shows mobile, pedunculated left atrial mass.	Atrial myxoma
60-y/o presents with chest pain relieved by sitting up and leaning forward; PE: pericardial friction rub; ECG: diffuse ST segment elevation; echocardiogram: pericardial effusion with thickening of the pericardium.	Acute pericarditis
65-y/o man presents with 1-week h/o fever, DOE, and orthopnea; PE: new, blowing holosystolic murmur at apex radiating into left axilla; W/U: blood cultures show *Viridans* spp. streptococci; echocardiogram: oscillating mass attached to mitral valve.	Acute infective endocarditis
60-y/o presents with dyspnea and palpitations; PE: 20 mm Hg decline in systolic BP with inspiration (pulsus paradoxus), $\downarrow$ BP, jugular venous distention, diminished S_1 and S_2; echocardiogram: large pericardial effusion.	Tamponade
58-y/o man with Marfan syndrome presents with the abrupt onset of "tearing" chest pain radiating to the back; PE: $\downarrow$ BP, asymmetric pulses, declining mental status; CXR: widened mediastinum.	Aortic dissection

70-y/o diabetic with hypercholesterolemia presents with angina, syncope, DOE, and orthopnea; PE: diminished, slowly rising carotid pulses, crescendo-decrescendo systolic murmur at second interspace at the right upper sternal border.	Aortic stenosis
80-y/o diabetic with HTN and a h/o rheumatic heart disease presents with left-sided weakness; PE: pulses are irregularly irregular; ECG: absence of P waves and irregularly irregular QRS complexes.	Atrial fibrillation (leading to embolic stroke)
70-y/o with h/o coronary artery disease (CAD) presents with worsening DOE, orthopnea, and paroxysmal nocturnal dyspnea; PE: jugular venous distention, S_3 gallop, positive hepatojugular reflex, bibasilar rales, and peripheral edema; CXR: cardiomegaly, bilateral pleural effusions.	Congestive heart failure (CHF)
50-y/o alcoholic presents with worsening DOE, orthopnea, and paroxysmal nocturnal dyspnea; PE: laterally displaced apical impulse; ECG: four-chamber dilation, mitral and tricuspid regurgitation.	Alcoholic dilated cardiomyopathy
35-y/o man with FH of sudden cardiac death presents with DOE and syncope; PE: double apical impulse, S_4 gallop, holosystolic murmur at apex and axilla; ECG: left ventricular hypertrophy and mitral regurgitation.	Hypertrophic cardiomyopathy
40-y/o black man with a h/o HTN presents with chest pain, dyspnea, and severe headache; PE: BP = 210/130 mm Hg in all four extremities, flame-shaped retinal hemorrhages, papilledema; W/U: negative vanillylmandelic acid (VMA), urine catecholamines, and cardiac enzymes.	Malignant hypertension
35-y/o woman with a h/o rheumatic fever presents with worsening DOE and orthopnea; PE: loud S_1, opening snap and low-pitched diastolic murmur at the apex; CXR: left atrial enlargement.	Mitral stenosis

65-y/o man presents with substernal pressure for the past hour with radiation of the pain into the jaw and left arm, nausea, diaphoresis, and dyspnea; PE: S$_4$ gallop; W/U: ↑ serum troponin and CK-MB; ECG: ST segment elevation in leads aVL, V$_1$ to V$_6$.

Anterior myocardial infarction

PULMONARY

7-y/o with h/o environmental allergies presents in acute respiratory distress; PE: tachypnea, expiratory wheezes, intercostal retractions, accessory muscle usage during respiration; CXR: hyperinflation; CBC: eosinophilia.

Bronchial asthma

60-y/o with a 50 pack-year h/o smoking presents with fever and cough productive of thick sputum for the past 4 months; PE: cyanosis, crackles, wheezes; W/U: Hct = 48, WBC = 12,000; CXR: no infiltrates.

Chronic bronchitis

60-y/o with a 50 pack-year h/o smoking presents with DOE and dry cough, but no chest pain; PE: ↓ breath sounds, ↑ heart rate (HR), hyperresonant chest, distant S$_1$ and S$_2$; CXR: hyperlucent lung fields.

Emphysema

60-y/o with 50 pack-year h/o smoking presents with fatigue, DOE, hoarseness, anorexia; PE: miosis, ptosis, anhydrosis, dullness to percussion at right apex; CXR: large, hilar mass extending into the right superior pulmonary sulcus.

Pancoast tumor (most likely bronchogenic squamous cell carcinoma, causing Horner syndrome)

60-y/o 4 days s/p total knee replacement has a sudden onset of tachycardia, tachypnea, sharp chest pain, hypotension; W/U: arterial blood gas (ABG) shows respiratory alkalosis; ECG: sinus tachycardia; lower extremity venous duplex ultrasound (U/S): clot in right femoral vein.

Pulmonary embolism (most likely from DVT)

30-y/o black woman presents with DOE, fever, arthralgia; PE: iritis, erythema nodosum; W/U: eosinophilia, ↑ serum ACE levels; PFT: restrictive pattern; CXR: bilateral hilar lymphadenopathy, interstitial infiltrates; lymph node biopsy: noncaseating granulomas.

Sarcordosis

40-y/o white man presents with chronic rhinosinusitis, ear pain, cough, dyspnea; PE: ulcerations of nasal mucosa, perforation of nasal septum; W/U: ↑ C-ANCA; U/A: red cell casts; biopsy of nasal lesions: necrotizing vasculitis and granulomas.

Wegener granulomatosis

GASTROENTEROLOGY

20-y/o woman presents with bloody diarrhea and joint pain; PE: abdominal tenderness, guaiac ⊕ stool; laboratory values: ↑ ESR and CRP, HLA-B27 +; colonoscopy: granular, friable muscosa with pseudopolyps throughout the colon.

Ulcerative colitis (UC)

28-y/o patient with h/o of UC presents with severe abdominal pain, distention, and high fever; PE: severe abdominal tenderness; CBC: leukocytosis; abdominal x-ray (AXR): dilated (> 6 cm) transverse colon.

Toxic megacolon

cirrhotic patient presents with massive hematemesis; PE: jaundice, ↓ BP, ↑ HR, ascites; W/U: stems pancytopenia, ↑ ALT and AST; EGD: actively bleeding vessel with numerous cherry red spots.

Esophageal varices

38-y/o man with recent h/o fatigue, excessive thirst, and impotence presents with hyperpigmentation of his skin; PE: cardiomegaly, HSM; W/U: ↑ glucose, ferritin, transferrin, and serum iron.

Hemochromatosis (hereditary)

19-y/o woman with recent h/o behavioral disturbance presents with jaundice and resting tremor; PE: pigmented granules in cornea and HSM; W/U: ↓ serum ceruloplasmin.

Wilson disease

29-y/o with h/o intermittent jaundice since receiving blood transfusion after motor vehicle accident (MVA) 2 years ago; PE: RUQ tenderness, hepatomegaly; W/U: negative HBV serology.

Hepatitis C infection

31-y/o woman presents with 10-month h/o foul-smelling, greasy diarrhea; PE: pallor, hyperkeratosis, multiple ecchymoses, and abdominal distention; W/U: abnormal D-xylose test.

Celiac disease

60-y/o white man presents with steatorrhea, weight loss, arthritis, and fever; small bowel biopsy shows PAS ⊕ macrophages and gram-positive bacilli.

Whipple disease

19-y/o Jewish woman with h/o chronic abdominal pain presents with recurrent UTIs and pneumaturia; PE: diffuse abdominal pain; CT: enterovesical fistula; colonoscopy: skip lesions of linear ulcers and transverse fissures giving cobblestone appearance to mucosa.

Crohn's disease

21-y/o man presents with hematemesis after ingestion of aspirin and seven shots of whiskey; PE: diaphoretic, ↑ HR, epigastric tenderness; EGD: edematous, friable, reddened gastric mucosa.

Acute gastritis

patient with h/o peptic ulcer disease (PUD) presents with melena; PE: ↑ HR, diaphoretic, diffuse abdominal pain; W/U: nasogastric tube (NGT) aspirate is bloody; EGD: visible bleeding vessel distal to the pylorus.

Bleeding duodenal ulcer

40-y/o obese, mother of four children presents with constant RUQ pain radiating to right scapula, N/V; PE: fever, tenderness, and respiratory pause induced by RUQ palpation, painful palpable gallbladder; W/U: ↑ WBC, ↑ ALP; U/S: thickened gallbladder wall, pericholecystic fluid with gallstones present.

Acute cholecystitis

39-y/o man presents with dull, steady epigastric pain radiating to the back after an alcohol binge, N/V; PE: fever, ↑ BP, epigastric tenderness, guarding, and distention; W/U: ↑↑ amylase/lipase, ↑ WBC; AXR: ⊕ sentinel loop and colon cutoff sign.	Acute pancreatitis
65-y/o black man with h/o smoking presents with anorexia, weight loss, pruritis, and painless jaundice; PE: palpable, nontender, distended gallbladder, migratory thrombophlebitis; W/U: ↑ direct BR, ALP, carcinoembryonic antigen (CEA), and CA 19-9.	Pancreatic adenocarcinoma
60-y/o black man with h/o gastroesophageal reflux disease (GERD) presents with weight loss and dysphagia; EGD: partially obstructing mass near GE junction.	Esophageal carcinoma
65-y/o presents with severe worsening left lower quadrant (LLQ) pain, N/V, and diarrhea; PE: fever, LLQ tenderness, local guarding, and rebound tenderness; W/U: ↑ WBC; abdominal CT: edematous colonic wall with localized fluid collection.	Diverticulitis
30-y/o woman presents with periumbilical pain which has now migrated to the RLQ followed by anorexia, N/V; PE: low-grade fever, local RLQ guarding, rebound tenderness, RLQ tenderness on LLQ palpation; W/U: β-hCG negative, ↑ WBC with left shift.	Appendicitis
55-y/o presents with colicky abdominal pain, small-caliber stools, and occasional melena; PE: cachexia, abdominal discomfort, guaiac ⊕ colonoscopy shows obstructing mass seen in ascending colon.	Right-sided colon carcinoma
80-y/o woman presents with halitosis, dysphagia, and regurgitation of undigested foods; W/U: barium swallow shows posterior midline pouch greater than 2 cm in diameter arising just above the cricopharyngeus muscle.	Zenker diverticulum

55-y/o Asian woman with h/o HBV presents with dull RUQ pain; PE: weight loss, painful hepatomegaly, ascites, jaundice; W/U: ↑ ALT/AST, ↑ α-fetoprotein; abdominal CT: mass seen in right lobe of liver.	Hepatocellular carcinoma
55-y/o with h/o choledocholithiasis presents with fever, chills, and RUQ pain; PE: jaundice; W/U: ↑ WBC, BR, and ALP; U/S: stone in common bile duct.	Cholangitis
43-y/o man presents with epigastric pain, diarrhea, and recurrent peptic ulcers; PE: epigastric tenderness; W/U: ↑ fasting gastrin levels, paradoxic ↑ in gastrin with secretin challenge; Octreotide scan: detects lesion in pancreas.	Zollinger-Ellison syndrome
72-y/o presents with recurrent, low-grade, painless hematochezia; PE: guaiac ⊕ stool; colonoscopy reveals slightly raised, discrete, scalloped lesion with visible draining vein in right colon.	Angiodysplasia
63-y/o Japanese man with h/o atrophic gastritis presents with weight loss, indigestion, epigastric pain, and vomiting; PE: supraclavicular lymph node; W/U: anemia, ⊕ fecal occult blood.	Gastric carcinoma
48-y/o with chronic watery diarrhea, hot flashes, and facial redness; PE: shows II/VI right-sided ejection murmur; W/U: ↑ 5-hydrocyindoleacetic acid (5-HIAA) in urine.	Carcinoid syndrome
40-y/o presents with dysphagia, regurgitation, and weight loss; W/U: barium swallow demonstrates dilated esophagus with distal narrowing (*bird beak* appearance).	Achalasia
16-y/o with strong FH of colorectal CA presents with rectal bleeding and abdominal pain; W/U: anemia; flexible sigmoidoscopy: > 100 adenomatous polyps visualized.	Familial adenomatous polyposis (FAP)

34-y/o bulimic presents with sudden-onset retrosternal pain after vigorous vomiting; upper GI series shows extravasation of contrast into mediastinum.	Boerhaave syndrome
44-y/o heavy smoker presents with heartburn and regurgitation that is worse when lying down and is relieved with antacids; upper GI series reveals mild hiatal hernia.	GERD
5-day-old infant presents with abdominal distention and failure to pass meconium until after a rectal examination; XR shows massively dilated colon.	Hirschsprung disease
39-y/o woman with h/o rheumatoid arthritis presents with fatigue and pruritus; PE: jaundice and HSM; W/U reveals ↑↑ ALP and γ-glutamyl transpeptidase (GGT) and presence of antimitochondrial antibodies.	Primary biliary cirrhosis
2-week-old first-born male infant presents with projectile vomiting and dehydration; PE: visible peristalsis and palpable knot in epigastrum.	Hypertrophic pyloric stenosis
50-y/o with long h/o retrosternal pain drinks and smokes despite undergoing treatment for GERD; biopsy of distal esophagus shows metaplasia.	Barrett's esophagus
34-y/o woman with factor V Leiden deficiency presents with abdominal distention and jaundice; PE: pitting pedal edema, markedly visible leg veins, HSM, and absent hepatojugular reflex; U/S shows obstruction of hepatic veins.	Budd-Chiari syndrome
7-month-old infant presents with vomiting and currant jelly-appearing stools; PE: right-sided, sausage-shaped, palpable mass in abdomen; barium enema (BE) shows telescoping of intestines.	Intussusception

REPRODUCTIVE/ENDOCRINE

31-y/o presents with loss of libido, galactorrhea, and irregular menses; PE: bitemporal hemianopia; W/U: negative β-hCG.

Prolactinoma

7-month-old with history of multiple infections turns cyanotic when aggravated; PE: abnormal facies, cleft palate, heart murmur; W/U: hypocalcemia, tetrology of Fallot.

DiGeorge syndrome (22qll)

Patient presents to clinic with polyuria and polydipsia; W/U: urine specific gravity < 1.005, urine osmolality < 200 mOsm/kg, hypernatremia.

Diabetes insipidus

30-y/o white woman presents with weight loss, tremor, and palpitations; PE: brisk DTRs, ophthalmopathy, pretibial myxedema; W/U: ↓ TSH, ↑ T_4, ↑ T_3 index.

Graves disease

40-y/o woman presents with fatigue, constipation, and weight loss; PE: puffy face, cold dry hands, coarse hair, and enlargement of thyroid gland; W/U: ↑ TSH, ↓ T_3 and T_4, ⊕ antimicrosomal and antithyroglobulin AB.

Hashimoto disease

32-y/o woman with h/o recurrent PUD presents with episodes of hypocalcemia and nephrolithiasis; W/U: fasting hypoglycemia, ↑ gastrin levels, and hypercalcemia.

Multiple endocrine neoplasia (MEN) 1

70-y/o presents with episodal hypertension, nephrolithiasis, and diarrhea; PE: ↑ BP, thyroid nodule; W/U: ↑ calcitonin levels, ↑ urinary catecholamines.

MEN 2

Female patient presents with bone pain, kidney stones, depression, and recurrent ulcers; W/U: hypercalcemia, hypophosphatemia, and hypercalciuria.

Hyperparathyroidism

35-y/o woman presents with weight gain, irregular menses, and HTN; PE: ↑ BP, ↑ weight in face and upper back, hirtuism, multiple ecchymoses; W/U: ↑ ACTH levels and suppression with high-dose dexamethasone suppression test.

Cushing disease

50-y/o woman presents with HTN, muscle weakness, and fatigue; W/U: hypokalemia, hypernatremia, and metabolic alkalosis.

Conn syndrome

30-y/o woman presents with progressive weakness, weight loss, N/V; PE: hyperpigmentation of skin, ↓ BP; W/U: hyperkalemia, hyponatremia, and eosinophilia.

Addison disease

40-y/o presents with episodes of HA, diaphoresis, palpitations, and tremor; PE: ↑ BP, ↑ HR; W/U: ↑ in urinary VMA and homovanillic acid.

Pheochromocytoma

17-y/o white adolescent with h/o diabetes mellitus (DM) presents with diffuse abdominal pain, N/V, and slight confusion; PE: ↓ BP, shallow, rapid breathing pattern; W/U: glucose = 300, hypokalemia, hypophosphatemia, and metabolic acidosis.

Diabetic ketoacidosis (DKA)-DM type 1

60-y/o diabetic obese patient found at home confused and disoriented; PE: ↓ BP, ↑ HR; W/U: glucose > 1000.

Hyperosmolar hyperglycemic non-ketotic (HHNK)-DM type 2

50-y/o woman presents with h/o weakness, blurred vision, and confusion several hours after meals, which improves with eating; W/U: ↑ fasting levels of insulin and hypoglycemia.

Insulinoma (with Whipple triad)

Newborn presents with ambiguous genitalia; PE: lethargy and ↓ BP; W/U: ↓ Na^+, ↑ K^+, ↑ 17 α-OH-progesterone, ↑ ACTH, and karyotype of 46,XX.

Congenital adrenal hyperplasia (21α-hydroxylase deficiency)

7-y/o girl presents with breast buds and monthly vaginal bleeding; PE: height and weight >> 95 percentile, full pubic and axillary hair; hand x-ray shows advanced bone age.

Precocious puberty

21-y/o woman presents with no h/o menarche; PE: normal breast tissue, no axillary or pubic hair, vagina ending in blind pouch, no palpable cervix or uterus; karyotype shows 46,XY.	Androgen insensitivity (testicular feminization) syndrome
45-y/o with recent h/o coarsening of facial features presents with headaches and states that his shoes no longer fit; PE: enlarged jaw, tongue, hands, and feet, and bitemporal hemianopia.	Acromegaly
65-y/o smoker with h/o lung cancer presents with fatigue and oliguria; W/U: ↓ Na⁺, ↓ serum osmolarity, ↑↑ urine osmolarity.	Syndrome of inappropriate antidiuretic hormone (SIADH)
22-y/o sexually active woman presents with dysuria, dyspareunia, vulvar pain for the past 3 days. PE: soft ulcer on labia majora, inguinal lymphadenopathy; W/U: culture grows *Haemophilus ducreyi*.	Chancroid
20-y/o sexually active woman presents with crampy abdominal pain and purulent vaginal discharge; PE: fever and adnexal tenderness; W/U: ↑ WBCs, ↑ ESR, and combined infection with *C. trachomatis* and *Neisseria gonorrhoeae*.	Pelvic inflammatory disease (PID)
18-y/o woman with 3 days of vaginal pruritis; PE: thick, white discharge; W/U: budding yeast on KOH preparation.	Vaginal candidiasis
28-y/o woman postpartum day 1 with excessive hemorrhage in labor becomes weak and loses consciousness. PE: hypotension; W/U: ↓ cortisol, ↓ TSH, ↓ fT₄, ↓ LH, ↓ FSH.	Sheehan syndrome (pituitary apoplexy)
31-y/o woman with h/o PID presents with sudden-onset nausea and LLQ pain; PE: ↓ BP, ↑ HR, rebound tenderness in LLQ; W/U shows ⊕ β-hCG and fluid in cul-de-sac on U/S.	Ruptured ectopic pregnancy
28-y/o man presents with gynecomastia and painless lump in his left testicle for 3 months; PE: firm 4 cm mass on left testis; W/U: ↑↑ serum hCG and AFP.	Testicular carcinoma

35-y/o man with sensation of heaviness in left scrotum; appears like a "bag of worms" on examination.	Varicocele
62-y/o obese nun with h/o menopause at age 57 presents with vaginal bleeding for the past 4 months; PE shows normal-sized uterus; Pap smear reveals abnormal endometrial cells.	Endometrial carcinoma
52-y/o obese patient presents with numbness in hands and feet; PE: ↑ BP and retinopathy; W/U: ↑ HbA_{1c} and glycosuria.	DM type 2
55-y/o woman presents with an itching, scaling, oozing rash over her left nipple; PE: serosanguinous discharge and eczematous redness of left nipple with axillary lymphadenopathy.	Paget disease of the breast
4-y/o girl presents with a "bunch of grapes" protruding from her vagina. W/U: desmin positive.	Sarcoma botryoides
37-y/o woman presents with dysmenorrhea, dyspareunia, menorrhagia, and pain coinciding with her menstrual cycle; PE: nodularity of uterosacral ligaments and cul-de-sac.	Endometriosis
22-y/o woman with 6-month h/o amenorrhea presents for infertility evaluation; PE: obesity, hirsutism; W/U: ↑ LH:FSH ratio, ↑ testosterone, and enlarged ovaries on U/S.	Polycystic ovarian syndrome (Stein-Leventhal syndrome)
44-y/o with recent h/o thyroidectomy presents with muscle cramping; PE: circumoral numbness, positive Trousseau and Chvostek signs.	Hypoparathyroidism
23-y/o woman marathon runner presents with lack of menses for 5 months; PE shows no signs of pregnancy; W/U: negative β-hCG, normal prolactin and thyroid hormones.	Secondary amenorrhea

28-y/o black woman at 35 weeks gestation in her first pregnancy presents with swollen legs; PE: ↑ BP and pitting pedal edema; W/U: 3+ proteinuria.	Preeclampsia
2-y/o child presents with developmental delay; PE: macroglossia, short stature, and protuberant abdomen; W/U: ↑ TSH, ↓ T_3 and T_4.	Congenital hypothyroidism (cretinism)
51-y/o woman with 9-month h/o amenorrhea presents with fatigue and flushing of skin; PE: atrophic vaginal mucosa; W/U: ↑ FSH and LH.	Menopause
24-y/o woman presents with painless lump in her left breast; PE: small, firm, palpable, and freely mobile, rubbery mass in the upper-outer quadrant of the breast.	Fibroadenoma
19-y/o man is brought to you for failure of pubertal maturation; PE: anosmia, ↓ muscle mass, no axillary or pubic hair, and hypogonadism; W/U: ↓ LH and FSH.	Kallmann syndrome
9-y/o girl presents with muscle cramps; PE: rounded face with flat nasal bridge, abnormal dentition, positive Trousseau and Chvostek sign, and shortened third and fourth metacarpals.	Albright hereditary osteodystrophy (pseudohypoparathyroidism)
22-y/o pregnant woman at 27 weeks with painless vaginal bleeding that stopped after an hour. W/U: placenta overlying the cervical os on ultrasound.	Placenta previa
19-y/o woman with h/o recent hydatidiform mole presents with vaginal bleeding, nausea, and vomiting; PE: vascular growth at cervical os and enlarged uterus; W/U: ↑↑ β-hCG.	Choriocarcinoma
35-y/o man presents for sterility evaluation; PE: eunuchoid body habitus, small testicles, and gynecomastia; karyotype reveals 47,XXY.	Klinefelter syndrome

RENAL AND GENITOURINARY

Patient hospitalized for CHF is started on an aminoglycoside for a UTI and develops oliguria, N/V, and malaise; PE: ↑ BP and asterixis; serum electrolytes: ↑ creatinine (Cr), K$^+$; UA: "muddy brown" casts, FeNa$^+$ > 3%.

Acute renal failure (drug-induced ATN)

70-y/o black man with h/o of life-long DM presents with peripheral edema, SOB, and oliguria; PE: auscultatory rales, pitting edema, myoclonus, and uremic frost; serum electrolytes: ↑ Cr, hyperkalemia, hypocalcemia, hyperphosphatemia.

Chronic renal failure

Teenage female presents with fever, chills, and flank pain; PE: costovertebral angle (CVA) tenderness; UA: leukocyte esterase ⊕, 30 WBC/hpf with WBC casts.

Pyelonephritis

32-y/o man presents with pain and hematuria; PE: ↑ BP, palpable kidney, and midsystolic ejection click; abdominal U/S: multiple cysts of renal parenchyma; cerebral angiogram: unruptured berry aneurysm.

Adult polycystic kidney disease

20-y/o man presents with significant blood loss following a trauma and begins to have decreased urine output. W/U: oliguria, FeNa < 1%, and BUN:Cr > 20.

Acute renal failure—prerenal

12-y/o girl with recent h/o sore throat presents with low urine output and dark urine; PE: periorbital edema; W/U: hematuria, ↑ BUN and Cr, ↑ antistreptolysin O (ASO) titer.

Poststreptococcal glomerulonephritis

45-y/o Asian man with h/o hepatitis B presents with malaise, edema, and foamy urine; PE: anasarca; W/U: proteinuria (> 3.5 g/day), hyperlipiduria; hyperlipidemia and hypoalbuminemia.

Membranous glomerulonephritis

Male infant is born with flattened facies, joint position abnormalities, and hypoplastic lungs. Oligohydramnios was noted prior to delivery.

Potter sequence—secondary to renal agenesis

80-y/o man presents with urinary hesitancy, nocturia, and weak urinary stream; PE: diffusely enlarged rubbery prostate; serum electrolytes: ↑ Cr, UA is WNL.

Benign prostatic hyperplasia (BPH)

68-y/o man, who is a smoker, presents with flank pain and hematuria; PE: fever, palpable kidney mass; W/U: hypercalcemia, polycythemia.

Renal cell carcinoma

20 y/o man presents with acute onset of left testicular pain and N/V; PE: swollen, tender testicle in transverse position, absent cremasteric reflex on left side; Doppler: no flow detected in left testicle.

Testicular torsion

65-y/o man, who is a smoker, presents with painless hematuria and occasional urinary urgency and frequency; PE: unremarkable; urine cytology positive for malignant cells.

Bladder—urothelial carcinoma

85-y/o man presents with back pain, weight loss, and weak urinary stream; PE: palpable firm nodule on digital rectal examination (DRE); W/U: ↑ PSA.

Prostate cancer

25-y/o Asian man presents with N/V and colicky right flank pain; PE: acute distress and CVA tenderness; W/U: hematuria and discrete radiopacities on abdominal XR.

Renal stones

45-y/o with documented h/o aortic atheromatous plaques presents with recent-onset, severe left flank pain, and hematuria; abdominal CT: wedge-shaped lesion in the left kidney.

Renal infarct

3-y/o boy presents with h/o flank mass found recently by his mother while bathing him; PE: palpable mass in left flank; abdominal CT: large mass growing out of left kidney.

Wilms tumor

55-y/o with long h/o DM presents with increasing fatigue and edema; PE: ↑ BP, retinopathy, and pitting edema; W/U: severe proteinuria and glycosuria.	Diabetic nephropathy (glomerulosclerosis)
21-y/o sexually active woman presents with frequency and dysuria; PE: suprapubic tenderness; W/U: *E. coli*-positive urine cultures.	Urinary tract infection (UTI)
25-y/o man presents with hemoptysis, dark urine, and fatigue; PE: bilateral crackles at lung bases; W/U: oliguria, hematuria, and anti-GBM antibodies.	Goodpasture syndrome
7-y/o presents in stupor after ingesting antifreeze; PE: Kussmaul respirations and mental status changes; W/U reveals anion gap of 21 mEq/L.	Metabolic acidosis (ethylene glycol toxicity)
6-y/o boy presents with hematuria and worsening vision; PE: corneal abnormalities, retinopathy, sensorineural hearing loss; W/U: hematuria with dysmorphic red cells.	Alport syndrome
3-y/o boy with h/o recent URI presents with facial edema; PE: ascitic fluid in abdomen and pedal edema; W/U reveals 4+ proteinuria and ↓ serum albumin.	Minimal change disease

HEMATOLOGY/ONCOLOGY

50-y/o with h/o bone marrow transplant for chronic myelogenous leukemia (CML) 3 weeks ago presents with severe pruritis, diarrhea, and jaundice; PE: violaceous rash on palms and soles; W/U: ↑ BR, ALT, and AST.	Graft-versus-host disease
1-y/o Greek child presents with pallor and delayed milestones; PE: skeletal abnormalities, splenomegaly; peripheral blood smear (PBS): hypochromic microcytic RBCs, target cells, fragmented RBCs; skull XR: "hair-on-end" appearance.	β-Thalassemia

10-y/o with a h/o recurrent chest pain presents with fever and bilateral leg pain; PE: febrile, multiple leg ulcers; PBS shows sickle-shaped erythrocytes; Hb electrophoresis shows HbS band.	Sickle cell anemia
60-y/o with headache, vertigo, blurry vision, pruritus, joint pain; PE: ↑ BP, plethoric splenomegaly; W/U: Hct = 60, mild leukocytosis, and hyperuricemia.	Polycythemia vera
4-y/o boy with a 1-week h/o fever, pallor, headache, and bone tenderness; PE: fever, HSM, and generalized, nontender lymphadenopathy; PBS reveals absolute lymphocytosis with abundant TdT+ lymphoblasts.	Acute lymphoblastic leukemia
27-y/o presents with 2-month h/o fatigue, oropharyngeal candidiasis, pseudomonal UTI, and epistaxis; PE: numerous petechiae and ecchymoses of skin, gingival mucosal bleeding, guaiac ⊕ stools; W/U: ↑ WBC; PBS shows >30% myeloblasts with Auer rods.	Acute myelocytic leukemia
17-y/o man presents with a 2-month h/o fever, night sweats, and weight loss; PE: nontender, cervical lymphadenopathy, and HSM; CBC: leukocytosis; CXR: bilateral hilar adenopathy; lymph node biopsy: Reed-Sternberg cells.	Hodgkin disease
60-y/o man presents with fatigue and anorexia; PE: generalized lymphadenopathy and HSM; W/U: WBC = 250,000, positive direct Coombs test; PBS: small, round lymphocytes predominate with occasional smudge cells.	Chronic lymphocytic leukemia
10-y/o African child presents with a 3-week h/o a rapidly enlarging, painless mandibular mass; CBC: mild anemia and leukopenia; cytogenetics reveal a t(8:14) translocation; excisional biopsy: "starry-sky" pattern.	Burkitt lymphoma

35-y/o presents with a 3-year h/o mild weight loss, anorexia, worsening DOE; PE: splenomegaly; CBC: mild anemia, WBC = 125,000; PBS: granulocytosis with < 10% myeloblasts; cytogenetics reveal a t(9:22) translocation.	Chronic myelocytic leukemia
55-y/o with a recent h/o streptococcal pneumonia presents with bone pain and weight loss; W/U: mild anemia, hypercalcemia; PBS: roleau formation; UA: Bence-Jones proteinuria; serum electrophoresis: M spike; XR: cranial "punched-out" lesions.	Multiple myeloma
18-y/o woman develops dyspnea and declining mental status 1 hour after a C-section complicated by excess blood loss; PE: mucosal bleeding, large clot in the vaginal vault; W/U: ↑ D-dimer, ↑ PT/PTT, ↓ antithrombin III, and thrombocytopenia.	Disseminated intravascular coagulation
7-y/o with h/o viral URI 1 week ago presents with epistaxis; PE: petechial hemorrhages of nasal mucosa and extremities; W/U: ↓ platelets, normal PT and PTT; bone marrow biopsy: ↑↑ megakaryocytes.	Idiopathic thrombocytopenic purpura
8-y/o with a h/o vomiting and diarrhea after eating a hamburger last week presents with fatigue, periorbital edema, and oliguria; PE: purpuric rash; CBC: ↓ platelets; PBS: burr cells, helmet cells; UA: RBC casts, proteinuria, hematuria.	Hemolytic uremic syndrome
8-y/o with a h/o environmental allergies presents with a painful rash on the legs, abdominal discomfort, joint pain; UA: hematuria and RBC casts; renal biopsy: glomerular mesangial IgA deposits.	Henoch-Schönlein purpura
8-y/o boy presents with a swollen painful knee; FH: maternal grandfather died from hemorrhage after a cholecystectomy; PE: cutaneous ecchymoses; W/U: gross blood in swollen knee joint, ↑ PTT, normal PT and platelet count, ↑ bleeding time.	Hemophilia A

2-y/o boy with a h/o recurrent epistaxis presents with the third episode of otitis media in 4 months; PE: eczematous dermatitis; W/U: thrombocytopenia, $\downarrow$ IgM, $\uparrow$ IgA.

Wiskott-Aldrich syndrome

Newborn develops jaundice rapidly during the first day of life; PE: HSM; W/U: severe anemia, $\oplus$ indirect Coombs test in both mother and newborn.

Rh incompatibility

16-y/o adolescent with a h/o menorrhagia presents with fatigue; PE: multiple cutaneous bruises; guiaic $\oplus$ stools; W/U: $\uparrow$ bleeding time, $\downarrow$ factor VIII, normal platelet count, PT, and PTT.

von Willebrand disease

SKIN AND CONNECTIVE TISSUES

30-y/o man with h/o recurrent sinusitis presents for sterility evaluation; PE: heart sounds are best heard over right side of chest.

Kartagener syndrome

9-y/o with h/o easy bruising and hyperextensible joints presents to the ER after dislocating his shoulder for the fifth time this year.

Ehlers-Danlos syndrome

5-y/o presents to the ER with his sixth bone fracture in the past 2 years; PE: bluish sclera and mild kyphosis; XR: fractures with evidence of osteopenia.

Osteogenesis imperfecta

8-y/o with a long h/o severe sunburns and photophobia presents to the dermatologist for evaluation of several lesions on the face that have recently changed color and size.

Xeroderma pigmentosum

6-y/o boy presents to the ophthalmology clinic with sudden $\downarrow$ visual acuity; PE: unusual body habitus, long and slender fingers, pectus excavatum, and superiorly dislocated lens.

Marfan syndrome

36-y/o with h/o celiac disease presents with clusters of erythematous vesicular lesions over the extensor surfaces of the extremities.	Dermatitis herpetiformis
5-y/o patient presents with honey-colored crusted lesions at the angle of his mouth; Gram stain of pus: gram-positive cocci in chains.	Impetigo
29-y/o HIV-positive patient presents with multiple painless pearly-white umbilicated nodules on the trunk and anogenital area.	Molluscum contagiosum
68-y/o fair-skinned farmer presents with large, telangiectatic, and ulcerated nodule on the bridge of the nose.	Basal cell carcinoma
11-y/o presents with bilateral wrist pain and a rash; PE: erythematous, reticular skin rash of the face and trunk with a "slapped-cheek appearance."	Erythema infectiosum
43-y/o woman presents with difficulty swallowing; PE: bluish discoloration of the hands and shiny, tight skin over her face and fingers.	Progressive systemic sclerosis (scleroderma)
5-y/o Asian boy presents with fever and diffuse rash including the palms and soles; PE: cervical lymphadenopathy, conjunctival injection, and desquamation of his fingertips; echocardiogram reveals dilation of coronary arteries.	Kawasaki syndrome (mucocutaneous lymph node syndrome)
33-y/o patient presents with itchy, purple plaques over her wrists, forearms, and inner thigh; PE: Wickham striae.	Lichen planus
25-y/o woman with h/o Raynaud phenomenon presents with arthralgias and myositis; W/U reveals esophageal hypomotility and ↑ anti-nRNP titers.	Mixed connective tissue disease

MUSCULOSKELETAL

25-y/o man presents with morning stiffness, heel pain, and photophobia; PE: ↓ lumbar spine extension and lateral flexion, tenderness on lumbar spinous processes and iliac crests; W/U: HLA-B27 ⊕ ; XR: bamboo spine.

Ankylosing spondylitis

7-y/o girl presents with a limp, anorexia, and spiking fevers; PE: salmon-pink linear rash on trunk and extremities and swelling of bilateral hip, knee, elbow, and wrist joints; W/U: ↑ ESR.

Juvenile rheumatoid arthritis

50-y/o woman presents with long-standing h/o morning stiffness and diffuse joint pain; PE: boutonierre and swan neck deformities of fingers, shoulder tenderness, and ↓ range of motion (ROM), symmetric and bilateral knee swelling; W/U: RF positive.

Rheumatoid arthritis

25-y/o man with a h/o urethritis 2 weeks ago presents with unilateral knee pain, stiffness, and eye pain; PE: conjunctivitis, edema, and tenderness of left knee, mucoid urethral discharge; W/U: urethral swab ⊕ for *Chlamydia*.

Reiter syndrome

45-y/o woman presents with dry eyes and dry mouth, PE: parotid gland enlargement, bibasilar rales; W/U: ⊕ ANA, RF, SS-A/Ro titers.

Sjögren syndrome

70-y/o woman presents with pain in hands that is worse with activity, PE: Heberden and Bouchard nodes, bony enlargement at DIP and PIP joints, bilateral knee effusions; W/U: negative RF, normal ESR; hand XR: joint space narrowing, osteophytes.

Osteoarthritis

72-y/o woman presents with a 6-week h/o morning stiffness in neck and shoulders; PE: low-grade fever, tenderness to palpation, and decreased ROM in neck, shoulder, hip joints; W/U: ↑ ESR and CRP, but negative RF.

Polymyalgia rheumatica

50-y/o man presents with acute onset of sharp pain in the left great toe; PE: severe tenderness, swelling, and warmth of the left MTP joint; synovial fluid analysis shows negatively birefringent crystals.	Gout
25-y/o woman with a 1-week h/o pain in several joints presents with swelling, redness, and pain in her right knee; PE: pustular lesions on palms, right knee shows erythema, tenderness, and ↓ ROM; W/U: gram-negative diplococci in synovial fluid.	Gonococcal arthritis
28-y/o woman presents with difficulty keeping her eyelids open and holding her head up during the day; PE: weakness of facial muscles, deltoids; W/U: anti-ACh titer +; CXR: anterior mediastinal mass.	Myasthenia gravis (associated with thymoma)
20-y/o black woman presents with fatigue, arthralgias, Raynaud phenomenon, and pleuritic chest pain; PE: butterfly malar facial rash; W/U: ↓ platelets, proteinuria, and ⊕ ANA, anti-dsDNA, and anti-Smith Abs.	Systemic lupus erythematosus (SLE)
20-y/o with a h/o developmental delay presents with facial weakness; PE: cataracts, marked weakness in muscles of hand, neck, and distal leg with sustained muscle contraction; genetic testing: CTG repeat expansion within *DMPK* gene.	Myotonic dystrophy

BEHAVIORAL SCIENCE

20-y/o woman presents with excessive anxiety about a variety of events for more than half of the days for the last 7 months.	Generalized anxiety disorder
8-y/o boy presents with a 5-month h/o regular bedwetting episodes; PE is unremarkable and fasting glucose is WNL.	Enuresis

28-y/o man who systematically checks each lock in his house every time before leaving, often causing him to be over an hour late for meetings.	Obsessive-compulsive disorder
29-y/o man presents with a 9-month h/o insatiable urges to rub himself against strangers, which he has regretably acted on several times.	Frotteurism
22-y/o woman college student who is 20% below her ideal body weight complains of not having any menstrual cycles and "feeling fat."	Anorexia nervosa
26-y/o woman medical student is convinced for the past 9 months that she has SLE and despite numerous negative workups, she fears she will have to drop out of school.	Hypochondriasis
17-y/o woman presents with complaints of "feeling fat" and h/o eating dinner alone in her bedroom; PE shows normal height and weight, dental erosions, and scars on the back of her hand.	Bulimia
21-y/o woman with no h/o trauma presents to the ER because she cannot feel or move her legs; W/U is WNL; detailed history reveals that her boyfriend left her this morning.	Conversion disorder
43-y/o alcoholic with h/o confabulation and amnesia presents to ER after falling down; PE shows nystagmus and ataxic gait; W/U reveals macrocytic anemia.	Wernicke-Korsakoff syndrome
6-y/o presents with 8-month h/o hyperactivity, inattentiveness, and impulsivity both at school and at home; PE and W/U are WNL.	Attention deficit hyperactivity disorder (ADHD)
33-y/o woman presents to your office distressed after turning down a lucrative job offer because of the requirement to speak in front of people.	Social phobia
9-y/o boy with 2-year h/o involuntary tics is brought to your office because he has recently been shouting obscenities.	Tourette syndrome

33-y/o woman nurse presents with recent occurrences of hypoglycemia; PE reveals multiple crossed scars on abdomen; W/U shows insulin/C-peptide ratio > 1.0.	Factitious disorder (Munchausen syndrome)
33-y/o is referred to you for reports of random episode of shouting and screaming during the night; he has no recollection of the event and denies having nightmares.	Sleep terror disorder
16-y/o with h/o sudden-onset daytime sleep attacks with loss of muscle tone and audiovisual hallucinations while waking and falling asleep.	Narcolepsy
19-y/o with an 8-month h/o deteriorating grades and social withdrawal presents with auditory hallucinations; PE shows odd thinking patterns, tangential thoughts, and flattened effects.	Schizophrenia
24-y/o with h/o depression presents with ↓ need for sleep and auditory hallucinations; PE reveals easy distractibility and pressured speech; W/U shows normal TSH and negative toxicology screen.	Bipolar disorder—type 1 (manic episode)
48-y/o woman presents with recent h/o early morning waking, ↓ appetite, feelings of guilt, and loss of interest in her usual hobbies over the past 3 months; PE and laboratory results are WNL.	Major depressive disorder
68-y/o veteran presents with complaints of vivid flashbacks, hypervigilance, and difficulty falling asleep for the past several years; patient appears very anxious during the PE.	Posttraumatic stress disorder
6-month-old child presents with unyielding crying; PE reveals multiple bruises in different stages of healing and bilateral retinal hemorrhages; XR shows multiple, healing fractures along posterior ribs.	Shaken baby syndrome

43-y/o woman from Boston finds herself   Dissociative fugue
in Utah, but does not remember
why she is there or how she got there;
PE and W/U are WNL; detailed history
reveals that her son suddenly died
1 week ago.

3-y/o boy with h/o of poor cuddling   Autism
presents with severely delayed
language and social development;
PE reveals below normal intelligence
with unusual calculating abilities
and repetitive behaviors.

Abbreviations

AA	amino acid		BM	basement membrane
Ab	antibody		BP	blood pressure
ABG	arterial-blood gas		BPG	bisphophoglycerate
ACE	angiotensin-converting enzyme		BPH	benign prostatic hyperplasia
ACEi	ACE inhibitor		BR	bilirubin
ACh	acetylcholine		BUN	blood urea nitrogen
ACL	anterior cruciate ligament		Bx	biopsy
ACTH	adrenocortiotropic hormone		CA	cancer/carcinoma
AD	autosomal dominant		CAD	coronary artery disease
ADH	antidiuretic hormone		cAMP	cyclic adenosine monophosphate
ADHD	attention deficit hyperactivity disorder		cANCA	cytoplasmic pattern of antineu trophil cytoplasmic antibodies
ADP	adenosine diphosphate		CBC	complete blood count
AFP	α-fetoprotein		CCK	cholecystokinin
Ag	antigen		CEA	carcinoembryonic antigen
AIDS	acquired immunodeficiency syndrome		CF	cystic fibrosis
ALL	acute lymphocytic leukemia		CFTR	cystic fibrosis transmembrane regulator
ALP	alkaline phosphatase		cGMP	cyclic guanosine monophosphate
ALS	amyotrophic lateral sclerosis		CHF	congestive heart failure
ALT	alanine transaminase		CIN	cervical intraepithelial neoplasia
AML	acute myelogenous leukemia		CK	serum creatine kinase
ANA	antinuclear antibody		CLL	chronic lymphocytic leukemia
ANOVA	analysis of variance		CML	chronic myelogenous leukemia
ANS	autonomic nervous system		CMV	cytomegalovirus
AR	autosomal recessive		CN	cranial nerve
ARB	angiotensin receptor blocker		CNS	central nervous system
ARDS	acute respiratory distress syndrome		CO	cardiac output
ASA	aspirin		CoA	coenzyme A
ASD	atrial septal defect		COMT	catechol-O-methyltransferase
ASO	antistreptolysin O		COPD	chronic obstructive pulmonary disease
AST	aspartate transaminase		COX	cyclooxygenase
ATN	ischemic acute tubular necrosis		C_p	concentration in plasma
ATP	adenosine triphosphate		CPK	creatine phosphokinase
ATPase	adenosine triphosphatase		Cr	creatinine
AV	atrioventricular		CRP	C-reactive protein
AXR	abdominal x-ray		CSF	cerebrospinal fluid
AZT	azidothymidine		CT	computed tomography
BAL	British anti-Lewisite		CV	cardiovascular

CVA	cerebrovascular accident or costovertebral angle	FSH	follicle-stimulating hormone
		FN	false negatives
CXR	chest x-ray	FP	false positives
D or DA	dopamine	FTA-ABS	fluorescent treponemal antibody-absorbed
d	day(s)		
d/o	disorder	Fx	fracture
DAG	diacylglycerol	G3P	glucose-3-phosphate
DES	diethylstilbesterol	G6PD	glucose-6-phosphate dehydrogenase
DHT	dihydrotestosterone		
DI	diabetes insipidus	GABA	γ-aminobutyric acid
DIC	disseminated intravascular coagulation	GBM	glomerular basement membrane
		GCT	germ cell tumor
DIP	distal interphalangeal joint	GFR	glomerular filtration rate
DKA	diabetic ketoacidosis	GGT	γ-glutamyl transpeptidase
DM	diabetes mellitus	GH	growth hormone
DNA	deoxyribonucleic acid	GI	gastrointestinal
DOE	dyspnea on exertion	G_i	G protein, inhibitory
DRE	digital rectal examination	GMP	guanosine monophosphate
ds	double stranded	GN	glomerulonephritis
DSM	diagnostic and statistical manual	GnRH	gonadotropin-releasing hormone
DTR	deep tendon reflex	G_s	G protein, stimulatory
DTs	delerium tremens	GSE	general somatic efferent
DVT	deep venous thrombosis	GTP	guanosine triphosphate
E	epinephrine	GU	genitourinary
EBV	Epstein-Barr virus	GVE	general visceral efferent
ECF	extracellular fluid	HA	headache
ECG	electrocardiogram	Hb	hemoglobin
ECT	electroconvulsive therapy	HBV	hepatitis B virus
EDV	end-diastolic volume	hCG	human chorionic gonadotropin
EEG	electroencephalogram	HDL	high-density lipoprotein
EF-2	elongation factor 2	HGPRT	hypoxanthine guanine phosphoryltransferase
EGD	esophagogastroduodenoscopy		
ELISA	enzyme-linked immunosorbent assay	HHV	human herpesvirus
		HIV	human immunodeficiency virus
EM	electron microscopy	HMG-CoA	hydroxymethylglutaryl-CoA
EOM	extraocular muscle	h	hour(s)
EPO	erythropoetin	h/o	history of
EPS	extrapyramidal symptoms	HPETE	hydroperoxyeicosatetraenoic acid
ER	endoplasmic reticulum or emergency room		
		HPV	human papillomavirus
ESR	erythrocyte sedimentation rate	HR	heart rate
ESV	end-systolic volume	HRT	hormone replacement therapy
ETOH	ethanol	HSM	hepatosplenomegaly
FAs	fatty acids	HSV	herpes simplex virus
FAD	flavin adenine dinucleotide (oxidized)	HTLV	human T-cell leukemia/lymphoma virus
$FADH_2$	flavin adenine dinucleotide (reduced)	HUS	hemolytic-uremic syndrome
		HTN	hypertension
FAP	familial adenomatous polyposis	IBD	inflammatory bowel disease
FEN_a^+	fractional excretion of sodium	ICAM	intracellular adhesion molecule
FFP	fresh frozen plasma	ICF	intracellular fluid
FH	family history	ICP	intracranial pressure

IF	intrinsic factor	NADH	nicotinamide adenine dinucleotide (reduced)
Ig	immunoglobulin		
IL	interleukin	NADP	nicotinamide adenine dinucleotide phosphate (oxidized)
IM	intramuscular		
IND	indication(s)	NADPH	nicotinamide adenine dinucleotide phosphate (reduced)
INH	isoniazid		
IOP	intraocular pressure	NE	norepinephrine
IP$_3$	inositol triphosphate	NSAID	nonsteroidal anti-inflammatory drug
IPV	inactivated polio vaccine		
IUGR	intrauterine growth retardation	N/V	nausea/vomiting
IV	intravenous	OAA	oxaloacetic acid
IVC	inferior vena cava	OCP	oral contraceptive pills
IVIG	IV immunoglobulin	OPV	oral polio vaccine
JG	juxtaglomerular	PABA	*para*-aminobenzoic acid
JVD	jugular venous distension	PAF	platelet activity factor
L	left	PAH	*para*-aminohippuric acid
LAD	left anterior descending	PALS	periarterial lymphoid sheath
LCA	left coronary artery	PAN	polyarteritis nodosa
LDH	lactate dehydrogenase	P-ANCA	perinuclear pattern of antineutrophil cytoplasmic antibodies
LDL	low-density lipoprotein		
LES	lower esophageal sphincter		
LFT	liver function test	PAS	periodic acid-Schiff (stain)
LH	leutinizing hormone	PBS	peripheral blood smear
LLQ	left lower quadrant	PCAM	platelet cell adhesion molecule
LLSB	left-lower sternal border	PCI$_2$	prostacyclin I$_2$
LMN	lower motor neuron	PCL	posterior cruciate ligament
LP	lumbar puncture	PCP	phencyclidine hydrochloride
LPS	lipopolysaccharide	PCR	polymerase chain reaction
LT	leukotriene	PCWP	pulmonary capillary wedge pressure
LUSB	left-upper sternal border		
LUQ	left upper quadrant	PDA	patent ductus arteriosus
LV	left ventricle	PDE	phosphodiesterase
MAOI	monoamine oxidase inhibitor	PDGF	platelet-derived growth factor
MCA	middle cerebral artery	PE	physical examination
MCP	metacarpel phalangeal	PFK	phosphofructokinase
MCL	medial collateral ligament	PFT	pulmonary function tests
MCV	mean corpuscular volume	PG	prostaglandin
MEN	multiple endocrine neoplasia	PID	pelvic inflammatory disease
MHC	major histocompatibility complex	PIP	proximal interphalangeal
MI	myocardial infarction	PIP$_2$	phosphatidylinositol-4,5-bisphosphonate
MLF	medial longitudinal fasciculus		
mm	millimeters or muscles	PK	pyruvate kinase
MMR	measles, mumps, rubella	PKU	phenylketonuria
MOA	mechanism of action	PMN	polymorphonuclear
MPTP	1-methyl-4-phenyl-1,2,3, 6-tetrahydropyridine	PNH	paroxysmal nocturnal hemoglobinuria
MRI	magnetic resonance imaging	PNS	peripheral nervous system
MS	multiple sclerosis	PPi	pronton-pump inhibitor
MTP	metatarsal-phalangeal	PPRF	parapontine reticular formation
MVA	motor vehicle accident	PSA	prostate-specific antigen
NAD	nicotinamide adenine dinucleotide (oxidized)	PT	prothrombin time
		PTH	parathyroid hormone

PTT	partial thromboplastin time	TIBC	total iron binding capacity
PVD	peripheral vascular disease	TMP	trimethoprim
R	right	TN	true negatives
RA	right atrium	TNF	tissue necrosis factor
RAA	Renin angiotensin aldosterone	TNM	tumor node metastasis
RBC	red blood cell	TOX	toxicity
RBF	renal blood flow	TP	true positives
RCA	right coronary artery	tPA	tissue plasminogen activator
REM	rapid eye movement	TPR	total peripheral resistance
RER	rough endoplasmic reticulum	TRH	thyrotropin-releasing hormone
RF	rheumatoid factor	TSH	thyroid-stimulating hormone
RLQ	right lower quadrant	TSS	toxic shock syndrome
ROM	range of motion	TTP	thrombotic thrombocytopenic purpura
RPF	renal plasma flow		
RPR	rapid plasma reagin	Tx	treatment/therapy
RR	respiratory rate	TXA	thromboxane
RSV	respiratory syncytial virus	UA	urinalysis
RUQ	right upper quadrant	UMN	upper motor neuron
RV	right ventricle	UGI	upper GI
RVH	right ventricular hypertrophy	URI	upper respiratory infection
s	second(s)	UTI	urinary tract infection
$S_{1(2, 3, 4)}$	1st heart sound (2nd, 3rd, 4th)	U/S	ultrasound
SA	sinoatrial	V_d	volume of distribution
SC	subcutaneous or sickle cell	VCAM	vascular cell adhesion molecule
SD	standard deviation	VDRL	venereal disease research laboratory
SEM	standard error of the mean		
SES	socioeconomic status	Vfib	ventricular fibrillation
SGOT	serum glutamic oxaloacetic transaminase	VHL	von Hippel-Lindau
		VLDL	very low-density lipoprotein
SGPT	serum glutamic pyruvate transaminase	VMA	vanillylmandelic acid
		V/Q	ventilation/perfusion ratio
SLE	systemic lupus erythematosus	VSD	ventricular septal defect
SMX	sulfamethoxazole	vWF	von Willebrand factor
SOB	shortness of breath	VZV	varicella-zoster virus
ss	single stranded	WBC	white blood cell
SSA	special somatic afferent	WNL	within normal limits
SSPE	subacute sclerosing panencephalitis	XL	x-linked
		XR	x-ray
SSRI	selective serotonin reuptake inhibitor	y/o	year-old
		ZE	Zollinger-Ellison
STD	sexually transmitted disease	5-FU	5-fluorouracil
SV	stroke volume	5-HIAA	5-hydroxyindoleacetic acid
SVA	special visceral afferent	5-HT	5-hydroxytryptamine (serotonin)
SVT	supraventricular tachycardia		
Sx	symptom(s)	↑	High or increases
s/p	status post	↓	Low or decreases
$t_{1/2}$	half-life	→	Leads to or causes
T_3	triiodothyronine	$1°/2°/3°$	primary/secondary/tertiary
T_4	thyroxine	~	Approximately
TB	tuberculosis	⊕	positive
TBW	total body water	>>>	much greater than
TG	triglyceride	<<<	much less than

Index